T0210329

MOSBY'S® PREP GUIDE *for the* CANADIAN PN EXAM

Practice Questions for Exam Success

FIRST EDITION

MOSBY'S® PREP GUIDE

for the CANADIAN PN EXAM

Practice Questions for Exam Success

FIRST EDITION

Marianne Langille RN, BScN, MEd
Fanshawe College, London, ON

Karen Katsademas RN, BScN, MN
Fanshawe College, London, ON

ELSEVIER

MOSBY'S® PREP GUIDE FOR THE CANADIAN PN EXAM:
PRACTICE QUESTIONS FOR EXAM SUCCESS

ISBN: 978-0-323-75914-4

Adapted from Mosby's Prep Guide for the Canadian RN Exam: Practice Questions for Exam Success, Second Edition by Janice Marshall-Henty et al.

Library of Congress: Control Number: 2021937142

Managing Director, Global ERC: Kevonne Holloway
Senior Content Strategist (Acquisitions, Canada): Roberta A. Spinosa-Millman
Director, Content Development: Laurie Gower
Content Development Specialist: Theresa Fitzgerald
Publishing Services Manager: Shereen Jameel
Senior Project Manager: Umarani Natarajan
Design Direction: Bridget Hoette

Last digit is the print number: 9 8 7 6 5 4 3 2

We dedicate this book to practical nursing students as they prepare for their examinations.

Marianne Langille & Karen Katsademas

Preface

Mosby's® Prep Guide for the Canadian PN Exam has been developed to provide practical nursing students with practice exams to aid in the preparation of completing the licensure exam. As nursing educators, we recognize that students not only require a broad knowledge of nursing theory, but they also need to feel confident answering the particular type of questions found on the licensure exam. For many, the problem is not a lack of nursing knowledge but rather a lack of ability to apply their knowledge in the exam situation.

You have probably purchased this text for the practice exams, but don't skip over the chapters on exam descriptions and tips for writing questions. They provide valuable guidelines for mastering multiple-choice questions.

Most students in their respective nursing education programs have not had sufficient experience with the specific format of the questions found on the licensure exam. The licensure exam is unique in several important ways:

- There is a high ratio of critical-thinking questions, where all options may be correct but one of the options is the most correct. Or many different aspects of a situation must be analyzed in order to select the most appropriate answer. This problem-solving process may be difficult for students who are used to cramming the night before an exam and then regurgitating memorized facts the next day.
- Most questions incorporate scope of practice, asking what the nurse would do in a particular situation, rather than testing knowledge of medical treatments.
- Questions are written within the framework of practical nursing practice in Canada. Most available review texts are published in the United States and are based on the National Council Licensure Examination for Practical Nurses (NCLEX-PN), which does not test the Canadian practical nurse competencies.

Questions included in this book are based on the 2020 entry-level/entry-to-practice competencies for practical nurses. They have been authored to include preventive and primary health care, teaching and learning, professional practice, therapeutic relationships, and current developments in health care. Each question has been authored by nursing experts, reviewed by nursing experts, and referenced to established resources.

This prep guide includes three complete practice exams. Each exam consists of 200 case and independent questions, for a total of 600 questions in the three exams. For each question, there is an explanation of why the incorrect answers are incorrect and why the correct answer is correct. You may want to write the first exam as a "diagnostic," to identify areas of weakness and get a feel for the exams. We recommend that for one of the exams, you, either by yourself or with a group of fellow students, approach it as a mock exam situation. Pretend that it is the real exam, prepare as you would for the actual day, and write the practice exam in a 4-hour time frame.

This book is intended to prepare candidates for the Canadian Practical Nurse Registration Exam (CPNRE) and those candidates in BC and ON who will be writing the Regulatory Exam-Practical Nurse (REx-PN) beginning in 2022. Although limited information about this new exam is available, we have included what is known at the time of this writing.

Evolve Resources for *Mosby's® Prep Guide for the Canadian PN Exam* are available to enhance student learning. Students have the option to use the Study Mode or Exam Mode to practice and perfect their understanding of the fundamental competencies.

- Three Practice Exams, along with Answers and Rationales from the core text
- Additional Practice Questions: 100 multiple choice questions with answers and rationales
- Practice Questions for the REx-PN Exam: 300 questions with answers and rationales; the question types include multiple choice, multiple response, and fill-in-the-blank calculation
- Printable Scoring Sheets to use with the Practice Exams

Acknowledgements

We would like to acknowledge and thank the following individuals for their time, support and expertise in the preparation of the text: Roberta Spinosa-Millman, Senior Content Strategist (Canada) and Theresa Fitzgerald, Content Development Specialist of Elsevier.

We would like to recognize the contribution of Janice Marshall-Henty and Jonathon Bradshaw, authors of *Mosby's Prep Guide for the Canadian RN Exam*. Their original work served as a foundation for our writing and set the standard of excellence we conscientiously followed.

Reviewers

Natasha Fontaine RN, BN, PID
Program Coordinator
School of Nursing
College of the Rockies
Cranbrook, BC

Cindy Pallister RN, BScN, MScN
Nursing Professor, Simulationist
Department of Nursing
St. Clair College
Chatham, ON

Sandra Parker RN, BScN, MA Ed-CC
Nursing Instructor-PND Program
Faculty of Continuing Education
Seneca College
Toronto, ON

Trina Propp RN, BSN
Nursing Instructor
Department of Health Sciences-Nursing Program
Vancouver Community College
Vancouver, BC

Valerie Sokolowski RN, MN
Faculty
Practical Nursing
College of New Caledonia
Prince George, BC

Contents

1 Introduction

BACKGROUND TO THE CANADIAN PRACTICAL NURSE LICENSURE EXAMINATIONS—REx-PN AND CPNRE

To practise as a practical nurse in Canada, you must be registered, or licensed. Nursing applicants across Canada except residents of the province of Quebec write the Canadian Practical Nurse Registration Exam (CPNRE). Beginning in 2022, nursing applicants in Ontario and British Columbia (BC) will write the Regulatory Exam – Practical Nurse (REx-PN). The licensure exams are administered by the individual provincial or territorial regulatory authorities. To write the exam, you must have completed an accredited nursing program or have foreign qualifications that have been assessed as being equivalent to a Canadian practical nursing education. Candidates who pass the exam in their home province or territory and meet all other requirements for registration qualify to apply for registration in all other jurisdictions in Canada.

Questions on the licensure exams are designed to evaluate the knowledge of generalist nurses who have just finished their education. Nursing specialties are not tested. Testable material is applicable whether in large cities with teaching hospitals or small towns with community clinics. When writing the exam, you need to be able to answer questions based on the knowledge, skills, and behaviours of any practical nurse, not just on what you or your colleagues might have experienced in a particular setting. Most questions you encounter on the exam contain only information found in textbooks or other authorized resources.

CPNRE

The development of the exam begins with a specific blueprint, or framework. Individual questions are authored by a team of nursing experts from across Canada. Each test item is reviewed, validated, and then piloted prior to being placed in a test bank. It takes more than a year to complete this process. Thus, most questions you encounter on the CPNRE were written several years ago and contain only information found in textbooks or other authorized resources.

For each CPNRE exam, questions are randomly chosen from a test bank. Individual exams are not exactly the same, so the June exam is different from the September, November, and January exams. Others you speak with may describe past exams as having been focused, for example, on pediatric, mental health, or maternal–child nursing, but you need to remember that your exam will be different.

Each exam has a different pass mark. Some versions of the exam may be considered more difficult than others. A panel of experts determines the pass mark depending on the assessed difficulty of a particular exam. Exams considered difficult will have lower pass marks than exams that are considered easier.

You receive a mark for each correct response. Marks are not deducted for incorrect answers. The results of the exam are reported as *Pass* or *Fail.* If, for example, the pass mark for a particular exam version is 125 and you scored 125 or higher, you would pass. If, however, you scored lower than 125, you would fail. There is no bell curve applied to the exam results. A frequent worry of students who are about to write the exam is, "What happens if I fail?" With proper preparation, including management of "test stress," this outcome should not occur. A candidate is allowed to write the exam a maximum of three times. Students who fail the exam may contact their regional regulatory bodies for information about having their paper regraded or about initiating an appeal.

REx-PN

The REx-PN is a newly developed exam based on data from a practice analysis completed in 2019, and which will be repeated every 5 years. This practice analysis was then used to develop a framework. Individual questions are authored by nursing experts in Ontario and BC. Each test item is reviewed, validated, and will be pretested by student volunteers who are preparing to graduate in 2020 and 2021 to determine the difficulty level for each item before being placed in an item bank.

The REx-PN will differ from the CPNRE in that it will use computerized adaptive testing (CAT). In this format, the system will determine the level of difficulty of the question it presents to you based on how well you responded to the preceding question. For example, if you responded correctly to a question of medium difficulty, the next question presented to you will be slightly more difficult. You must achieve a certain ability level on the exam to pass. If you do not pass the REx-PN exam, you will have no limit on the number of times you can write the exam. However, you will have to wait a minimum of 60 days before writing again, up to a maximum of six attempts per year. After a fail, students will receive a breakdown of results, including areas of knowledge deficits. Students can then use this information to identify areas to focus on for further study (CNO, 2020).

HOW TO USE THIS BOOK

Mosby's Prep Guide for the Canadian PN Exam is designed to provide you with practice exams that are similar in content to the CPNRE and REx-PN licensure exams. The value of the practice exams is that they give you the opportunity to apply your knowledge to the multiple-choice type of questions you will experience in the exam. You can choose to write each exam as a whole to mimic a 4-hour exam condition, or you can answer each question individually.

Once you have answered the questions, review the correct answers and rationales. Were there knowledge gaps? Did you misread the question? Did you add information that was not in the question? Did you misunderstand the question? Identify the frequency with which you made particular errors, and use this information as a database for further study. Perhaps you need to review certain topics, practise your math skills, or increase your reading comprehension. Remember, you are not expected to get a perfect score. If you correctly answer about 70% of the questions, you demonstrate the potential for success on the actual licensure exam.

Do not use this prep guide as a source for studying content, and do not attempt to memorize any of the information from the questions in this guide. All test items on the licensure exams are secure and have never been published, so the questions found in this book will not appear on the licensure exams.

2 Description of the Canadian Practical Nurse Licensure Examinations—REx-PN and CPNRE

REx-PN AND CPNRE

The Canadian Practical Nurse Exam (CPNRE) consists of 165–70 questions, including experimental questions that are not scored, in multiple-choice format. Writing time is 4 hours. Questions are written at different cognitive levels: knowledge/comprehension, application, and critical thinking. The knowledge–comprehension level requires recollection of facts. The application level of the intellectual process requires not only knowing and understanding information but also being able to apply it to a new situation. Critical thinking questions ask you to analyze, evaluate, problem-solve, or interpret data from a variety of sources before you respond to them.

The REx-PN exam is a variable length computerized adaptive test and can range from 90 to 150 items, including 30 pretest items that are not scored. Question format may include multiple choice, multiple response, fill-in-the-blank calculation, exhibit, and graphics. Writing time is 4 hours. Test items are categorized by the level of difficulty, and the difficulty level of a question you receive is based on your previous answer.

ENTRY-TO-PRACTICE COMPETENCIES

The licensure exam focuses on testing entry-level competencies that are essential to providing safe care at the beginning of your practical nurse career. Competencies include knowledge, skills, behaviours, attitudes, and judgements that a practical nurse is expected to demonstrate in order to provide safe, professional care. In the licensure exam, competencies are applied to various health situations and clients. For example, what are the safety hazards for the mental health client, the infant, or the older person? How do you prevent the spread of infection in a hospital, a day care centre, or to an immunocompromised client? Practical nurses learn these competencies in their education programs. There are 79 competencies in BC and Ontario and 76 competencies in the rest of Canada. The competencies are organized in five categories. See the Appendix for a complete list of the entry-to-practice competencies.

COMPETENCY CATEGORIES

Professional Practice

Professional practice means that the practical nurse is accountable for safe, competent, ethical nursing care. Professional practice includes professional conduct and evidence-informed practice.

Sample Competency

Initiates, maintains, and terminates the therapeutic nurse–client relationship.

Related Sample Question

What is the most therapeutic response to Mr. Smith's question, "Am I going to die?"

1. "No, of course not."
2. "You have a very serious illness."
3. "Do you think you are going to die?"
4. "What have you been told about your illness and prognosis?"

The correct answer is 4.

This response invites Mr. Smith to discuss his understanding of his illness and provides the nurse with baseline information for further dialogue.

Ethical Practice

Practical nurses use ethical frameworks when making professional judgements and practice decisions. Ethical practice involves understanding the impact of personal values, beliefs, and assumptions in the provision of care.

Sample Competency

Establishes and maintains professional boundaries

Related Sample Question

Ms. Jasper, a client newly admitted to a mental health facility, asks the practical nurse, "Do you have a boyfriend?" What is the most appropriate response by the nurse?

1. "Let's talk about you. Do you have a boyfriend?"
2. "I am not allowed to tell you about my personal life."
3. "Yes I do. We have been together for three wonderful years."
4. "This interview is about you, not me."

The correct answer is 4.

This response refocuses the conversation to the client and does not cross professional boundaries.

Legal Practice

Practical nurses adhere to applicable legislation and regulations, standards, and policies that direct practice. Practical nurses have knowledge of the relevant laws and legal boundaries within which they practice.

Sample Competency

Documents according to established legislation, practice standards, ethics, and organizational policies.

Related Sample Question

Mrs. Leung was found by the nurse at 0100 hours lying on the floor beside her bed. What should the nurse document in the health record?

1. Mrs. Leung fell out of bed at 0100.
2. At 0100 hours, Mrs. Leung was found by the nurse on the floor beside her bed.
3. Mrs. Leung got out of bed at 0100 hours, slipped, and fell on the floor.
4. Mrs. Leung apparently fell out of bed at approximately 0100 hours.

The correct answer is 2.

This notation provides factual and objective documentation about the nurse's observation.

Foundations of Practice

Foundational knowledge includes nursing theory, health sciences, humanities, pharmacology, and ethics.

Sample Competency

Demonstrates knowledge of nursing theory, pharmacology, health sciences, humanities, and ethics.

Related Sample Question

Which of the following lunch menus would be most appropriate and nutritious for a healthy 2-year-old child?

1. Hamburger and French fries
2. Jelly sandwich and grape soda
3. Cheese sandwich and fruit slices
4. Macaroni and cheese and cookies

The correct answer is 3.

This menu provides healthy nutrients and would appeal to a toddler.

Collaborative Practice

Collaborative practice involves mutual respect and effective communication when working collaboratively with clients and other members of the health care team.

Sample Competency

Demonstrates leadership, direction, and supervision to unregulated health workers and others.

Related Sample Question

The practical nurse checks on a client who was admitted to the hospital with pneumonia. He has been coughing profusely and has required nasotracheal suctioning. He has an intravenous infusion of antibiotics. He is febrile. Which of the following tasks may the practical nurse delegate to the support worker assigned to the client today?

1. Assessing vital signs
2. Changing intravenous dressing
3. Nasotracheal suctioning
4. Administering a bed bath

The correct answer is 4. The practical nurse may delegate this task to the support worker.

MULTIPLE-CHOICE QUESTIONS

The CPNRE and the REx-PN both contain multiple-choice questions. The multiple-choice questions on the CPNRE are written as either case-based or independent questions. Case-based questions present a health care situation along with approximately 3–5 questions related to the scenario. Independent, or stand-alone, items contain all the information necessary to answer the question.

Each multiple-choice question is made up of two components. The part of the item that asks the question or poses a problem is called the *stem*. The alternatives from which you are asked to select the best answer are called the *options*. There are four options; only one of the options is the correct answer. The other three options are called *distractors*. Distractors may seem to be reasonable answers but are, in fact, incorrect or incomplete.

Only one answer is correct. There are no combination options such as "1 and 2," "all of the above," or "none of the above." All questions are worth one mark. Marks are not deducted for wrong answers.

Sample Question

While receiving a blood transfusion, Mr. Ryan develops chills and a headache. What would be the practical nurse's initial action?

1. Notify the physician stat.
2. Stop the transfusion immediately.
3. Cover Mr. Ryan with a blanket and administer ordered acetaminophen (Tylenol).
4. Slow the blood flow to keep the vein open.

The correct answer is 2. Mr. Ryan is experiencing a transfusion reaction, thus the blood infusion must be stopped immediately.

The REx-PN contains many multiple-choice questions. You may also be asked questions that are multiple response, fill-in-the-blank calculation, exhibit, and graphics. See Evolve for further information.

3 Study and Exam Tips

Although you may be academically well prepared to write the licensure exam, strategies for studying, stress management, and test taking will increase your chances of success and help to alleviate anxiety.

STUDY TIPS

It is easy to become overwhelmed as you prepare to study for the licensure exam. Remember, though, that you know a lot more than you think you do. While studying is crucial, much learning is not a conscious activity. The first key to developing successful study strategies is to be realistic. Identify where you have incomplete knowledge or the need to refresh your learning.

Keep in mind that most of the questions on the exam do not merely test recalled facts, so you should try to understand the material that you read, rather than memorize it. The focus of your studies should be on principles of care and nursing interventions within a particular health situation, that is, what should the practical nurse do or say?

One of the best strategies for learning is to form a study group. Self-testing and peer testing have proven to be the most effective methods for consolidating material. Have each member of the group choose a topic to teach the other members. This way, you stimulate discussion and get different perspectives on the subjects, which will help you in understanding and remembering them. If you are unable to participate in a study group, try teaching yourself the information. Rephrase or reword the written information to aid in understanding rather than memorizing.

Repetition works well for many people. If you are having trouble remembering some knowledge material, it may help to record it so that you can play it aloud while performing other activities.

Schedule your studying. Start reviewing content several months prior to the exam so that you do not feel rushed or panicked at the volume of material you need to learn. Cramming or "all-nighters" may be useful for memorizing facts, but the licensure exam is an exam that requires problem-solving based on a comprehensive knowledge base. It is better to think through and analyze the material, make judgements, and determine how the subject relates to nursing. By performing these analytical and reflective processes, you are more likely to commit the information to long-term memory, which is much more reliable than your short-term memory.

To remember the strategies for studying, you can use the initialism *PQRS*, which stands for *p*lanning, *q*uestions practice, *r*epetition, and *s*elf- and peer testing.

While you study, remember to stay hydrated, eat sensibly, build in exercise breaks, and get plenty of sleep. It is also important to pursue other activities and not be involved solely in study. Research has shown that both sleep and "time out," in the form of exercise, social activities, or nutrition breaks, help to consolidate learned information.

MANAGING STRESS

STUDENT QUOTATION

> "If I answer one more multiple-choice question, I think I may become physically ill. I won't be able to help myself. Can't they think of any other way of assessing how much we know?"

The student quoted above is setting himself up for failure because of his negativity toward the format of the test.

It is perfectly normal to feel nervous and anxious about the licensure exam. You have worked hard to be successful in your nursing program, and now all that effort comes down to passing one exam. As you prepare for the exam, empower yourself by developing a positive mental attitude. Henry Ford said, "Whether you think you can or think you can't… you're right."

Challenge your negative thoughts! Do not let them guide you.

TIPS

Become active and positive about your learning and your preparation. The more actively you plan and prepare, the more likely you will be successful. The following tips will help you manage stress:

- Try to avoid fellow students who feel overly anxious about the exam. Anxiety is like a communicable disease. You can catch it.
- Use the power of positive thinking. Build up your self-confidence by repeating to yourself, "I am well prepared. I will pass this exam."
- Practise yoga or other forms of exercise; they are great stress relievers.
- Try aromatherapy—lavender works well to promote relaxation. Sometimes just the smell will help you remember to relax and breathe.
- Eat a well-balanced diet, and get plenty of rest.

THE EVENING BEFORE THE EXAM

STUDENT QUOTATION

> "The night before a test, I can't sleep. Then I worry because I can't sleep. Then I can't sleep because I'm worrying that I'm worried that I can't sleep. By morning, I'm glad to get out of bed just to stop the terrible racket in my head."

The evening before the exam, organize your clothes and exam supplies (e.g., identification, bottle of water). Make sure you know the location of the exam and have arranged your transport to the exam.

Then be nice to yourself. Do something you enjoy and get a good night's sleep. Information is processed during sleep, so sleep will help you retain what you have studied. Last-minute cramming may have aided you in past test situations but is helpful only for memorizing facts. It actually decreases your ability to problem-solve the application and critical-thinking types of questions that are on the licensure exam.

THE DAY OF THE EXAM

Eat a healthy breakfast of protein and carbohydrates. Engage in moderate exercise if possible. If you absolutely cannot eat, try drinking a sports electrolyte solution. Although you need to be adequately hydrated, do not drink too many fluids or cups of coffee. Dress in comfortable clothes, preferably in layers, so that you can add or take off articles depending on the temperature of the exam room.

Plan to arrive at the test location at least 30 minutes ahead of the exam start time. This cushion will allow you time to relax, visit with friends, and prepare yourself mentally. However, avoid talking about the exam with your friends as conversations about it will only make you more anxious. Arriving early also gives you time for that last-minute washroom trip—stress is a potent diuretic. When you sit down in the exam room, make a conscious effort to relax and continue your positive thinking.

AFTER THE EXAM

After the exam, you will likely feel a sense of relief that it is over, but you may also feel the need to review questions in your head and discuss answers with your peers. Try not to dwell on this activity for too long. These postmortems can bring you down. Remember, you have probably done better than you think!

CONTENT TO STUDY

Mosby's Comprehensive Review for the Canadian PN Exam is the most valuable resource for your licensure exam studying. This uniquely Canadian-based review text has content created specifically for Canadian practical nurses, providing all you need to know about practical nursing in Canada—and to pass the licensure exam—in one text.

Your first step in preparing for the exam is to review the Competencies in the Appendix. Notice the wording: *advocates, collaborates, supports, takes action, engages, facilitates, promotes,* and *integrates.*

PROFESSIONAL PRACTICE

The topics of the Professional Practice competencies include accountability, scope of practice, self-awareness, adherence to regulatory requirements, competence, therapeutic nurse–client relationship, nonjudgemental care, sensitivity to spiritual beliefs and cultural practices, supporting clients in making informed decisions, self-reflection and continuous learning, integration of relevant evidence, role in practice and policy, continuous quality improvement, professionalism, fitness to practice, maintaining current knowledge of relevant trends and issues, professional misconduct, action with near misses, errors and adverse events, and distinguishing mandates of regulatory bodies, professional associations and unions.

Other resources for this competency include provincial standards of practice and related websites; Potter et al., *Canadian Fundamentals of Nursing*, sixth edition; and Arnold and Boggs, *Interpersonal Relationships*, eighth edition.

ETHICAL PRACTICE

The topics of the Ethical Practice competencies include professional boundaries, personal values, respect for clients, ethics, truth and reconciliation, dignity, sensitivity to diversity, and advocacy. Adherence to the duty to provide care is a competency in ON and BC only.

Other resources for this competency include provincial standards of practice and related websites; Potter et al., *Canadian Fundamentals of Nursing*, sixth edition; and Keatings and Adams, *Ethical and Legal Issues in Canadian Nursing*, fourth edition.

LEGAL PRACTICE

The topics of the Legal Practice competencies include adherence to legislation and regulations, promoting safe practice, adherence to duty to report, confidentiality and privacy, documentation, and informed consent.

Other resources for this competency include Potter et al., *Canadian Fundamentals of Nursing*, sixth edition and Keatings and Adams, *Ethical and Legal Issues in Canadian Nursing*, fourth edition.

FOUNDATIONS OF PRACTICE

The topics of the Foundations of Practice competencies include comprehensive health assessment; technology application; research and response to relevant clinical data; evidence-informed practice; comprehension, response to, and report of assessment findings, formulation of clinical decisions, identification of nursing diagnosis, care plans; appropriate interventions; intervention prioritization; health literacy; teaching and learning; health education; client safety; quality improvement and risk management; evaluation of nursing interventions; care plan revision and appropriate communication; assessment of implications of own decisions; critical thinking, critical inquiry and clinical judgement; professional judgement in utilization of technology and social media; safe care; prevention, de-escalation and management of disruptive, aggressive, violent behaviour; recognition and response to client's deteriorating condition; and knowledge of nursing theory, pharmacology, health sciences, humanities, and ethics. ON and BC have an additional competency: application of knowledge of pharmacology and principles of safe medication practice.

Other resources for this competency include Potter et al., *Canadian Fundamentals of Nursing*, sixth edition and Jarvis et al., *Physical Examination and Health Assessment*, third Canadian edition.

COLLABORATIVE PRACTICE

The topics of the Collaborative Practice competencies include client engagement; collaborative communication; providing essential client information; promoting effective interpersonal interaction; conflict resolution; role articulation; role determination; advocating for use of Indigenous health knowledge in collaboration with the client; leadership, direction and supervision of unregulated health workers; emergency preparedness and disaster management; quality practice environment; encouraging questioning and exchange of information; mentoring; group process; leadership; and time management. Additionally, ON and BC have the competency: preparing client and collaborating with health care team in transitions and transfer of responsibility of care.

Other resources for this competency include provincial standards of practice and related websites; Potter et al., *Canadian Fundamentals of Nursing*, sixth edition; Arnold and Boggs, *Interpersonal Relationships*, eighth edition; and Wadell and Walton, *Yoder-Wise's Leading and Managing in Canadian Nursing*, second edition.

Although the licensure exam is based on competencies, most resources you will be using for study are organized by topic or clinical area. The following sections outline the most common subjects within these traditional topic areas. *Mosby's Comprehensive Review for the Canadian PN Exam* contains all the necessary information in each section. However, should you choose to conduct further research, alternative resources are provided. When reviewing specific conditions and diseases, focus on the related nursing implications and remember to think about community-based aspects of care.

MEDICAL–SURGICAL NURSING

You cannot know all diseases. Try to think globally and consider all problems associated with a system, rather than studying specific diseases. Remember that it is unlikely that you will be asked to recall specifics of disease pathology. Rather, you will need to understand effective therapies, including associated clinical skills and interventions.

- Endocrine: diabetes Type 1 and 2
- Cardiovascular: stroke, myocardial infarction, heart failure, peripheral vascular disease
- Hematology: anemia, leukemias
- Gastrointestinal: Crohn's, colitis, diverticulitis, colorectal cancer, constipation, diarrhea, ulcers, appendicitis
- Renal: urinary tract infections, renal failure, dialysis, incontinence
- Liver: cirrhosis, hepatitis, pancreatitis
- Respiratory: chronic obstructive pulmonary disease (COPD), asthma, pneumonia, lung cancer, tuberculosis, common cold, atelectasis, pneumothorax/hemothorax
- Musculoskeletal: arthritis, osteoporosis, fractures, chronic fatigue syndrome, scoliosis, multiple sclerosis
- Immune: human immunodeficiency virus (HIV), inflammation
- Infections: methicillin-resistant *Staphylococcus aureus* (MRSA), vancomycin-resistant enterococci (VRE), *Clostridium difficile* (*C. diff.*), influenza, common cold, sepsis, epidemics, pandemics
- Sensory: cataracts, glaucoma, hearing loss
- Integumentary: burns, infestations, allergies
- Neurological: seizures, intracranial pressure, Parkinson's, multiple sclerosis, spinal cord injuries
- Women's and men's health: menopause, birth control, sexually transmitted infections, breast and prostate cancers
- Emergency: shock, hemorrhage, anaphylaxis
- Fluid and electrolyte, acid–base imbalance

Resources include Lewis et al., *Medical-Surgical Nursing in Canada*, fourth Canadian edition, and www.sexandu.ca.

MATERNAL–CHILD NURSING

- Health in child-bearing years
- Fertility
- Prenatal care
- Fetal development
- Pregnancy risks and complications
- Labour and birth
- Apgar scoring
- Newborn assessment
- Preterm and newborn health problems
- Postpartum care
- Breastfeeding
- Bonding

Resources include Perry et al., *Maternal Child Nursing Care in Canada*, second edition and Leifer and Keenan-Lindsay, *Leifer's Introduction to Maternity and Pediatric Nursing in Canada*.

PEDIATRIC NURSING

- Family and parenting; child development, infancy to adolescence; play; safety
- Respiratory: asthma, respiratory syncytial virus (RSV), croup, cystic fibrosis
- Gastrointestinal: gastroenteritis, reflux, cleft lip and palate, appendicitis, pyloric stenosis
- Cardiovascular: atrial septal defect (ASD), ventricular septal defect (VSD)
- Hematology: sickle cell, leukemias, anemia
- Immune: human immunodeficiency virus (HIV)
- Infections and immunization: common childhood infectious diseases, schedule of vaccines
- Genitourinary: urinary tract infections
- Neurological: head injury, seizures, meningitis, hydrocephalus

- Endocrine: diabetes
- Integumentary: infestations, allergies
- Musculoskeletal: trauma, fractures, sprains and strains, arthritis, scoliosis
- Neuromuscular: cerebral palsy

Resources include Hockenberry et al., *Wong's Essentials of Pediatric Nursing*, eleventh edition and Leifer and Keenan-Lindsay, *Leifer's Introduction to Maternity and Pediatric Nursing in Canada.*

MENTAL HEALTH NURSING

- Legal, ethical, interpersonal, communication, and therapeutic approaches
- Mood disorders: depression, bipolar
- Anxiety disorders: phobias, obsessive compulsive disorder
- Schizophrenia spectrum and other psychotic disorders
- Personality disorders
- Substance-related and addictive disorders
- Cognitive disorders: dementias, Alzheimer's
- Sexual and identity disorders
- Eating disorders, body dysmorphic disorder
- Psychiatric emergencies

Resources include Halter, *Varcarolis' Foundations of Psychiatric Mental Health Nursing*, eighth edition.

DIAGNOSTIC TESTS

Understand the reason for the test and the appropriate health teaching for the client.

- Biopsies
- X-rays, computed tomography (CT) scans, magnetic resonance imaging (MRI), ultrasounds, nuclear scans
- Mammograms
- Gastrointestinal scopes, bronchoscopes
- Allergy tests
- Oxygen saturation, pulmonary function tests
- Fetal tests

Resources include Pagana et al., *Mosby's Canadian Manual of Diagnostic and Laboratory Tests*, second edition.

LABORATORY TESTS

Note the normal ranges and test implications.

- Complete blood count (CBC)
- International normalized ratio (INR)
- Blood glucose
- Blood urea nitrogen (BUN)
- Creatinine
- Glycosylated hemoglobin (HbA_{1c})
- Glomerular filtration rate (GFR)
- Electrolytes
- Cholesterol
- Urinalysis
- Culture and sensitivity (C & S)
- Stool
- Low-density lipoprotein (LDL), high-density lipoprotein (HDL)

Resources include Pagana et al., *Mosby's Canadian Manual of Diagnostic and Laboratory Tests*, second edition.

PHARMACOLOGY

Note classifications, common drugs within each classification, therapeutic effects, and precautions. You will need to know about frequently prescribed and over-the-counter drugs. Knowledge regarding common herbal preparations may also be tested. Keep in mind lifespan considerations.

- Analgesics and anti-inflammatories: narcotic and non-narcotic (e.g., Tylenol, nonsteroidal anti-inflammatory drugs [NSAIDs], morphine, and Demerol)
- Antacids
- Antidepressants (e.g., selective serotonin reuptake inhibitors [SSRIs])
- Antibiotics (e.g., penicillin, ampicillin)
- Anticoagulants (e.g., Coumadin, heparin)
- Antidiabetics (e.g., insulin, oral hypoglycemics)
- Antivirals
- Cardiac drugs (e.g., nitroglycerin, digoxin, antihypertensives)
- Corticosteroids (e.g., prednisone)
- Diuretics (e.g., furosemide [Lasix])
- Hormones
- Respiratory drugs (e.g., bronchodilators, inhaled steroids)
- Stool softeners and laxatives (e.g., psyllium [Metamucil], docusate sodium [Colace])
- Statins (e.g., atorvastatin [Lipitor])
- Vitamins and minerals
- Alternative, complementary, or herbal preparations

Resources include Sealock, *Lilley's Pharmacology for Canadian Health Care Practice*, fourth Canadian edition; Skidmore-Roth, *Mosby's Nursing Drug Reference*, thirty-fourth edition.

CLINICAL SKILLS

To test your clinical skills, the exam may include questions about any or all of the following: vital signs, infection control, medication administration, body mechanics, hygiene, positioning, suctioning, chest tubes, oxygen therapy, tracheostomy, intravenous initiating and maintaining, urine specimens, urinary catheters, enemas, wound care, ostomies, and first aid.

Resources include Potter et al., *Canadian Fundamentals of Nursing*, sixth edition, and Perry et al., *Canadian Clinical Nursing Skills and Techniques.*

TIPS FOR WRITING MULTIPLE-CHOICE EXAMS

Listed below are some tips for completing the multiple-choice questions particular to the licensure exam:

A. Read and listen to the instructions carefully.

B. Plan your time and pace yourself. Keep track of time. You should answer approximately 25 to 30 questions in each half-hour.

C. Reading comprehension is crucial to success. Read the stem of each question carefully and make sure that you understand exactly what it asks. One of the most common test-taking errors is misreading the question. Identify words such as *initial* or *most important* or *priority*. Take special note of any negatives such as *never* or *except*.

> *Sample Question*
>
> Ms. Chang's surgical dressing is saturated in blood. What would be an early sign of hemorrhagic shock?
>
> 1. Increased blood pressure
> 2. Pallor
> 3. Increased pulse
> 4. Shallow breathing
>
> The key word is *early*; thus the correct answer is 3.

D. Be prepared to problem-solve *every* question.

E. Try to answer the question before looking at the multiple-choice options.

F. Read all the options before choosing one. Do not immediately assume a response is correct without looking at all the other options; another answer may be *more correct* than the one you choose first.

G. Read each option carefully, mentally crossing out the options you know are incorrect. Choose the best option out of the ones remaining.

H. Some questions that appear to be trick questions may, in reality, measure your ability to think critically. If you believe all the options are correct, choose the one that is most comprehensive, makes the most common sense, or is the most professional answer.

> *Sample Question*
>
> Which of the following is most important when performing a preoperative assessment?
>
> 1. Physical assessment
> 2. Cardiac assessment
> 3. Assessment of vital signs
> 4. Auscultation of breath sounds
>
> All options are valid, but answer 1 is the most inclusive.

I. To choose the most important nursing action when all of the answers appear to be correct, take the following steps:

- Read the situation and question very carefully.
- In almost all cases, consider the mnemonic *ABC* (*a*irway, *b*reathing, *c*irculation), with *airway* being the most important.
- Remember the "nursing process": collecting and validating information before acting.
- Consider safety—for the client and for yourself.
- Choose an action that can be completed quickly and safely, almost at the same time as other actions.
- Do not necessarily look for fancy answers.
- Choose simple, common-sense, safe actions.
- Choose the sickest, most unstable client as the priority.

J. A common error students make is choosing a response that might have been applicable in a specific client situation that they have experienced. Always answer according to "textbook," or standard, nursing principles.

K. Answer as you believe the perfect "textbook practical nurse" would answer.

L. Do not assume any information that is not given. Choose your answer based only on information in the question asked.

M. Do not panic if you have never heard of a particular disease or client situation. Apply general nursing principles to each question—the particular client health state may not matter. Candidates for the exam come from various academic backgrounds, and curricula are not identical in all education institutions. You are not expected to know all the answers, nor are you expected to write a perfect exam!

> *Sample Question*
>
> Ms. Townsend is suffering from Hick's asymmetrical dementia. Which of the following activities would be appropriate for her condition?
>
> 1. Vigorous exercise
> 2. Competitive games

3. Social stimulation in group activities
4. Solitary reading

Hick's asymmetrical dementia is a fictitious disorder. The care needs for a client with dementia are fundamental, so the correct response is answer 3. This is a "trick question" for the purpose of illustration. The licensure exam, however, contains no trick questions.

N. Your first answer choice is usually correct. You may have learned some information subconsciously, and your first impression is often an automatic response to what you have learned. Do not second-guess yourself unless you are absolutely sure that you have misunderstood the question or provided a wrong answer.

O. Select answers that are therapeutic, show respect, involve the client in care, and focus on nursing judgement rather than hospital rules or orders from other health team members.

Sample Question

Jessica tells the practical nurse, "I am tired of waiting for you to brush my hair. You're never here when I want you." Which of the following responses is the most appropriate for the practical nurse to give?

1. "I'm sorry you've had to wait. I'll get your hairbrush out for you and be back in 15 minutes to do your hair."
2. "That's not fair. I spent my lunch break with you yesterday."
3. "Jeremy down the hall is really sick, and he needs me more than you do right now."
4. "I'm doing my best, but I have a really busy assignment today."

Option 1 acknowledges the client's feelings, shows respect, and provides a clear, factual response.

Sample Question

Ms. Steele asks the practical nurse when she can start eating after surgery. What is the most appropriate response for the practical nurse to give?

1. "You'll have to ask the doctor."
2. "Tell me about your appetite."
3. "You'll likely start on clear fluids once bowel sounds can be heard."
4. "I'll have the dietitian consult with you about the most nutritious postsurgery menus."

Option 3 involves nursing judgement and directly answers the client's question.

P. Most questions will ask about actions that are based on nursing judgement rather than physician orders. However, some questions may test your knowledge of the scope of nursing practice and have as a correct response "contact the doctor." Examples of such situations include unclear or illegible orders, a specific request from a client, deteriorating client condition, and a client emergency.

Q. In the case of communication questions, answers that demonstrate the practical nurse asking the client open-ended questions are most often correct.

Sample Question

Which of the following would elicit the best information from Mr. Loates about his pain?

1. "Do you have severe pain?"
2. "Do you have any pain?"
3. "Is your pain throbbing or stabbing?"
4. "Describe your pain to me."

Option 4 is open-ended—that is, it requires the client to give more than a one- or two-word answer. Phrasing questions in an open-ended fashion is a key component of therapeutic nursing communication.

R. Do not choose an answer because you have seen that question before and think you recall the answer. Questions on the exam may look similar to ones you have encountered during practice but will not be exactly the same. Therefore, the answer may also not be the same.

S. There is no pattern to the assigned answers. Do not change an answer because you have had too many answers in the same position.

T. If all else fails, guess. Never leave a question unanswered. You have at least a 25% chance of getting it correct.

Tips for Guessing

1. If two of the options are similar except for one or two words, choose one of those.

Example

Take the apical pulse
Take the radial pulse

2. If two options have opposite meanings, choose one of those.

Example

Vasodilation
Vasoconstriction

3. If two quantities or mathematical calculations are similar, choose one of those.

Example

0.14 mL
0.014 mL

4. Choose the longest answer.
5. While there is no pattern to the answers, some studies say that in multiple-choice exams, option b or 2 is correct most of the time.

U. Answering many questions can be boring and tiring. You may find yourself becoming confused about what information relates to the question. Throughout the exam, take a mini-exercise break every 20 minutes; sip water, do neck rolls, and flex your arms and legs.

V. Do not panic if someone leaves when you have completed only 20 questions. The time taken to complete the exam is not an indication of performance on the exam.

COMPUTER ADAPTIVE TESTING

The REx-PN uses a computer adaptive testing format. "Examination items are presented to the candidate one at a time on a computer screen. There is no time limit for a candidate to spend on each individual item. Once an answer to an item is selected, the candidate has the ability to consider the answer and change it, if necessary. However, once the candidate confirms the answer and proceeds to the next time by pressing the <NEXT> button, the candidate will no longer have the ability to return to a previous item. The computer will not allow the candidate to proceed to the next item without answering the current item on the screen. The best advice is to maintain a reasonable pace (one item every minute or two), and carefully read and consider each item before answering. During the administration of the REx-PN, candidates will be required to respond to items in a variety of formats. These formats may include multiple-choice, multiple response, fill-in-the-blank calculation, exhibit, and graphics." (National Council of State Boards of Nursing. (2020). 2022 REx-PN Test Plan).

SUMMARY

Preparing for the exam well in advance, ensuring comprehensive content review, following the exam-taking tips, developing your reading comprehension, and maintaining a positive outlook will equip you with the necessary abilities to be successful in the licensure exam.

4 Practice Exam 1

INTRODUCTION TO PRACTICE EXAMS

The practice exam questions are designed to be similar to those you will encounter in the licensure exam.

INSTRUCTIONS FOR PRACTICE EXAM 1

You will have 4 hours to complete the exam. The questions are presented as nursing cases or as independent questions. Read each question carefully, and then choose the answer that you think is the best of the four options presented. If you cannot decide on an answer to a question, proceed to the next question and return to this question later if you have time. Try to answer all the questions. Marks are not subtracted for wrong answers. If you are unsure of an answer, it will be to your advantage to guess.

Answers to Practice Exam 1 appear on page 44.

CASE-BASED QUESTIONS

CASE 1

A practical nurse works in a medical–surgical unit of a hospital administering medication to her clients. Medications are dispensed through automated dispensing system.

QUESTIONS 1 to 6 refer to this case.

1. What is the most accurate method for the practical nurse to determine she is administering the correct medication to Mr. Rickhelm?

1. Compare the name of the drug on the medication prepackage with the prescriber's order.
2. Ask Mr. Rickhelm to confirm he is receiving the correct medication.
3. Contact the agency pharmacy to confirm Mr. Rickhelm's medication profile.
4. Check the medication identified on the medication prepackage against information from a drug reference text or agency intranet site.

2. Mr. Ogalino has been taking a brand name oral anti-infective medication at home for 6 months prior to being admitted to hospital. When the practical nurse brings his medications to him for the first time, he states, "What is this pink pill? I have never taken that one before." Which of the following responses by the practical nurse indicates safe medication administration?

1. "This is a generic form of your regular anti-infective."
2. "I don't know, but I'll check your medication record."
3. "This is what your doctor has prescribed for you."
4. "If you wish, you may refuse the medication."

3. Ms. Jasmin is a newly admitted client to the unit. The practical nurse prepares to administer long-acting insulin to her at 1800 hours. Ms. Jasmin tells the practical nurse that at home she takes this insulin at bedtime, around 2300 hours. How should the practical nurse respond?

1. "I will test your blood sugar to make sure this is the best time to inject your insulin."
2. "What is the reason you take your insulin at bedtime?"
3. "Generally the schedule for administering insulin is different when you are in hospital than when you are at home."
4. "Bedtime is not the best time for administration of long-acting insulin."

4. Ms. Corel is admitted to the unit with a diagnosis of deep vein thrombosis. Which of the following categories of drugs is likely to be ordered?

1. A statin
2. An antibiotic
3. An analgesic
4. An anticoagulant

5. The pharmacy technician comes to the unit to add some narcotics to the narcotic draw on the unit. The pharmacy technician asks the practical nurse to sign as a witness for the added medications to the narcotic draw count. Who may legally sign the narcotics administration count sheet?

1. A registered nurse (RN)
2. An RN or registered/licensed practical nurse (RPN/LPN)
3. An RN or a physician
4. Any registered or regulated health care provider

6. Mrs. Aina is ordered digoxin (Lanoxin) 0.075 mg. The pharmacy dispenses digoxin, three tablets of 0.25 mg for the above order. The practical nurse administers the provided three tablets of digoxin. Evaluate this action.

1. Correct, as the digoxin has been calculated by the pharmacy.
2. Correct, as the digoxin is the same dose that the physician has ordered.
3. Incorrect, as the ordered dose of digoxin is below the therapeutic level.
4. Incorrect, as the dose administered is too high.

END OF CASE 1

CASE 2

Mr. Smadu, age 19 years, was diagnosed with a schizophrenia disorder 8 months ago. His symptoms include hallucinations, delusions, flat affect, and grossly disorganized behaviour. He lives at home with his mother and his sister Shannon, both of whom work full time. His father and extended family live in another country and are not involved in his care. His mother has asked for a visit from the community nurse to discuss concerns she has regarding her son's management at home. The practical nurse visits with Mr. Smadu, his mother, and his sister.

QUESTIONS 7 to 13 refer to this case.

7. Mr. Smadu's mother and sister ask the practical nurse what the best way is to respond when he is hearing voices. What should the practical nurse advise them to say?

1. "I do not hear the voices that you hear."
2. "Who is talking to you?"
3. "There are no voices talking to you."
4. "Why do you say you are hearing voices?"

8. Mr. Smadu asks for suggestions to help him cope with the voices he hears. What might the practical nurse suggest?

1. To tell the voices to go away
2. To listen to music on his headphones
3. To distract himself by going for a walk
4. To increase his dose of antipsychotic medication

9. Mr. Smadu's mother tells the practical nurse some of the neighbours are concerned that her son will be violent. They are afraid of him when he yells at the voices. What should the practical nurse advise Mr. Smadu's mother to tell the neighbours?

1. "My son has a disease that causes him to hear voices, but he will never be violent."
2. "Call the police if my son is acting in a strange manner."
3. "Engage my son in conversation to distract him."
4. "Do not crowd my son or get too close to him if he appears agitated."

10. Mr. Smadu is being treated with risperidone (Risperdal) 40 mg intramuscularly (IM) every 2 weeks to help manage his psychotic behaviours. What is the primary reason this drug is given to him by the intramuscular rather than oral route?

1. It is not absorbed from the gastrointestinal tract.
2. There is better compliance when given every 2 weeks by injection.
3. There is greater therapeutic response with the IM route.
4. The IM route decreases the incidence of tardive dyskinesia.

11. Mr. Smadu's mother asks if her son will ever get better. What is the practical nurse's best response to this question?

1. "While there is no cure for a schizophrenia disorder, people can and do improve. The exact course and impact of a schizophrenia disorder is unique to each person."
2. "One half of people diagnosed with a schizophrenia disorder recover completely ten years from their first episode."
3. "A schizophrenia disorder is a lifelong illness that can be managed, but he will never get better."
4. "If he doesn't get better, there are community supports to help you with his care."

12. Mr. Smadu's mother and sister tell the practical nurse that Mr. Smadu seems to have no interest in the world, has not followed through on his plan to return to school, and is generally not motivated to do anything. The practical nurse recognizes these behaviours as typical of people with a schizophrenia disorder. What is the term for these behaviours?

1. Alogia
2. Anhedonia
3. Avolition
4. Attention impairment

13. Several days after the practical nurse's home visit, Mr. Smadu's sister calls her because Mr. Smadu is saying that the voices are telling him to buy a gun and kill himself. How should the practical nurse advise Mr. Smadu's sister?

1. "Find out why he wants to commit suicide."
2. "Call 9-1-1."
3. "Take him to the mental health clinic or the hospital."
4. "I understand your concern, but although many people with schizophrenia say they are going to commit suicide, they almost never follow through."

END OF CASE 2

CASE 3

A practical nurse works at a large teaching hospital. The hospital has recently had an outbreak of methicillin-resistant Staphylococcus aureus (MRSA).

QUESTIONS 14 to 16 refer to this case.

14. The practical nurse is concerned about the spread of MRSA. Which of the following examples would be a likely mode of transmission?

1. Direct contact of an open wound with contaminated hands
2. Inhalation of aerosol particles from a person with MRSA pneumonia
3. Ingestion of contaminated food
4. Contact with blood or body fluids from a person with poor hygiene

15. Which of the following hospitalized clients has the greatest risk for acquiring MRSA?

1. Mrs. Andrews, age 65 years: pacemaker insertion
2. Andria, age 4 months: investigation of vomiting and failure to thrive
3. Mr. Anneke, age 87 years: diagnosis and assessment of possible dementia
4. Ms. Gary, age 35 years: chronic urinary tract infections secondary to spinal cord injury

16. The practical nurse has an open cut on his finger and is concerned about becoming infected with MRSA from his clients. What should the practical nurse do?

1. Keep the cut clean and cover with an occlusive adhesive bandage or tape
2. Refrain from caring for any clients with MRSA
3. Cover the cut with occlusive tape and wear gloves when performing care
4. Wash his hands before and after client contact

END OF CASE 3

CASE 4

Denika, age 2 years, is admitted to a hospital paediatric unit. She has a severe case of eczema, which has resulted in many infected lesions. She will be receiving intravenous (IV) antibiotics.

QUESTIONS 17 to 21 refer to this case.

17. Denika has scratched her eczema to the point that she is bleeding. The practical nurse has repeatedly told her to stop, but she continues to scratch. The practical nurse decides to restrain her arms to the sides of the crib. Which explanation best describes the practical nurse's action?

1. She has acted with professional accountability.
2. She has used actions that can be interpreted as assault and battery.
3. Denika's skin had to be protected, so the practical nurse acted in a prudent manner.
4. The practical nurse should have asked Denika's parents for permission to restrain her.

18. Denika visits the hospital playroom. At her age, which of the following behaviours will she likely display?

1. Building houses with blocks
2. Being possessive of toys
3. Attempting to stay within the lines when colouring
4. Amusing herself with a picture book for 15 minutes

19. Denika is to receive 1 L of IV fluid per 24 hours. Using a minidrip IV set, with a drop rate of 60 drops/mL, at what rate should the IV infuse?

1. 16 drops per minute
2. 26 drops per minute
3. 42 drops per minute
4. 48 drops per minute

20. Denika is about to be discharged. The practical nurse advises Denika's mother to increase her fluids for several days. Her mother says Denika consistently says "no" every time she is offered fluids. What might the practical nurse advise Denika's mother to do?

1. "Distract her with some food."
2. "Be firm and hand her the glass."
3. "Offer her a choice of two things to drink."
4. "Explain to Denika why she needs to drink a lot of fluids."

21. Denika's mother asks the practical nurse when it would be appropriate to take her to the dentist for dental prophylaxis. What is the practical nurse's most appropriate response?

1. Before starting primary school
2. Between 2 and 3 years of age
3. When Denika begins to lose deciduous teeth
4. The next time another family member goes to the dentist

END OF CASE 4

CASE 5

A practical nurse is working on a postpartum unit at the hospital. One of her clients, Ms. Oliver, just delivered a healthy baby.

QUESTIONS 22 to 27 refer to this case.

22. Four hours after a vaginal delivery, Ms. Oliver still has not voided. What should be the practical nurse's initial action?

1. Palpate her suprapubic area to check for distention
2. Encourage voiding by placing her on a bedpan frequently
3. Place her hands in warm water to encourage micturition
4. Inform the physician of her inability to void

23. Why will the practical nurse encourage Ms. Oliver to ambulate shortly after delivery?

1. It promotes respiration.
2. It increases the tone of the bladder.
3. It maintains abdominal muscle tone.
4. It increases peripheral vasomotor activity.

24. Ms. Oliver is breastfeeding her newborn. What are the expected characteristics of the infant's stool for the first 24 hours?

1. Pale yellow to light brown, firm in consistency with a mild offensive odour
2. Mustardy yellow, soft and seedy in appearance
3. Blackish-green tarry stool
4. Brown with pebble like consistency

25. Ms. Oliver states her breasts feel engorged between feedings. What action would the practical nurse encourage Ms. Oliver to do to help relieve her engorged breast?

1. Only breast feed every 4 hours
2. Gently massage the breast from chest wall to nipple area
3. Apply warm compresses frequently
4. Restrict fluid intake

26. While checking Ms. Oliver on the second postpartum day, the practical nurse observes that Ms. Oliver's fundus is at the umbilicus and displaced to the right. What is the likely cause of this finding?

1. A slow rate of uterine involution
2. A full, over-distended bladder
3. Retained placental fragments in the uterus
4. Overstretched uterine ligaments

27. The practical nurse observes Ms. Oliver's lochia. What type of lochia is expected on the second postpartum day?

1. Lochia serosa
2. Lochia rubra with large clots
3. Lochia alba
4. Lochia rubra

END OF CASE 5

CASE 6

Mr. Richard, age 21 years, is brought to the emergency department by the police. He has been involved in a house fire caused by his mixing volatile chemicals to make illegal street drugs. Mr. Richard has a history of intravenous drug use. He has sustained burns to his face and body. He is uncoordinated in his movements and verbally combative.

QUESTIONS 28 to 31 refer to this case.

28. Mr. Richard is shouting and agitated and demands to see the doctor immediately. What is the most appropriate practical nursing intervention?

1. Talk with him to de-escalate the behaviour
2. Monitor his behaviour to see if he becomes more agitated
3. Inform him that he will be asked to leave if he does not behave
4. Offer to take him to a quiet examination room where you would continue to monitor him closely

29. Mr. Richard is admitted to a medical unit. Which of the following observations by the practical nurse is a priority during the first 24 hours?

1. Wound sepsis
2. Pulmonary distress
3. Pain
4. Fluid and electrolyte imbalances

30. Mr. Richard requires an analgesic for the pain from his burns. What is the most important reason for the practical nurse to administer the drugs via the IV route rather than via IM injection?

1. IM injections increase the risk for tissue irritation.
2. IM injections are more painful than IV administration.
3. IV administration will ensure more effective absorption.
4. IV administration provides more prolonged relief of pain.

31. Mr. Richard has been charged by the police for his illegal drug possession and manufacturing. A lawyer comes to visit Mr. Richard and tells the practical nurse that he would like to read Mr. Richard's health record. What is the most appropriate response by the practical nurse?

1. "You may read the chart if you get permission from Mr. Richard."
2. "You will have to get permission from the doctor."
3. "You are allowed to read the health record because Mr. Richard has been charged with a criminal offence."
4. "I am not allowed to let you read Mr. Richard's health record."

END OF CASE 6

CASE 7

Mr. Wilmot, age 23 years, has been diagnosed with cancer in his left testicle. He is admitted to hospital for the surgical removal of the testicle. Mr. Wilmot is engaged to be married in 6 months.

QUESTIONS 32 to 35 refer to this case.

32. Mr. Wilmot asks the practical nurse if he will still be able to father children after having his testicle removed. Which of the following responses by the practical nurse would be most therapeutic?

1. "The important thing is that you become healthy again. You can always adopt if children are important to you."
2. "I understand your fears. Any intervention for cancer is likely to cause infertility."
3. "I can see you are very concerned about this. Although you will still have one functioning testicle, perhaps you would like to discuss sperm banking before the surgery."
4. "There is a possibility that the surgery will make you unable to maintain an erection, which would lead to an inability to father children."

33. Mr. Wilmot tells the practical nurse that he feels he will not be a "real man" after the surgery, and he worries about losing his ability to perform sexually. How should the practical nurse respond to these concerns?

1. Tell Mr. Wilmot that he is still a man even with one testicle.
2. Reassure Mr. Wilmot there is very little chance that he will have any problems.
3. Ask Mr. Wilmot if he would like to talk with a therapist to discuss his concerns.
4. Tell Mr. Wilmot the prognosis for this type of cancer is excellent and he need not worry.

34. Which of the following topics would the practical nurse include in his client teaching?

1. Once surgery and chemotherapy are completed, Mr. Wilmot can expect to lead a normal life, free of cancer.
2. Mr. Wilmot will have to take low-dose testosterone for the rest of his life.
3. Mr. Wilmot must have regular physical exams with his oncologist.
4. The likelihood of a relapse is quite high, so Mr. Wilmot must be tested every 3 months.

35. Mr. Wilmot is ready for discharge. The practical nurse teaches self-examination of the remaining testicle. Which of the following statements is correct?

1. Once a month in the shower, roll the testis between the thumb and first three fingers to cover the entire surface.
2. Lie flat on a bed and use circular motions with the fingers to detect any unusual lumps.
3. Shine a flashlight through the testis from the side to highlight any lesions.
4. The testis will feel like a soft-boiled egg, with the epididymis feeling smoother than the testis.

END OF CASE 7

CASE 8

A practical nurse is in charge on the evening shift at a long-term care facility. She is the only registered practical nurse working with unregulated care providers (UCPs) who have been trained to perform basic hygiene care and take vital signs. The practical nurse is responsible for administering medications to the 20 clients on her unit.

QUESTIONS 36 to 39 refer to this case.

36. Mr. Lok has a history of hypertension, treated with a variety of antihypertensive medications. The physician's order directs the practical nurse not to administer the regularly scheduled nifedipine (Adalat) if Mr. Lok's blood pressure is below 100 systolic. The UCP records a blood pressure of 94/72 for Mr. Lok. What should the practical nurse do?

1. Hold the nifedipine.
2. Check with the doctor before holding the nifedipine.
3. Ask the UCP if the blood pressure reading was accurate.
4. Check Mr. Lok's blood pressure before holding the nifedipine medication.

37. Enteric-coated Aspirin (ECASA) q6hr prn is ordered for Ms. Bystriska. Which of the following is a correct nursing action related to the administration of the ECASA?

1. Obtain verbal consent from Ms. Bystriska at the time of administration of the ECASA.
2. Crush the tablet if she is unable to swallow it.
3. Leave the ECASA at her bedside for her to take as necessary.
4. Obtain a written consent that covers all medication administration.

38. Mr. Gileppo is to receive insulin subcutaneously. Which would be an incorrect action by the practical nurse when administering the insulin?

1. Injecting it into subcutaneous abdominal tissue
2. Using a 29-gauge needle
3. Massaging the area to increase absorption
4. Pinching the tissue of the lateral aspect of the thigh

39. Ms. Banwait, a client with dementia related to Alzheimer's disease, is ordered donepezil (Aricept) to slow the progress of her disease. When the practical nurse offers her the donepezil, Ms. Banwait refuses to take it, stating that it upsets her stomach too much. Her husband, Mr. Banwait, insists that she take the medication. What should the practical nurse do?

1. Give the medication, as Ms. Banwait has dementia.
2. Give the medication, as Mr. Banwait is the next of kin and is authorized to make treatment decisions.
3. Do not give the medication, as it is producing adverse effects.
4. Do not give the medication, as Ms. Banwait has withdrawn her consent.

END OF CASE 8

CASE 9

A practical nurse works in a family planning clinic. She provides teaching about reproductive and sexual health and birth control to a variety of clients.

QUESTIONS 40 to 44 refer to this case.

40. Ms. Eigo, age 27 years, consults the practical nurse regarding family planning. Ms. Eigo asks the practical nurse about the contraceptive diaphragm as a form of birth control. What should the practical nurse tell Ms. Eigo about the contraceptive diaphragm?

1. Use a vaginal lubricant to assist with the insertion of the diaphragm.
2. Leave the diaphragm in place once inserted as it does not require removal after each use.
3. Receive an annual gynecologic examination to assess the fit of the diaphragm.
4. Do not use a spermicide with this form of contraception.

41. Sarah, a 16-year-old single adolescent, finds out that she is 4 weeks pregnant. She asks the practical nurse, "Do you think I should have an abortion?" Which of the following statements by the practical nurse is the most appropriate?

1. "It would probably be best for the baby and you."
2. "Do you think you would feel guilty if you had an abortion?"
3. "What do you think would be the best thing for you to do?"
4. "What do your parents want you to do?"

42. Ms. Lee is a sex worker. She asks the practical nurse what she should use for contraception and prevention of sexually transmitted infections (STIs). Which of the following methods of prevention would be recommended by the practical nurse?

1. A diaphragm
2. A spermicide
3. A cervical cap
4. A female condom

43. Ms. McLeod has a positive test result for human papilloma virus (HPV). What should the practical nurse discuss with Ms. McLeod regarding future health care?

1. The need to have routine Papanicolaou (Pap) tests
2. The importance of finishing her prescribed antibiotics
3. That she should abstain from sexual intercourse to prevent transmission
4. If her treatment involves cryotherapy, that she will no longer be infectious to her sexual partners

44. A cardiologist has recommended to Ms. Ahmadi, age 42 years, that she should never become pregnant due to her severe heart failure. Ms. Ahmadi has complied with this recommendation and asks the practical nurse what form of birth control would be the best option for her. What information should the practical nurse provide?

1. "Your best option is the oral birth control pill."
2. "A tubal ligation is almost 100% effective."
3. "I'd suggest your partner have a vasectomy."
4. "An intrauterine device is easily inserted and is an effective birth control method."

END OF CASE 9

CASE 10

The World Health Organization has predicted that a pandemic form of influenza will spread to Canada. A vaccine has been rapidly manufactured, and health care providers are preparing for mass immunizations and caring for acutely ill, infected people.

QUESTIONS 45 to 50 refer to this case.

45. Health care workers are a priority group to receive the vaccine. A practical nurse is concerned about receiving this new vaccine, as the media have reported that it is not safe. What should the practical nurse do?

1. Not have the vaccine because safety is in question
2. Research reputable resources for information on the safety of the vaccine
3. Have the vaccine in order to protect the practical nurse and her clients from the flu
4. Discuss with nursing colleagues their opinions about the vaccine

46. A practical nurse cares for her older adult mother and has two young children. She feels that if a pandemic occurs, she will have to make a choice between caring for her clients and protecting the health of her family. What term relates to this situation?

1. Ethical dilemma
2. Ethical theory
3. Moral distress
4. Nonmaleficence

47. A practical nurse is aware that this pandemic situation will result in limited resource allocation. She wonders who will receive priority treatment if many acutely ill people require intensive hospital care. Which of the following guidelines would most likely be recommended?

1. Older, frail adults receive priority care, as they are more at risk.
2. Healthy adults receive the resources, as they are most likely to survive.
3. The federal government legislates who the at-risk groups are for treatment.
4. Local, provincial, federal, and international pandemic planning committees identify priorities.

48. A practical nurse is participating in a large community influenza vaccine clinic. The vaccine is to be delivered by injection in a 0.5 mL volume per dose. How would the practical nurse landmark to inject in the most appropriate muscle for older children and adults?

1. Midpoint of the lateral aspect of the upper arm, about 3 to 5 cm below the acromion process
2. The centre of the triangle of the index finger pointing to the anterior superior iliac spine and middle finger along the iliac crest toward the buttock
3. Divide the buttocks into quadrants; the site is in the middle of the upper outer quadrant
4. Middle third of the anterior lateral aspect of the thigh

49. Which of the following questions would the practical nurse ask prior to administering the influenza vaccine to a 20-year-old man?

1. "Have you ever had an allergic reaction to the influenza vaccine?"
2. "Are you sexually active?"
3. "Have you ever had influenza?"
4. "Are your childhood immunizations up to date?"

50. A mother brings her priority-listed asthmatic daughter to be immunized at the vaccine clinic. She also brings in her teenage son and requests that he receive the vaccine. At this time, well adolescents are not on the priority list for the vaccine. What should the practical nurse do?

1. Give the vaccine to the adolescent son
2. Tell the mother her teenage son is not allowed to have the vaccine
3. Inform the mother her teenage son is not at risk for getting the pandemic influenza, so he does not need to have the vaccine
4. Explain to the mother why her adolescent son is not in a priority group at present and tell her that he will likely be able to be vaccinated at a later date

END OF CASE 10

CASE 11

A practical nurse is working in a long-term care facility. Ms. Smith, age 87, is admitted to the facility.

QUESTIONS 51 to 53 refer to this case.

51. Ms. Smith tells the practical nurse that she might as well die now, as she has no family left to care for her. Which of the following responses by the practical nurse would be most therapeutic?

1. "Don't worry; you will soon make new friends here."
2. "I know it must be hard for you, but you will soon settle in."
3. "Let me get us some tea, and we can talk about how you are feeling."
4. "Why don't we go down to the lounge, and I will introduce you to some other residents."

52. Ms. Smith is mobile but spends most of her day sitting in a chair. Staff members have told her on many occasions that she needs to exercise and have explained the benefits of regular exercise for her mobility and cognitive function. Ms. Smith has said, "I am aware of the benefits of exercising, but I have never been one to enjoy exercise, and I am not going to start now." What should the practical nurse do?

1. Move the chair from her room so she is not able to sit in it
2. Take her to the agency exercise classes
3. Assess Ms. Smith's cognitive abilities and need for a substitute decision maker (SDM)
4. Respect her decision and continue to encourage exercise

53. Ms. Smith tells the practical nurse she appreciates her care and concern so much that she would like to give her a gift as a thank-you. She hands the practical nurse a diamond and emerald brooch. What should the practical nurse do?

1. Accept the gift if Ms. Smith is cognitively intact and aware of the value of the brooch.
2. Tell Ms. Smith that since the gift is quite valuable, it is best to leave it to the practical nurse in her will.

3. Thank Ms. Smith but explain it is against professional ethics to accept expensive gifts from clients.
4. Tell Ms. Smith agency policies do not permit nurses to accept any type of gift from clients.

END OF CASE 11

CASE 12

Mr. Hudson is a 53-year-old man who has been diagnosed with type 2 diabetes. He is referred to the practical nurse for education about his disease. He is somewhat overweight and requires education about nutrition for weight loss and diabetes management.

QUESTIONS 54 to 60 refer to this case.

54. After developing a rapport with Mr. Hudson, what would be the most appropriate initial strategy for the practical nurse to use with Mr. Hudson at his first learning session?

1. Provide him with a list of "dos and don'ts" about his diet
2. Explain the need for a balanced diet to regulate his blood sugar and lose weight
3. Ask him what behaviours he would like to change
4. Ask him what he would like to learn from nutrition counselling

55. Which of the following would be a key concept in meal planning for Mr. Hudson?

1. Smaller meals at frequent intervals
2. Decreased carbohydrate intake
3. Vitamin and mineral supplements to replace deficiencies in food intake
4. Reduced total fat

56. Baked beans, whole grain cereals, flax seed, brown rice, and soybeans are recommended for a healthy diet. They are examples of which of the following types of carbohydrates?

1. Simple carbohydrates
2. Complex carbohydrates
3. Monounsaturated carbohydrates
4. High-glycemic-index carbohydrates

57. Mr. Hudson asks the practical nurse how he can lower his intake of saturated fats. Which of the following foods would the practical nurse recommend that Mr. Hudson avoid?

1. Fish
2. Canola oil
3. Whole milk
4. Omega 3 trans-fat-free soft margarine

58. Mr. Hudson asks the practical nurse what would be a good breakfast for him, considering his diabetes and that he would like to lose weight. Which of the following menus would be the most appropriate?

1. One bran muffin with margarine, half a grapefruit, and a glass of orange juice
2. A poached egg, one slice of whole-wheat toast, a glass of skim milk, and an apple
3. Two slices of crisp bacon, scrambled eggs, and green tea
4. One cup of raisin bran cereal with lactose-free milk and a glass of grapefruit juice

59. One month after Mr. Hudson's visit to the diabetes clinic, he calls the practical nurse to say that he is sick with gastroenteritis and had vomited a small amount of emesis once earlier in the morning. He wants to know what to do about his medications and food. How should the practical nurse advise Mr. Hudson?

1. Not to take his oral hypoglycemic pills and to drink as much sweetened juice as he is able
2. Maintain his normal diabetes medications, monitor his blood sugar every 3 to 4 hours, and drink frequent sips of carbohydrate fluids as required
3. Contact his doctor for instructions
4. Take half the usual dose of his oral hypoglycemic pills and sip fluids every hour

60. Mr. Hudson comes back to the clinic 3 months after his first visit. Which of the following would be the best criterion for evaluating the status of his type 2 diabetes?

1. A weight loss of 5 kg
2. A fasting blood-sugar reading of 6.5 mmol/L
3. A glycosylated hemoglobin (HbA_{1c}) test reading of 5.9%
4. A statement by Mr. Hudson that he feels well and is managing the disease

END OF CASE 12

CASE 13

Tiffany, age 15 years, is admitted to an eating disorders unit at a general hospital because of severe malnutrition. She has a history of self-restricted food intake and excessive exercising over the past 2 years. She is assessed to be below 60% of the expected normal body weight for her height. Her practical nurse performs an admission health history.

QUESTIONS 61 to 67 refer to this case.

61. The practical nurse asks Tiffany about her health history. What might the practical nurse expect Tiffany to tell her?

1. "I feel really hot sometimes."
2. "I stopped menstruating when I was 14."

3. "My skin is really oily."
4. "I get diarrhea quite often."

62. Which of the following blood tests would be most important for Tiffany?

1. Sodium
2. Potassium
3. Electrolytes
4. Chloride

63. The practical nurse interviews Tiffany's parents. Which of the following descriptions might her parents use for Tiffany?

1. "We suspect she is promiscuous."
2. "Tiffany openly discusses her anorexia with us."
3. "She often acts out and is difficult to manage."
4. "Tiffany is a high achiever at school."

64. The practical nurse takes Tiffany's vital signs later that night while Tiffany is sleeping. She discovers that Tiffany's apical rate is 41 beats per minute. What is the appropriate initial nursing intervention?

1. Immediately notify the on-call physician
2. Monitor the apical rate every hour until it increases and stabilizes
3. Wake Tiffany and have her drink a glass of juice or water
4. Bring Tiffany a snack of her preferred food

65. When Tiffany's vital signs stabilize, she is permitted to walk around the unit. The practical nurse plans to monitor Tiffany's physical activity. What is the primary rationale for this intervention?

1. Adolescents with anorexia may secretly exercise as a weight-loss activity.
2. Tiffany is so malnourished that physical activity will be harmful.
3. Regular physical activity is an important component of the therapeutic plan.
4. Exercise will improve Tiffany's ability to tolerate the increased nutritional intake.

66. Tiffany is scheduled to attend group sessions with the other adolescent girls on the unit who have anorexia. Tiffany says, "I don't want to sit around with a bunch of silly girls. Do I have to go?" What would be the best response from the practical nurse?

1. "I think you need their support."
2. "Let's talk about your feelings about not going to these meetings."
3. "No, it is best to wait until you feel you really need to talk with other girls."
4. "Yes, because the group sessions will help you cope with your anorexia."

67. Which of the following dietary goals would be appropriate for Tiffany?

1. Tiffany will consume a high-calorie diet to promote rapid weight gain.
2. Tiffany will eat a prescribed diet to ensure gradual weight gain.
3. Tiffany will drink 3 L of water a day to ensure adequate hydration.
4. Tiffany will gain 1 kg per week.

END OF CASE 13

CASE 14

A practical nurse works at a community health clinic. She receives a call from Ms. McColm, the mother of a 3-week-old infant.

QUESTIONS 68 to 71 refer to this case.

68. Ms. McColm is worried that her 3-week-old infant might be sick. What would be a significant manifestation of illness in an infant of this age?

1. A red, papule-type rash on the face
2. Long periods of sleep
3. Grunting and rapid respirations
4. Desire for increased fluids during the feedings

69. Ms. McColm tells the practical nurse her infant "feels warm." By which of the following methods would the practical nurse recommend that Ms. McColm take the infant's temperature?

1. Oral
2. Rectal
3. Axillary
4. Tympanic

70. Ms. McColm determines that the infant's temperature is 38.9°C. What should the practical nurse recommend?

1. "Give the infant extra fluids."
2. "Bring the infant to the clinic to see the physician."
3. "Monitor the temperature every 4 hours for the next several days."
4. "Administer infant acetaminophen (Tempra)."

71. The practical nurse documents this telephone consultation using computer charting. Which of the following is an accurate statement regarding computerized documentation?

1. Each nurse must have an individual and secret password.
2. Clients are not allowed to view their computerized health records.
3. Client permission is required prior to accessing any health record.
4. Research has shown that more documentation errors occur with computer charting.

END OF CASE 14

CASE 15

A rural community has a program to provide support to older persons to enable them to live independently for as long as possible in their own homes. A practical nurse leads this community initiative.

QUESTIONS 72 to 75 refer to this case.

72. Many of the practical nurse's clients do not have a great deal of money. What is the most important factor to consider when caring for clients who have limited financial resources?

1. They will have decreased access to the health care system.
2. They may have low self-esteem related to the stigma of poverty.
3. Their basic physical needs may not be met.
4. There is often a lack of client compliance with recommended treatment.

73. The practical nurse visits the home of Ms. Gash, an active 84-year-old client. Which of the following would most concern the practical nurse about Ms. Gash's home environment?

1. It is a wood-frame house.
2. There is a small throw rug on the hardwood floor.
3. It has a microwave oven.
4. There is electric heating from baseboard heaters.

74. Many of the practical nurse's clients are concerned about "moving their bowels." Which of the following recommendations would the practical nurse suggest to help prevent constipation in an older client?

1. Fibre in the form of bran and fresh fruits
2. Cellulose in the form of corn on the cob and rice
3. Natural laxatives in the form of bananas and milk
4. Peristalsis stimulators in the form of echinacea

75. The local health department has issued a pollution alert on a hot, humid day. Mr. Scanlon, who has chronic obstructive pulmonary disease (COPD), phones the practical nurse to ask what he should do. What should the practical nurse advise?

1. To stay inside his air-conditioned house
2. To carry on with his ordinary activities
3. To contact his respiratory therapist for advice
4. To increase his inhaled medications

END OF CASE 15

CASE 16

Ms. Merkel, a woman who lives in a self-sufficient religious community, has been admitted to hospital with severe pulmonary fibrosis.

QUESTIONS 76 to 78 refer to this case.

76. When providing care for Ms. Merkel, how should the practical nurse assess and treat her?

1. In accordance with known religious beliefs
2. According to her individually expressed needs
3. In compliance with guidelines that her family has provided
4. No differently from the other clients on the unit

77. Ms. Merkel refuses to allow Alex, a male nurse, to care for her as she says it would be considered inappropriate in her community. She insists that she have a female nurse. What should Alex do?

1. Arrange for a change-of-client assignment to a female nurse
2. Discuss with Ms. Merkel why she wishes not to have a male nurse
3. Tell Ms. Merkel that in Canadian society the rights of male nurses are respected
4. Tell Ms. Merkel she must accept him as her nurse because the charge nurse assigned him

78. Due to the severity of her illness, Ms. Merkel dies. Before performing end-of-life care for the body, what should the practical nurse do?

1. Arrange for Ms. Merkel's relatives to see her
2. Ensure Ms. Merkel's wishes regarding organ donation have been discussed with the family
3. Identify any cultural death rites that must be respected
4. Avoid touching the body until the religious leader has provided permission

END OF CASE 16

CASE 17

Ms. Lesley is admitted to the postpartum unit with her full-term newborn son Lee, after having a caesarean section.

QUESTIONS 79 to 82 refer to this case.

79. Ms. Lesley received a caesarean section due to untreated genital herpes. What would be the danger to the infant if she were to have delivered vaginally?

1. Thrush
2. Systemic herpes
3. Ophthalmia neonatorum
4. Neurological complications

80. The practical nurse obtains an oxygen saturation reading of 87% on 2-hour-old Lee, who is not experiencing respiratory distress. What initial action should he take?

1. No action is required
2. Contact the physician
3. Administer ordered oxygen
4. Place the infant in a humidified Isolette

81. During the examination of newborn baby Lee, the practical nurse notes that he has asymmetric gluteal folds. Which of the following conditions does this indicate?

1. Central nervous system damage
2. A dislocated hip
3. An inguinal hernia
4. Peripheral nervous system damage

82. Baby Lee has had a circumcision. What is the most essential nursing observation during the immediate period after the circumcision?

1. Manifestations of infection
2. Hemorrhage
3. A shrill, piercing cry
4. Decreased urinary output

END OF CASE 17

CASE 18

Ms. Canseco, age 64, is admitted to hospital with a diagnosis of anginal pain.

QUESTIONS 83 to 85 refer to this case.

83. The practical nurse provides teaching to Ms. Canseco about angina. What will the practical nurse include in the teaching?

1. "The pain from angina indicates that your heart cells are being damaged."
2. "The pain of a myocardial infarction is more severe than angina pain."
3. "Sublingual nitroglycerin usually relieves pain within 15 minutes."
4. "Rest and nitroglycerin relieve pain from angina."

84. The practical nurse counsels Ms. Canseco about cholesterol in relation to atherosclerosis. What information should be included in the counselling?

1. "Cholesterol is provided to the body entirely by dietary intake."
2. "Cholesterol is found in many foods, from both plant and animal sources."
3. "Cholesterol has no function in the body so must be controlled to prevent atherosclerosis."
4. "Cholesterol is naturally produced by the body but can increase with a high dietary intake."

85. A nitroglycerin transdermal patch is prescribed for Ms. Canseco's anginal pain. Which of the following statements should be included in health teaching for Ms. Canseco?

1. "Remove the patch at bedtime to prevent tolerance to the drug."
2. "There are no adverse effects since the drug is delivered so slowly."
3. "Before strenuous exercise, another patch may be cut in half and applied to prevent pain."
4. "Used patches should be disposed of in the toilet or with biodegradable recyclable waste."

END OF CASE 18

CASE 19

Mr. Bangay, age 88 years, is a resident of an older-people's retirement home. Mr. Bangay's wife has advanced Alzheimer's disease and is a client in a long-term care facility in another part of the city. Mr. Bangay misses his wife and lately has shown manifestations of depression.

QUESTIONS 86 to 89 refer to this case.

86. One morning Mr. Bangay says to the practical nurse, "I feel terrible today." What would be the practical nurse's most appropriate response?

1. "You look fine."
2. "Do you feel ill?"
3. "You'll feel better tomorrow."
4. "Tell me about how you feel."

87. Mr. Bangay says to the practical nurse, "I wish you could have known my wife." Which response would be the most therapeutic at this time?

1. "There are many lady residents here who would appreciate your company."
2. "We have counsellors available to speak with you."
3. "Her move to the long-term care facility must have made you feel very sad."
4. "My mother had Alzheimer's, so I understand your sadness."

88. Several days later, the practical nurse notes Mr. Bangay's oral temperature at 0800 hours is 37.8°C. Protocol at the retirement centre is that vital signs are to be monitored every 8 hours. Which nursing action is most appropriate?

1. Take his temperature at 1600 hours as per agency policy
2. Take his temperature again in 2 to 4 hours
3. Call his physician for a more frequent vital signs order
4. Retake his temperature using the axillary route

89. There is a lot of conflict among the team at the retirement home concerning the length of time some nurses take for their evening breaks. How should the nurses best resolve their conflict?

1. Encourage each other not to take excessive time for breaks
2. Mandate the length of breaks
3. Report the issue to the nurse manager
4. Collaborate on a mutually agreeable length of time for breaks

END OF CASE 19

CASE 20

Olivia, age 11 years, is taken to her physician by her parents because she has developed severe headaches. Her physician admits her to hospital for tests to rule out a brain tumour.

QUESTIONS 90 to 95 refer to this case.

90. The practical nurse performs a physical assessment on Olivia, which she documents on the health record. What would be the most accurate description of Olivia's general behaviour?

1. "Behaviour appropriate for age"
2. "Drowsy but awake and oriented to conversation"
3. "Behaves well"
4. "Complaining of headaches"

91. Olivia is scheduled to have a computed tomography (CT) scan. Her parents ask, "What is a CT scan?" How should the practical nurse answer?

1. "A CT scan records the electrical activity of the brain."
2. "Pulses of ultrasonic waves are sent through the brain."
3. "A dye is injected into the brain, and images are viewed on a computer."
4. "X-ray pictures are assembled by a computer and displayed as images."

92. Olivia is diagnosed with a medulloblastoma, a type of malignant brain tumour, and is scheduled for surgery. She asks the practical nurse if her bad headaches will go away after the operation. What is the best response by the practical nurse?

1. "The operation will cure your headaches."
2. "How bad is your headache today?"
3. "We hope the surgery will cure the headaches, but there is a chance you will still continue to have headaches."
4. "Are you afraid of the surgery?"

93. Olivia has surgery and is brought postoperatively to the neurology floor. How should the practical nurse position Olivia after surgery?

1. It depends on the location of the operative site
2. Flat with body and head in the midline
3. Trendelenburg's position
4. On the operative side to prevent excess bleeding

94. The practical nurse notices the presence of colourless drainage on Olivia's scalp dressing. What should be the initial action by the practical nurse?

1. Circle the drainage area with a pen every hour
2. Report the drainage to the surgeon immediately
3. Document normal drainage on the postsurgical record
4. Change the dressing and note any blood on the soiled gauze

95. Olivia does not recover from surgery. She becomes comatose and is transferred to a palliative care unit in the hospital. She is expected to die, and her parents do not wish resuscitation. Two weeks later at 0200 hours, the practical nurse finds Olivia with absent vital signs, skin discoloration, and a fixed stare. What action should the practical nurse take?

1. Pronounce death
2. Certify death
3. Call the physician to pronounce death and complete the death certificate
4. Remove Olivia's body to the morgue

END OF CASE 20

CASE 21

A practical nurse arrives at the long-term care facility for her 8 hour evening shift. She receives the report on her clients from the 8 hour day-shift practical nurse.

QUESTIONS 96 to 98 refer to this case.

96. The practical nurse has arrived on the unit to replace the day shift nurses. Which of the following situations should the practical nurse attend to first when she begins her evening shift?

1. A client who rings the call bell to request a sponge bath
2. The narcotics count with the day-shift nurse
3. A physician who requests assistance with reinsertion of a gastrostomy tube (G-tube)
4. A client who is returning from having a CT scan at the local hospital

97. Ms. David is a client who is receiving palliative therapy for her end-stage cardiac disease. During the night, the physician telephones Ms. David's family to inform them that her vital signs are deteriorating, and she is having episodes of apnea. They are advised to come immediately to the unit. At Ms. David's bedside, the son asks the practical nurse, "Do you think she will die tonight?" What is the most appropriate response by the practical nurse?

1. "Why do you think she is going to die?"
2. "You'll have to ask the doctor if she is going to die."
3. "Would you like me to call the chaplain?"
4. "We cannot say for sure, but it appears that she will die soon."

98. Mr. Marshall has heart failure and pulmonary edema. Which of the following nursing actions would help to alleviate his respiratory distress due to these conditions?

1. Elevate his lower extremities
2. Encourage frequent coughing
3. Place him in an orthopneic position
4. Prepare him for modified postural drainage

END OF CASE 21

CASE 22

Mr. Camponi is experiencing an acute exacerbation of right-sided heart failure and has been admitted to the acute medical unit.

QUESTIONS 99 to 100 refer to this case.

99. Which of the following nursing actions would most accurately assess the degree of Mr. Camponi's edema?

1. Checking for pitting in his extremities
2. Weighing Mr. Camponi
3. Measuring the diameter of his ankles
4. Monitoring fluid intake and output

100. Which of the following independent nursing actions should the practical nurse implement to limit the spread of Mr. Camponi's ankle edema?

1. Restricting his fluids
2. Elevating his legs
3. Applying elastic bandages
4. Performing range-of-motion exercises

END OF CASE 22

INDEPENDENT QUESTIONS

QUESTIONS 101 to 200 do not refer to a particular case.

101. Each day a practical nurse writes about her activities and experiences on the social networking site Facebook. Which of the following statements best reflects professional judgement concerning her participation in Facebook?

1. The practical nurse must take care never to write about clients, client care, and the organization.
2. The practical nurse should not participate in Facebook.
3. Participation in a social networking site is an optimum use of technology for professional development.
4. The practical nurse may write about clients if she receives their verbal permission.

102. Christopher, age 16 years, has a patient-controlled analgesia (PCA) device postsurgery. Choose the statement that best indicates that his family has understood the teaching about the PCA.

1. "We will push the button for him when he needs it."
2. "The PCA will provide variable blood levels of the pain medication."
3. "We should tell the practical nurse when we think Christopher needs to push the button."
4. "The PCA will help Christopher have some control over his pain."

103. Ms. Levis is a newly graduated francophone nurse. Although she wrote and passed the English version of the licensure exam, she does not feel comfortable speaking or understanding English. What is her professional responsibility when accepting employment as a practical nurse in Canada?

1. She has passed the licensure exam in English; therefore, she is legally able to work in an English-speaking environment.
2. She should obtain employment at a francophone agency until she feels confident communicating in English.
3. She must not accept employment in a bilingual environment until she has passed a recognized English communications course.
4. She may obtain employment at an English-speaking agency but should accept only French-speaking clients.

104. Mrs. Smirnoff, age 83 years, has advanced dementia and is not able to communicate verbally. She sustained a fractured hip, which required surgery. What is the best method of managing her postoperative level of pain?

1. Provide her with a pediatric pain-rating scale
2. Provide her with a PCA and show her how to use it
3. Provide an analgesic and comfort measures as per agency protocol
4. Provide analgesics at regular intervals and observe her behaviour

105. A young hockey player has been admitted to an observational unit after being hit hard on the head by another player's stick. How would the nurse position this client?

1. Supine
2. Sims
3. Semi-Fowler
4. With the head of the bed lowered by 15 to 30 degrees

106. Ms. William has just had a below-the-knee amputation as a result of severe peripheral vascular disease. Nursing staff has ensured she has received the knowledge and support to make informed decisions. Although she understands the role smoking has contributed to her disease and that she will likely face further amputation if she continues to smoke, she leaves the unit regularly to go outside for a cigarette. The practical nurses feel helpless with her noncompliance. What nursing action is appropriate?

1. Continue to advise and support Ms. William but do not judge her decisions
2. Suggest to Ms. William's family that they find a substitute decision maker
3. Consult with the health care team to obtain the assistance of a mediator
4. Refuse to care for Ms. William since she is being noncompliant

107. Mr. Seaberg has a tracheotomy, which requires frequent suctioning. What is the most important action by the practical nurse before performing suctioning?

1. Ensure he is well hydrated
2. Provide increased oxygen
3. Provide oral care
4. Ensure that clean tracheotomy ties are at the bedside

108. A practical nurse works on a surgical unit of a hospital. On the night shift, she is "floated" to the palliative care unit, where she is assigned to a woman who is scheduled for medical assistance in dying (MAID). The nurse does not believe in MAID. What should she do?

1. Ask the unit manager if there is another client she could be assigned to who is not having MAID
2. Refuse to care for the woman on the grounds that it is against her ethics
3. Tell the manager of her surgical unit that she is not able to float to the palliative care unit
4. Care for this woman, using the time as an opportunity to provide health teaching about the better options for palliative care instead of MAID

109. Which of the following clients would be most likely to meet the criteria to be eligible for medical assistance in dying (MAID)?

1. An 81-year-old female suffering from dementia and asks to die.
2. A 10-year-old child with an incurable brain tumour who is now blind and no longer wants to live.
3. A 37-year-old male with rapid progression of amyotrophic lateral sclerosis (ALS) who states he no longer wants to live in a helpless state waiting for death.
4. A 47-year-old female suffering a major depression disorder and no longer wants to live.

110. A practical nurse working in the community setting visits a client who is taking a variety of complex medications. The client requires more education about the medications. What is the most appropriate action by the practical nurse?

1. Arrange a consultation with the client's pharmacist
2. Suggest that the client discuss the medications with the ordering physician
3. Research the medications and conduct a teaching session with the client
4. Obtain manufacturer's package inserts for the client to read

111. The practical nurse is providing teaching to a client about deep breathing and coughing techniques to use postoperatively after her surgery. The practical nurse senses the client does not understand the information she is delivering. What would be the best action by the practical nurse?

1. Continue with the information because the client will understand as she develops the topic.
2. Demonstrate to the client how to do the deep breathing and coughing exercises and have the client repeat the exercise back to the nurse.
3. Change to another topic and not continue with breathing techniques because it is too confusing for the client.
4. Stress to the client that this is very important information that will help her postoperatively.

112. An older adult client in a long-term care facility often gets out of bed during the night. She has advanced osteoporosis and is unsteady on her feet. Which of the following actions by the practical nurse would help ensure the client's safety?

1. Ensure both side rails are up at all times
2. Ask the physician to increase her medications taken at bedtime
3. Place the bed in the lowest position and check on the client frequently
4. Place the bed against a wall, keeping the open side bed rail raised

113. A practical nurse is caring for Mr. Green, who has recently been diagnosed with Parkinson's disease. What will the practical nurse teach Mr. Green's family about the early manifestations of the disease?

1. He may experience mood swings.
2. Tremors will not be noticeable with rest.
3. He may not recognize his caregivers from day to day.
4. His appetite will increase.

114. Mr. Mason, age 19 years, is a resident in a hostel for homeless people. The practical nurse at the hostel suspects that he is dependent on fentanyl which he obtains illegally. During an initial interview, which of the following questions would be appropriate for the practical nurse to ask?

1. "How much fentanyl do you take, and what is its effect on you?"
2. "How do you get the fentanyl?"
3. "Are you aware of the legal and health implications of taking fentanyl?"
4. "Why did you start to take fentanyl?"

115. While the practical nurse is administering an enema, the client complains of abdominal cramping. What should be the practical nurse's initial action?

1. Slow the rate
2. Discontinue the procedure
3. Stop until his cramps have subsided
4. Lower the height of the container

116. A practical nurse in a walk-in clinic performs a health assessment on Mr. Nascad, age 81 years, and observes that he has a hand tremor. What should the practical nurse initially do?

1. Question Mr. Nascad about his past history and present symptoms
2. Notify the physician
3. Document this finding but recognize that most tremors are benign
4. No action is necessary as this is a common finding in older persons

117. Ms. Evans states that her last menstrual period began on June 11, but she experienced some spotting on July 8. Which date represents the practical nurse's calculation of Ms. Evan's expected date of delivery?

1. March 10
2. March 18
3. April 12
4. April 15

118. Ms. Gary, a breastfeeding mother, has developed mastitis. What should the practical nurse explain to Ms. Gary?

1. "Only breastfeed from the unaffected breast"
2. "Limit your fluid intake"
3. "Stop breastfeeding until your symptoms have resolved"
4. "Continue breastfeeding from both breasts"

119. A practical nurse observes another nurse hitting a confused client. What should be the practical nurse's first action?

1. Intervene in the situation
2. Report the occurrence to the nurse manager
3. Tell the nurse to leave the unit
4. Document the incident

120. Mr. Benjamin has type 1 diabetes. He asks the practical nurse what insulin does in the body. Which of the following statements would be the best response by the practical nurse?

1. "Insulin helps block extra glucose from entering the bloodstream."

2. "Insulin is necessary to help glucose get into the cells to provide energy."
3. "Insulin works with the liver to control the amount of glucose released for energy."
4. "Insulin blocks the absorption of glucose in the small intestine."

121. A community practical nurse who consults at a secondary school is concerned that the teenagers are consuming a lot of high-calorie, high-sugar-content soft drinks and snacks bought from vending machines in the cafeteria. What would be the most appropriate action by the practical nurse?

1. Make posters to educate the teenagers about the dangers of the snacks and pop
2. Tell the school administration they must remove the vending machines
3. Host a parent–teacher meeting to promote teenagers' bringing lunches from home to eat at school
4. Consult with school administration to have the snacks and pop in the machines replaced with nutritional choices

122. An older woman is admitted to a busy medical unit. All client rooms are full, so she is placed in a bed in the hall. The woman is hard of hearing. What strategy could the practical nurse use to maintain confidentiality when interacting with the woman?

1. Speak in a low voice
2. Use pen and paper to communicate with the woman
3. Refrain from communicating with the woman
4. Use body language to convey information

123. An 89-year-old woman is admitted to the acute medical unit during the night with a diagnosis of pneumonia. She is accompanied by four adult children, all of whom say they are determined to stay at her bedside. The acute medical unit is very busy, and there is a rule that no more than one visitor may stay at the client's bedside. What should the practical nurse say to the family?

1. "You don't need to stay; your mother will be fine. I'll call if she gets worse."
2. "Only one visitor is allowed. The rest of you will have to go home."
3. "The rules of the hospital state that only one visitor is allowed."
4. "I suggest you rotate visits, ensuring one bedside visitor at a time overnight."

124. Ms. Morrissey has just been diagnosed with genital herpes. At this time, which of the following would be a priority nursing action?

1. Ensure Ms. Morrissey is tested for other sexually transmitted infections (STI)
2. Counsel Ms. Morrissey about her sexual activities
3. Discuss with Ms. Morrissey the action of ordered antiviral medication
4. Perform a mouth exam to check for oral herpes

125. Mr. Constantine is scheduled to have a sigmoidoscopy and will be performing his own preparation for the test. What will the practical nurse direct him to do?

1. Self-administer an enema the morning of the exam
2. Collect any stool specimens he passes prior to the procedure
3. Not have any fluids or foods for 24 hours before the exam
4. Drink the chalklike substance that will be provided to him

126. Mr. Ross required a mid-thigh amputation of his left leg after a farming accident. Postoperatively, what should the practical nurse explain to Mr. Ross when he is observed elevating the surgical limb on pillows.

1. This position helps promote molding and shaping the limb for a prosthesis.
2. This position decreases phantom limb discomfort.
3. The flexed position can lead to permanent muscle shortening.
4. Moving the extremity will increase the risk of infection at the incision site.

127. A student nurse asks an antenatal clinic practical nurse how smoking during pregnancy affects the baby. How should the practical nurse respond?

1. "The placenta is permeable to specific substances but not nicotine."
2. "Nicotine is addictive, and this will cause withdrawal in the fetus."
3. "Nicotine causes vasoconstriction, which will affect both fetal and maternal blood vessels."
4. "The effect is minimal as fetal circulation is separated from maternal circulation by the placental barrier."

128. The practical nurse working in the pre-op clinic is conducting a health history of a client whom she is preparing for surgery in 2 weeks. Of the following, which would be the most important question for the practical nurse to ask?

1. "What country are you from?"
2. "Are you taking any herbal supplements or over-the-counter medicines?"
3. "Does your diet provide adequate nutrition?"
4. "Do you have any sleep problems that might interfere with your recovery?"

129. Mr. Mehmet has metastatic lung cancer. He is refusing chemotherapy and radiation, stating his wish to use alternative therapies that do not use "poisons." What might the practical nurse say to Mr. Mehmet?

1. "This is not a wise decision. You are endangering your life."
2. "It is your right to decide what type of treatment you prefer."
3. "According to Canadian law, the doctor can make you take the chemotherapy."
4. "Would you like to be provided with more information about scientific medical therapies and alternative treatments?"

130. Mr. Ciavello is admitted to the medical unit with atherosclerosis and hypertension. He has been placed on a low sodium-diet. He complains that low-sodium food is flavourless. What would be the practical nurse's best response?

1. "I'll get the dietitian to consult with you about strategies to improve the flavour of your food."
2. "You miss your favourite foods?"
3. "Salt can be very harmful to your health."
4. "Ask the doctor if you can indulge occasionally."

131. Mr. Kiros is admitted to hospital with diarrhea, anorexia, weight loss, and abdominal cramps. A diagnosis of colitis is confirmed. Which of the following early manifestations of fluid and electrolyte imbalance should the practical nurse anticipate?

1. Skin rash, diarrhea, and diplopia
2. Extreme muscle weakness and tachycardia
3. Tetany with muscle spasms
4. Nausea, vomiting, and leg and stomach cramps

132. The practical nurse must tally a client's fluid intake and output for 8 hours. At the time of calculation, there was 650 mL left from a 1000-mL bag of dextrose 5% in water. The client had three gastrostomy tube (G-tube) feedings of 200 mL each, plus a 50-mL flush of water at every feed. The practical nurse emptied the catheter bag twice, of 290 mL and 320 mL, respectively. The client had a small emesis of 25 mL. What is the intake and output?

1. Intake 930 mL, output 650 mL
2. Intake 1000 mL, output 680 mL
3. Intake 1080 mL, output 595 mL
4. Intake 1100 mL, output 635 mL

133. The practical nurse assesses a client's IV site and determines it is interstitial. What would be the initial action by the practical nurse?

1. Elevate the IV site
2. Discontinue the infusion
3. Attempt to flush the tube
4. Apply warm saline soaks to the site

134. Mr. Stephanopoulos has been admitted to the hospital with heart failure. The practical nurse walks into his room and finds him cyanotic and unresponsive. What is the priority nursing action?

1. Call for help
2. Assess for breathing
3. Administer oxygen
4. Assess for a pulse

135. A community health practical nurse counsels Mr. Carter about smoking cessation. He has smoked two packages of cigarettes a day for 20 years. He says he wants to quit, but he has concerns about withdrawal symptoms. Which of the following responses by the practical nurse is most therapeutic?

1. "After 24 hours, your body will be free of the physical dependency."
2. "Increasing your intake of vitamin B and vitamin C will reduce any withdrawal symptoms."
3. "You can always call the support group if your cravings get too hard to handle."
4. "I will refer you to a physician for medications to help with the symptoms of withdrawal."

136. Which of the following is a risk factor for abruptio placentae?

1. Cardiac disease
2. Hyperthyroidism
3. Cephalopelvic disproportion
4. Pregnancy-induced hypertension

137. Most nursing jurisdictions have a quality assurance program for their members. Which of the following statements is most important concerning nursing quality assurance (QA) programs?

1. It is a formal process that practical nurses engage in once each year.
2. It is an ongoing process of practical nurses reflecting on their practice.
3. It is a tool used by employers to evaluate their nursing employees.
4. It is a necessary component for maintaining registration.

138. Ms. Helena has been found to have an indeterminate lesion on a breast ultrasound, and her physician schedules her for a biopsy. She says to the practical nurse, "Why am

I having a biopsy? Do I have breast cancer?" What is the best response by the practical nurse?

1. "Don't worry—the biopsy is being done just to make sure everything is okay."
2. "You probably do have breast cancer, and the biopsy will confirm it."
3. "Your ultrasound showed a suspicious lesion in your breast: a biopsy will determine if it is cancer."
4. "Your physician ordered the biopsy, so I don't really know why you are having it."

139. A practical nurse has been working alternating 12-hour day and night shifts in a busy medical surgical unit for 12 years. She is the mother of three young children. Lately, she has been experiencing nightmares about making errors in care and feels tired and overwhelmed all the time. What should be the practical nurse's first action?

1. Ask her manager to change her to only either day or night shifts
2. Reflect on areas of her personal and work life that can be changed
3. Make a decision to change to part-time work rather than full-time work
4. Implement healthier living habits such as sufficient sleep and improved nutrition

140. Ms. Tang, who has type 1 diabetes, is in the second half of pregnancy. Which of the following therapeutic interventions is she most likely to require?

1. Decreased caloric intake
2. Increased dosage of insulin
3. Administration of pancreatic enzymes
4. Decreased dosage of insulin

141. The practical nurse has been reading research articles concerning the emotional aspects of pregnancy and childbirth. Research concerning the emotional factors of pregnancy indicates which of the following reactions?

1. A rejected pregnancy will result in a rejected infant.
2. Ambivalence and anxiety about mothering are common.
3. Maternal love is fully developed within the first week after birth.
4. Most mothers experience neither ambivalence nor anxiety about mothering.

142. Mr. Patrick brings his 18-month-old son, Colm, to the clinic. He asks the practical nurse why his son is so difficult to please, has temper tantrums, and annoys him by throwing food from the table. What would the practical nurse explain to Mr. Patrick?

1. "Toddlers need to be disciplined at this stage to prevent the development of antisocial behaviours."
2. "The child is learning to assert independence, and his behaviour is considered normal for his age."
3. "This is the usual way that a toddler expresses his needs during the initiative stage of development."
4. "It is best to leave the child alone in his crib after calmly telling him why his behaviour is unacceptable."

143. Kathleen, age 2 years, is hospitalized with laryngotracheobronchitis (croup). Which would be the highest-priority nursing action when caring for Kathleen?

1. Measures to reduce fever
2. Assessment of respiratory status
3. Provision of comfort to reduce crying and bronchospasm
4. Delivery of ordered humidified oxygen

144. A 14-year-old boy is in a rehabilitation centre following a skateboard accident that caused musculoskeletal damage. He develops muscle weakness because he refuses to move. What should the practical nurse do to promote mobility?

1. Encourage his friends to visit every day
2. Explain that, as with sports, some pain is inevitable
3. Set strict limits to increase his compliance with the mobility plan
4. Permit him to make decisions regarding the type of activity or exercise he engages in

145. Ms. Sloane has been seen by the nurse practitioner, who diagnosed that she has a bacterial infection. Which criterion would the nurse practitioner use when selecting an effective drug for the bacterial infection?

1. Ms. Sloane's toleration of the drug
2. Cost-effectiveness of the drug
3. Sensitivity of the causative organism
4. The prescriber's preference of drug

146. Mr. McCormick, a 58-year-old Indigenous male, is admitted to the acute medical floor with type 2 diabetes. He has not been following his diabetic diet and he suffers from hyperglycemia. What is the most appropriate action for the practical nurse to support him in following a diabetic diet?

1. Stress he needs to follow the diabetic diet as ordered by the physician.
2. Ask him what types of healthy foods he likes to eat and arrange for the diabetic educator to meet with him to review meal planning and preparation.

3. Encourage him to follow Canada's Food guide for First Nations, Inuit, and Métis.
4. Tell him he cannot continue to eat the way he has been if he wishes to get better.

147. Ms. Price, a resident of British Columbia, develops appendicitis while on vacation in Saskatchewan. What services will the Saskatchewan health service cover for Ms. Price?

1. All hospital-provided services including medications and standard ward
2. All hospital-provided services excluding medications
3. All standard hospital services excluding specialists and intensive care
4. All health services whether or not provided by a hospital and regardless of the health care provider

148. Which of the following is an example of the implementation of primary health care by a practical nurse?

1. Advanced diagnostic testing
2. Correction of dietary deficiencies
3. Establishing goals for rehabilitation
4. Assisting in immunization programs

149. During labour, Ms. Jasmin becomes very restless, flushed, and irritable and perspires profusely. She states that she is going to vomit. Which stage of labour is this?

1. Late stage
2. Third stage
3. Second stage
4. Transition stage

150. Which of the following symptoms may occur in a client with atelectasis?

1. Slow, deep respirations
2. Rales and crackles in lower lobes
3. A dry, unproductive cough
4. Diminished breath sounds

151. Baby Sabrina is born at 32 weeks' gestation following a difficult delivery. She develops muscle twitching, convulsions, cyanosis, abnormal respirations, and a short, shrill cry. These manifestations may be due to which of the following conditions?

1. Tetany
2. Spina bifida
3. Hyperkalemia
4. Intracranial hemorrhage

152. Mrs. Manns has recently been diagnosed with kidney failure and hemodialysis has been recommended. Which statement by Mrs. Manns would demonstrate an understanding of hemodialysis?

1. "I will be coming to the kidney dialysis unit 3 to 4 times a week to have my blood filtered through the dialyzer."
2. "I can drink as much fluid as I want because the dialyzer will remove the excess fluid I drink."
3. "One treatment of hemodialysis is required."
4. "I can do the treatment at home with a catheter attached to my abdomen."

153. Ms. Mullis sustained a fractured mandible from a motor vehicle incident. Her jaw is surgically immobilized with wires. What is a potential life-threatening problem?

1. Infection
2. Vomiting
3. Osteomyelitis
4. Bronchospasm

154. Ms. Griffin is admitted with an exacerbation of multiple sclerosis and is prescribed medical cannabis for muscle spasms. The practical nurse has a moral objection to participating in the administration of cannabis. What should the practical nurse do?

1. Refuse to care for the client because it is against her ethical beliefs.
2. Ask the unit coordinator if she could be assigned to a different client who does not take cannabis.
3. Care for the client and take this as an opportunity to reinforce her personal beliefs of refraining from cannabis to the client.
4. Write an order to administer some other medication to treat the client's spasms.

155. A practical nurse is the clinical preceptor for Wai, a foreign-educated nurse. The practical nurse notices that Wai does not look her clients in the eye and does not introduce herself to her clients. What should the practical nurse say to Wai?

1. "In Canada, we introduce ourselves to the clients."
2. "It is considered rude in Canada not to look people in the eye."
3. "Why don't you look your clients in the eye or introduce yourself?"
4. "The next time we go into a client room, let's make sure we introduce ourselves."

156. A mother decides that her son Lawrence, age 5 years, no longer requires hospitalization for his asthma because he is not experiencing respiratory distress. The attending physician has not discharged him. The mother arrives at the nursing station with Lawrence, saying she does not care if he has not been discharged; she is taking him home. What is the appropriate nursing action?

1. Explain to the mother that if she takes Lawrence home, the appropriate child welfare authorities will be notified.
2. Tell the mother that because Lawrence is a minor, she is not allowed to discharge him against medical orders.
3. Inform the mother that agency policy does not allow them to release Lawrence into her care.
4. Ensure that the mother receives health teaching as necessary about asthma and document the situation as per agency policies.

157. Mr. Hassan has just returned to the unit from the postanaesthetic care unit after surgery. He has an IV of dextrose 5% in water and 0.9% NaCl at 100 mL per hour, O_2 at 4 L per nasal cannula, a nasogastric tube set to low suction via a Gomco pump, and a urinary catheter to straight drainage. He was medicated with morphine sulphate 1 hour ago and is reporting nausea. Which of the following components of assessment is the priority of the practical nurse when Mr. Hassan returns to the unit from the postanaesthetic care unit?

1. Ensure patency of the nasogastric tube and urinary catheter
2. Monitor the IV site
3. Check that the oxygen is set at the correct flow rate
4. Assess Mr. Hassan's pain and nausea

158. What is the most common cause of mortality in the adolescent years?

1. Motor vehicle accidents
2. Suicide
3. Cancers
4. Sports-related accidents

159. Mr. Edward, age 83 years, has moved into a retirement home. Mr. Martin, his life partner, visits him regularly. Which of the following statements is true regarding their sexuality?

1. They will have no sexual inhibitions because they are homosexual.
2. They will enjoy companionship more than sex.
3. They probably have become disinterested in sexual activities.
4. They will likely have an interest in sexual activity if privacy is available.

160. A second year practical nursing student obtained a manual blood pressure of 200/120 on an 8-year-old child. She assumed that she had made a mistake in taking the blood pressure and did not report her finding to anyone. Who is responsible for this error in care?

1. The student practical nurse
2. The nurse working with the practical nursing student
3. The teacher responsible for the practical nursing student
4. Both the student and her teacher

161. What is the practical nurse's initial responsibility in teaching the pregnant adolescent client?

1. Informing her of the benefits of breastfeeding
2. Advising her about the proper care of an infant
3. Instructing her to watch for danger signs of pre-eclampsia
4. Discussing the importance of consistent prenatal care

162. Which of the following statements is the correct description of hemiplegia?

1. Paresis of both lower extremities
2. Paralysis of one side of the body
3. Paralysis of both lower extremities
4. Paralysis of upper and lower extremities

163. Ms. Townsend has unresolved edema in her legs. Which of the following complications should the practical nurse assess for?

1. Proteinemia
2. Contractures
3. Tissue ischemia
4. Thrombus formation

164. Ms. Polaska has a diagnosis of systemic lupus erythematosus (SLE). Which of the following manifestations commonly occur with SLE?

1. A butterfly rash
2. Firm skin fixed to tissue
3. Muscle mass degeneration
4. An inflammation of small arteries

165. Mr. Scales expresses concern about radiation therapy for his cancer because he has heard that being exposed to radiation can cause him to develop other types of cancer. What should the practical nurse explain to Mr. Scales?

1. Dosage of radiation is strictly controlled.
2. Radiation doses are lowered if problems arise.
3. Good physical condition prevents problems.
4. Optimum cellular nutrition is protective.

166. Peter, age 15 years, asks his practical nurse why his testes are suspended in his scrotum. What would be the most appropriate response by the practical nurse?

1. To protect the sperm from the acidity of urine
2. To help with the passage of sperm through the urethra
3. To protect the sperm from high abdominal temperatures
4. To enable the testes to mature during embryonic development

167. A practical nurse is counselling Mr. Olan following his vasectomy surgery. Which of the following components of health teaching is most important prior to discharge?

1. Sterilization is permanent and cannot be reversed.
2. Some impotency is to be expected for several weeks.
3. Unprotected coitus is allowed within a week to 10 days.
4. At least 10 ejaculations are required to clear the tract of sperm.

168. Ms. Angelo, age 20 years, tells the practical nurse her menstrual periods are extremely painful, making her feel nauseated and keeping her in bed for several days. What should the practical nurse recommend?

1. Maintain her daily activities as much as possible
2. Make an appointment with a gynecologist
3. Take an over-the-counter drug such as ibuprofen
4. Practise relaxation of her abdominal muscles

169. Ms. McMahon is scheduled to undergo pelvic ultrasonography. What is the required preparation for this test?

1. Tell the patient no sedation or fasting required.
2. A laxative the evening before and an enema the morning of the test
3. Drinking 1 200 to 1 500 mL of water 1 hour before the test
4. An injection of radiopaque dye immediately before the test

170. A unit nurse coordinator believes that consultation with her staff is unnecessary and serves only to confuse and slow down decision making on the unit. Which of the following terms would indicate her leadership style?

1. Situational
2. Laissez-faire
3. Autocratic
4. Positional

171. A practical nurse prepares a client for coronary angiography. The client asks the reason for this test. Which of the following statements is the best response by the practical nurse?

1. "This test will look at the patency of the heart valves in your coronary blood flow."
2. "This exam will ensure that your heart's electrical system is operating as it should."
3. "This exam will determine the amount of blood flow through the coronary arteries to nourish your heart muscle."
4. "This exam will evaluate the strength of the left ventricle's contractions."

172. A practical nurse is working on an adolescent unit. One of the clients informs her that she has had multiple male and female sexual partners in the last year. She has not used anything for prevention of sexually transmitted infections (STIs) or contraception. What would be the most appropriate response by the practical nurse?

1. "Once you decide your sexual orientation, we can figure out how to help you."
2. "I suggest you make friends with a group of different girls so they can help you with being a female."
3. "Your actions are putting you at a high risk for sexually transmitted infections and perhaps unwanted pregnancy. Let's discuss what is the best method for protecting yourself."
4. "Have you discussed this with your parents?"

173. Mr. Brendan has a substance use disorder and is addicted to intravenous heroin. He works in the sex industry to pay for his heroin. What would be the most important topic for health teaching?

1. Safety
2. Nutrition
3. Self-esteem
4. Legal issues

174. Ms. Hoang, who has type 2 diabetes, hypertension, and high cholesterol, tells the practical nurse that she takes herbal remedies. What is the most important aspect related to herbal preparations that the practical nurse should discuss with Ms. Hoang?

1. Most herbal preparations are not formulated in standardized doses.
2. Herbal preparations are not regulated by Health Canada.
3. Some herbal preparations interact with prescription medications.
4. She should purchase herbal remedies from a recognized pharmacy rather than a traditional herbalist.

175. A practical nurse is attending an education session on the potential therapeutic uses for cannabis. Which statement by the practical nurse would indicate a need for further teaching?

1. "Cannabis may improve multiple sclerosis side effects."
2. "Cannabis may be helpful in alleviating the symptoms of inflammatory bowel disease."
3. "Cannabis may provide relief of a wide variety of palliative care symptoms."
4. "Postoperative pain is managed well with the use of cannabis."

176. A client is pregnant and tells the practical nurse, "This is the fourth time I have been pregnant. I had an abortion when I was a teenager and then delivered a baby girl when I was 20. Last year, I had a miscarriage when I was 10 weeks pregnant." How would the practical nurse record the client's pregnancy status?

1. G.3, P.1, A.1
2. G.3, P.0, A.2
3. G.4, P.1, A.2
4. G.4, P.1, A.1

177. Ms. Gilles, age 40 years, has just been admitted to hospital. She has bipolar disorder and is experiencing a manic episode. Her language becomes vulgar and profane. What would be the most appropriate nursing response?

1. State, "We do not allow that kind of talk here."
2. Ignore it since the client is using it only to get attention.
3. Recognize the language as part of the illness but set limits on it.
4. State, "When you can talk in an acceptable way, I will talk to you."

178. Maher is a 15-month-old infant who has a chronic renal disorder that has resulted in numerous prolonged hospitalizations since he was born. His parents visit infrequently because they live far away; both work; and they have other children. Maher's practical nurse is aware that studies have shown that children who have suffered prolonged maternal deprivation early in life may demonstrate difficulty in which of the following behaviours?

1. Trusting others
2. Recalling past experiences
3. Developing age-appropriate cognitive development
4. Establishing relationships with caregivers

179. Mr. Jain, age 23 years, has a history of dependence to narcotics and is receiving methadone hydrochloride. He has undergone an emergency appendectomy. For which of the following signs of narcotic withdrawal should Mr. Jain be closely observed?

1. Piloerection
2. Agitation
3. Skin dryness
4. Lethargy

180. What is the most appropriate way to help a client with generalized anxiety disorder decrease his excessive apprehension and fear?

1. Suggest he avoid unpleasant objects and events.
2. Suggest he purposefully expose himself to fearful situations.
3. Help him develop specific coping skills.
4. Explore ways to introduce an element of pleasure into fearful situations.

181. Ms. Alley tells the practical nurse that she wants to lose weight. She says she weighs 225 lbs. and she wants to be 180 lbs. How many kilograms does Ms. Alley want to lose?

1. 45 kg
2. 24 kg
3. 20 kg
4. 12 kg

182. Isabelle, a toddler, is an unstable client in the emergency room. Her mother reports that Isabelle developed sudden hoarseness and unintelligible speech. The practical nurse notes that Isabelle is very distressed and anxious. What might be the first question the practical nurse asks Isabelle's mother?

1. "Did Isabelle have breathing problems at birth?"
2. "Has Isabelle shown previous signs of an upper respiratory tract infection (a cold)?"
3. "Is there a family history of breathing or throat problems?"
4. "Could she have aspirated something she put in her mouth?"

183. Mrs. George, an Indigenous patient, is receiving treatment on the subacute medical unit for a pressure injury. She asks to have a spiritual ceremony in which sweet grass is burned. What is the best response by the practical nurse?

1. "This is not allowed in the hospital because of our 'no smoking' policies."
2. "I will find out where you may have a sweet grass ceremony at the hospital."
3. "I am sure our fire policies would not allow this."
4. "It will be easier for you to do this in your own home once you are discharged."

184. What self-care measures should the practical nurse advise for a 15-year-old female who experiences occasional outbreaks of acne?

1. "Scrub your face vigorously once a day."
2. "Don't eat foods such as chocolate and French fries."
3. Always use an oil-based sunscreen when you are outside."
4. "Wash your face with mild soap and water twice a day."

185. Ms. Coutinho, a client on a long-term care unit, is immobilized. How would the practical nurse demonstrate the application of good body mechanics when caring for Ms. Coutinho?

1. Bending at the waist to provide power for lifting
2. Placing her feet at shoulder-width apart to increase the stability of her body
3. Keeping her body straight when lifting to reduce pressure on her abdomen
4. Relaxing her abdominal muscles and using her extremities to prevent strain.

186. What assistive device would be the most appropriate for early ambulation after hip-replacement surgery?

1. A walker
2. A cane
3. Crutches
4. A wheelchair

187. Following orthopedic surgery, Mr. Ferguson complains of pain. His practical nurse administers 50 mg of tramadol which has been ordered PO, q4 hr prn. Two hours later, Mr. Ferguson tells the practical nurse he is still experiencing severe pain. What should the practical nurse do?

1. Report that Mr. Ferguson has an apparent idiosyncrasy to tramadol.
2. Tell Mr. Ferguson additional tramadol cannot be given for 1 more hour.
3. Request that the physician evaluate Mr. Ferguson's need for additional medication.
4. Administer another dose of tramadol within 15 minutes since it is a relatively safe drug.

188. Moses is ordered ampicillin 200 mg/kg/d. He weighs 45 kg. What dose should Moses receive every 6 hours?

1. 9.0 g
2. 4.5 g
3. 3.2 g
4. 2.3 g

189. Which of the following analgesic dosage regimens is most likely to provide optimum pain relief for a client who is 1 day postoperative from abdominal surgery?

1. "Around the clock," at intervals dependent on the length of action of the analgesic.
2. "As needed" (prn), at intervals of 3 to 4 hours.
3. As requested by the client and within accepted time frames.
4. As assessed by the practical nurse.

190. A practical nurse is teaching a group of adolescents about aspects of human sexuality. Which of the following statements is the most correct referring to gender identity?

1. Preference for a partner of either the male or female sex
2. How one considers one's own sexual orientation
3. The internal sense of being either male or female or both male and female
4. The way one chooses to present one's gender to the world through dress and mannerisms

191. Mr. Akland, age 74, tells the practical nurse that because of his arthritis he is having difficulty caring for his feet. Mr. Akland has had type 2 diabetes for 7 years. Which of the following actions by the practical nurse would be initially most beneficial to Mr. Akland?

1. Assess Mr. Akland's movement and ability to manage his own hygiene
2. Arrange for a home care nurse to visit him
3. Ask Mr. Akland if there is a family member who could assist him
4. Suggest to Mr. Akland that he make regular appointments with his physician to monitor the condition of his feet

192. Mr. James, age 24, is HIV positive. He has been started on a new medication regimen and admits he has not been compliant with taking his drugs. Which of the following actions by the practical nurse would be most helpful to get Mr. James to take his medications?

1. Give him a fact sheet about human immunodeficiency virus/acquired immune deficiency syndrome (HIV/AIDS) medications so that he can understand the importance of the drugs.
2. Arrange with the pharmacy to "bubble-pack" all of his medications so that he could be sure that he had taken his proper dose.
3. Discuss with Mr. James how his medications might be changed to fit in with his lifestyle.
4. Ask Mr. James what his reasons are for not taking his medications.

193. The family of a 92-year-old man who has advanced dementia would like to care for him at home but are overwhelmed by the care he requires. The practical nurse realizes they will need extensive assistance from community agencies and resources. What is the most appropriate action by the practical nurse?

1. Arrange a consultation with a social worker
2. Suggest that the family discuss community resources with the physician
3. Research the community agencies and conduct a teaching session with the family
4. Provide a community services pamphlet to the family

194. Which of the following procedures is correct when obtaining a throat culture from a client?

1. Have the client sit erect and swab the tonsillar area, making contact with inflamed or purulent areas but not touching the teeth, lips, or tongue
2. Have the client deep-breathe and cough, and then swab the mucus that the client has loosened
3. Have the client lie in a supine position and turn his or her head to the side; insert the swab and move it from side to side to cover as much area as possible
4. Place the client in a high Fowler position and ask him or her to lean forward with the mouth open while the swab is inserted and rotated in a clockwise movement.

195. The practical nurse attends a conference and hears about a new type of incontinence product. She would like to try this new product and compare it with what is currently used on the unit. What is the most appropriate initial step for the practical nurse?

1. Compile all available data on the new product
2. Ask the physician on the unit if she would consider ordering the new product
3. Write a research proposal and present it to the nurse manager
4. Obtain a sample of the new product and use it with clients who have provided consent

196. A client is going to the diagnostic imaging department for a magnetic resonance imaging (MRI) scan. He has an IV running at 75 mL per hour. The practical nurse observes that there is 100 mL of solution remaining to be absorbed. What would be the practical nurse's most appropriate action to ensure that the IV is maintained while he is having the MRI?

1. Accompany the client to the MRI and change the IV solution bag when required
2. Ensure that a new IV bag of solution is sent with the client for the MRI department
3. Reduce the drip rate of the IV to 25 mL per hour before the client leaves for the MRI
4. Change the IV solution to a new bag just prior to the client leaving the unit for the MRI

197. Mr. Balasingham was identified 1 year ago to be incompetent to make decisions regarding his care. When a care decision occurs, what will happen?

1. The substitute decision maker (SDM) will make the decision.
2. His next of kin will be contacted.
3. The physician will assume responsibility for care decisions.
4. Mr. Balasingham will be provided with the opportunity to make his decision.

198. Ms. Lewis is admitted to the hospital with fever, productive cough, shortness of breath, and fatigue. A dialysis client occupies the only private room on the unit. What should the practical nurse do?

1. Move the dialysis client from the private room and admit Ms. Lewis to it
2. Admit Ms. Lewis to a semi-private room with a postoperative client
3. Admit Ms. Lewis to a semi-private room with a client who has cancer
4. Refuse to admit Ms. Lewis due to infection control concerns

199. A student practical nurse is working with an experienced practical nurse preceptor on a postpartum unit. The preceptor recommends supplementing breastfeeding with formula to a first-time mother of a full-term healthy 1-day-old infant. The student practical nurse is aware that supplementing breastfeeding with formula is not recommended by lactation experts. What should the student practical nurse do?

1. Speak with the mother in private about the benefits of breastfeeding
2. Discuss with the preceptor the best-practice research concerning not supplementing breastfeeding with bottles
3. Complain to the nursing manager about the preceptor's lack of knowledge of breastfeeding
4. Comply with the advice of the preceptor to the new mother since the preceptor is an experienced postpartum practical nurse

200. The nursing team leader tells the practical nurse that his client requires a two-way Foley catheter to be inserted. What would be the first action taken by the practical nurse?

1. Wash his hands
2. Collect the equipment for the procedure
3. Check the physician's orders
4. Inform the client of the procedure

END OF PRACTICE EXAM 1

5 Answers and Rationales for Practice Exam 1

CASE–BASED QUESTIONS ANSWERS AND RATIONALES

CASE 1

1\.

1. In order to comply with the rights of medication administration, the practical nurse must compare the medication prepackage with the prescriber's (usually a physician) order to confirm that the pharmacy has prepared the correct medication for Mr. Rickhelm.

2. Mr. Rickhelm may not know all of the medications he is receiving. The prescriber's order is the most valid resource.
3. This action is not necessary, although if a discrepancy were discovered with the prescriber's order, the pharmacy should be contacted.
4. This action will provide information about the drug but would not confirm it is the correct drug for Mr. Rickhelm.

CLASSIFICATION
Competency:
Professional Practice
Taxonomy:
Critical Thinking

2\.

1. This response answers Mr. Ogalino's question and indicates that the practical nurse is aware of what drug is being administered and that it is an accepted generic form of the drug.

2. It is not responsible for the practical nurse to administer a drug without knowing the name of the drug nor the reason it has been prescribed.
3. This does not answer Mr. Ogalino's question, and it is potentially dangerous for the practical nurse to disregard his questioning of an unfamiliar medication.
4. This does not answer Mr. Ogalino's question, and it is potentially dangerous for him not to take a medication.

CLASSIFICATION
Competency:
Professional Practice
Taxonomy:
Application

3\.

1. A blood sugar reading at 1800 hours has no value in deciding optimum time for administration of long-acting insulin.

2. This response validates Ms. Jasmin's comment and may provide important information to the practical nurse for the dosing schedule.

3. Reliance on hospital routines or policies is not an accountable response.
4. This is incorrect; if the insulin were given at 1800 hours, the peak action and potential hypoglycemia may occur in the middle of the night.

CLASSIFICATION
Competency:
Professional Practice
Taxonomy:
Application

4\.

1. Statins reduce serum cholesterol levels, which are not aspects of the pathology of deep vein thrombosis.
2. Antibiotics are used to treat bacterial infections, which are not an aspect of the pathology of deep vein thrombosis.
3. Analgesics are used to treat pain and reduce fever. There is no indication Ms. Corel requires either.

4. Anticoagulants, or blood thinners, are used to treat and prevent deep vein thrombosis.

CLASSIFICATION
Competency:
Foundations of Practice
Taxonomy:
Knowledge/Comprehension

5\.

1. A registered nurse (RN) is not the only health care provider who can legally sign the narcotics count sheet.
2. Licensed/registered practical nurses are able to sign the count sheet but are not the only health care providers who can.

3. An RN or a physician are not the only health care providers legally able to sign a narcotics count sheet.
4. **Regulated health care providers, such as nurses, physicians, dentists, chiropractors, pharmacist/technicians, and so on, are legally able to sign narcotics count sheets.**

CLASSIFICATION
Competency:
Legal Practice
Taxonomy:
Knowledge/Comprehension

6.
1. Practical nurses are responsible for ensuring the correct dose of medication whether or not it has been calculated by the pharmacy.
2. The digoxin administered is not the same dose as was ordered.
3. The administered digoxin is an overdose.
4. **The dose of digoxin is 10 times the ordered dose. It is a nursing responsibility to calculate and ensure the correct dose of every drug administered.**

CLASSIFICATION
Competency:
Professional Practice
Taxonomy:
Application

CASE 2

7.
1. **This response helps to identify it as a unique experience for Mr. Smadu, without getting into a discussion of whether it is a symptom of his schizophrenia disorder.**
2. It is not helpful to pretend to believe in the hallucination, even though it may be helpful for the practical nurse to find out more about the hallucinations.
3. It is not helpful to Mr. Smadu to argue reality with him.
4. Exploring with Mr. Smadu the reasons he hears voices is not helpful to him. The hallucinations are a symptom of his disease.

CLASSIFICATION
Competency:
Professional Practice
Taxonomy:
Application

8.
1. This action will not help, as Mr. Smadu cannot control the hallucinations.
2. **Some individuals find that listening to music on headphones helps to decrease the effect of voices.**
3. Physical activity may help decrease some symptoms over time, but a walk is unlikely to reduce particular episodes of hearing voices.
4. This option is unsafe.

CLASSIFICATION
Competency:
Foundations of Practice
Taxonomy:
Application

9.
1. Some people with a schizophrenia disorder may become violent, particularly if they are experiencing severe paranoia.
2. There is no need to call the police unless Mr. Smadu's behaviour is threatening. The word *strange* does not adequately describe the behaviour.
3. This action would not eliminate his hallucinations.
4. **With any person in distress they could strike out to protect themselves.**

CLASSIFICATION
Competency:
Foundations of Practice
Taxonomy:
Application

10.
1. Risperidone can be given orally and is absorbed from the gastrointestinal tract.
2. **Compliance with medication is a problem with clients who have a schizophrenia disorder. Administering the antipsychotic in a form that will provide therapeutic levels for 2 weeks aids in compliance.**
3. There is not a better response with the IM route.
4. Tardive dyskinesia is a risk regardless of the route of administration.

CLASSIFICATION
Competency:
Foundations of Practice
Taxonomy:
Application

11.

1. **Recovery may involve learning ways to maintain wellness, decrease the impact of problems, and work around obstacles. Some people experience periods of wellness between episodes, while others may experience episodes that last a longer period of time.**
2. Ten years after their first episode, one quarter, not one half of people, recover and live fairly independent lives. The impact of the disorder is unique to each individual.
3. Approximately one half of people diagnosed with a schizophrenia disorder will either improve to a degree or recover.
4. This response does not address Ms. Smadu's question.

CLASSIFICATION
Competency:
Foundations of Practice
Taxonomy:
Critical Thinking

12.

1. Alogia involves decreases in thought, speech, and fluency.
2. Anhedonia is the inability to feel pleasure or happiness.
3. **Avolition is the inability to act on plans.**
4. Attention impairment is the inability to keep attention focused on a particular thought or activity.

CLASSIFICATION
Competency:
Foundations of Practice
Taxonomy:
Knowledge/Comprehension

13.

1. The voices have told Mr. Smadu to commit suicide. The most important action is to keep him safe.
2. This situation is not necessarily an emergency unless Mr. Smadu possesses a gun.
3. **Suicide precautions need to be put into effect, which means that Mr. Smadu may need to be admitted to hospital for close observation.**
4. Ten percent of all people with a schizophrenia disorder commit suicide due to feelings of torment or the voices commanding them to kill themselves.

CLASSIFICATION
Competency:
Foundations of Practice
Taxonomy:
Critical Thinking

CASE 3

14.

1. **MRSA is spread by direct contact with skin that has the bacteria or with contaminated surfaces.**
2. MRSA is not spread through the air by aerosol or droplet transmission.
3. MRSA is not spread via the fecal–oral route.
4. Such contact could be a possible mode of transmission; however, there is no evidence in this question that persons who did not wash their hands were colonized or infected with MRSA.

CLASSIFICATION
Competency:
Foundations of Practice
Taxonomy:
Application

15.

1. Open wounds are a risk factor, but hers would be a small incision. A surgical incision should not be colonized with bacteria.
2. Being an infant and the possible decreased immunity due to failure to thrive are possible risk factors but are not as great as those in answer 4.
3. Advanced age is a risk factor for MRSA, but there are no other risks.
4. **Ms. Gary has several risk factors. Those who are most at risk have chronic diseases that have been treated frequently with antibiotics. With a spinal cord injury, there is a possible increased risk for tissue breakdown and MRSA colonization on the skin.**

CLASSIFICATION
Competency:
Foundations of Practice
Taxonomy:
Critical Thinking

16.

1. These actions should be taken, but, in addition, the practical nurse should wear gloves.
2. If the cut is appropriately managed, the practical nurse has no reason to refrain from caring for clients with MRSA.

3. **Occlusive tape will cover the open cut. All nurses should wear gloves when caring for clients with MRSA.**
4. This action should be done with all clients and does not provide for additional precautions for the open cut.

CLASSIFICATION
Competency:
Foundations of Practice
Taxonomy:
Critical Thinking

CASE 4

17. 1. The practical nurse's behaviour is unprofessional and does not account for the growth and developmental needs of children of this age.
2. **When a client is restrained inappropriately and without exploring other alternatives, the action could be considered assault and battery. If necessary, mittens are much more appropriate.**
3. Although the behaviour (scratching) needs to be decreased, the practical nurse can address it with the use of mittens, rather than immobilizing a child of this age.
4. Restraining Denika's hands is inappropriate whether the parents give permission or not.

CLASSIFICATION
Competency:
Ethical Practice
Taxonomy:
Application

---

18. 1. This task is too advanced for toddlers and more accurate for preschoolers.
2. **Common developmental norms of the toddler, who is struggling for independence, are inability to share easily, egotism, egocentrism, and possessiveness.**
3. This exercise is true of 4-year-olds.
4. One characteristic of toddlers is their short attention span; 15 minutes is too much to expect.

CLASSIFICATION
Competency:
Foundations of Practice
Taxonomy:
Application

---

19. 1. This would be too slow to infuse the desired amount.
2. Same as answer 1.
3. **Correct calculation:**
Amount to Administer = Available Dosage × Ordered Dosage

$$x\frac{\text{drop}}{\text{min}} = \frac{60\,\text{drop}}{\text{mL}} \times \frac{1\text{L}}{24\,\text{hr}}$$

$$x\frac{\text{drop}}{\text{min}} = \frac{60\,\text{drop}}{\text{mL}} \times \frac{1{,}000\,\text{mL}}{24\,\text{hr}}$$

$$x\frac{\text{drop}}{\text{min}} = \frac{60\,\text{drop}}{\text{mL}} \times \frac{1{,}000\,\text{mL}}{24 \times 60\,\text{min}}$$

$$x\frac{\text{drop}}{\text{min}} = \frac{\cancel{60}\,\text{drop}}{\cancel{\text{mL}}} \times \frac{1{,}000\,\cancel{\text{mL}}}{24 \times \cancel{60}\,\text{min}}$$

$$x\frac{\text{drop}}{\text{min}} = \frac{1{,}000\,\text{drop}}{24\,\text{min}}$$

$$x\frac{\text{drop}}{\text{min}} = 41.67\frac{\text{drop}}{\text{min}} = 42\frac{\text{drop}}{\text{min}}$$

4. This would be too rapid; the fluid would run out before 24 hours had elapsed.

CLASSIFICATION
Competency:
Foundations of Practice
Taxonomy:
Application

20.
1. This action will not achieve the goal of giving fluids.
2. This action will not likely be successful with a toddler.
3. **Children who are expressing negativism need to have a feeling of control. One way of achieving this, within reasonable limits, is for the parent or caregiver to provide a choice of two items, rather than force one on the child.**
4. A toddler would not respond to intellectual reasoning, particularly regarding an activity that she does not want to do.

CLASSIFICATION
Competency:
Foundations of Practice
Taxonomy:
Application

21.
1. This is too late.
2. **Denika should be taken to the dentist between 2 and 3 years of age, when most of the 20 deciduous teeth have erupted.**
3. Same as answer 1.
4. This is too indefinite.

CLASSIFICATION
Competency:
Foundations of Practice
Taxonomy:
Knowledge/Comprehension

CASE 5

22.
1. **The practical nurse must determine if there is a distended bladder. This physical assessment is a form of data collection and is the first step in planning care. In agencies where it is available, the practical nurse may also assess for urinary retention with a bladder scanner.**
2. This action may be a nursing intervention but is not the initial action.
3. Same as answer 2.
4. Bladder distension is fairly common after delivery. It is too soon for medical intervention; other nursing measures should be tried first.

CLASSIFICATION
Competency:
Foundations of Practice
Taxonomy:
Critical Thinking

23.
1. Vaginal deliveries should not lead to respiratory problems.
2. Bladder tone is improved by regular emptying and filling of the bladder.
3. Abdominal muscle tone is not important this soon after delivery.
4. **There is extensive activation of the blood-clotting factor after delivery. This, together with immobility, trauma, or sepsis, encourages thromboembolization, which can be limited through activity.**

CLASSIFICATION
Competency:
Foundations of Practice
Taxonomy:
Critical Thinking

24.
1. This is the expected consistency of stool of an infant that is formula fed.
2. Mustardy yellow, soft and seedy in appearance is the expected consistency of stool of an infant that is breast fed who is a few days old.
3. **This is the expected consistency of the first stool of an infant after delivery. Meconium stool can occur for first 12 to 24 hours.**
4. This is the consistency of stool of an infant with constipation.

CLASSIFICATION
Competency:
Foundations of Practice
Taxonomy:
Knowledge and Comprehension

25.
1. Breastfeeding needs to be encouraged more frequently and on demand, not restricted. Breastfeeding helps to drain the milk ducts.
2. **Gentle breast massages from the chest wall to the nipple is helpful prior to and during milk expression. This will help reduce congestion and start the milk flow.**

CLASSIFICATION
Competency:
Foundations of Practice
COMPETENCY:
Application

3. Heat to breasts between feedings will increase swelling and inflammation. Warm compresses should be limited to only a few minutes prior to feeding to help with milk flow.
4. This action does not reduce engorgement.

26.
1. Slow uterine involution would be manifested by suboptimum uterine descent into the pelvis.
2. **A distended bladder will easily displace the fundus upward and laterally.**
3. If placental fragments were retained, in addition to being displaced, the uterus would be soft and boggy, and vaginal bleeding would be heavy.
4. From this assessment, the practical nurse cannot make a judgement about overstretched uterine ligaments.

CLASSIFICATION
Competency:
Foundations of Practice
Taxonomy:
Application

27.
1. Lochia serosa occurs from the third day postpartum until the tenth day postpartum.
2. Dark red with clots is abnormal and should be reported.
3. Lochia alba occurs a few weeks after delivery.
4. **Lochia rubra is dark red and is a normal vaginal discharge for day 2 postpartum.**

CLASSIFICATION
Competency:
Foundations of Practice
Taxonomy:
Knowledge and Comprehension

CASE 6

28.
1. Trying to talk Mr. Richard out of his behaviour is unlikely to be effective.
2. Other clients need to be protected from this client. Waiting to see if the behaviour worsens is dangerous and may cause further agitation.
3. This action may further aggravate Mr. Richard.
4. **This action separates Mr. Richard from the other clients and places him in a less stimulating environment. Staying with the client allows for close observation regarding the burns.**

CLASSIFICATION
Competency:
Professional Practice
Taxonomy:
Application

29.
1. Wound sepsis is a possible complication but would not be evident until the third to fifth day.
2. **Inhalation burns are usually present with facial burns, regardless of their depth; the threat to life is asphyxia from irritation and edema of the respiratory passages and lungs. Breathing is the most important priority in this situation, and difficulties are most likely to occur within the first 24 hours.**
3. Pain is certainly a concern but is not the most important one within the first 24 hours.
4. Fluid and electrolyte imbalances are a danger but do not reach their maximum until the fourth day.

CLASSIFICATION
Competency:
Foundations of Practice
Taxonomy:
Critical Thinking

30.
1. This statement may be true in the case of some injectable substances but is not an important consideration in this situation.
2. While repeat intramuscular (IM) injections are more painful than intravenous (IV) administration of drugs, this is not the most important concern for Richard at this time.
3. **Damage to tissues from the burns interferes with the stability of peripheral circulation and with the effectiveness of intramuscular medications.**
4. IV administration provides more consistent blood levels of analgesic but does not necessarily provide longer pain relief than IM administration.

CLASSIFICATION
Competency:
Foundations of Practice
Taxonomy:
Critical Thinking

31.
1. **The client may give permission to any other person to read the health record. The only other circumstance that would allow a legal official to read the chart is the issuance of a court order.**
2. The doctor may not give permission to read the health record.
3. Being charged with a criminal offence does not change the legislation with regard to privacy of health information.
4. This statement is true, but it is not the most appropriate response.

CLASSIFICATION
Competency: **Legal Practice**
Taxonomy: **Application**

CASE 7

32.
1. This response dismisses Mr. Wilmot's concern.
2. This response is not necessarily true, and Mr. Wilmot will still have one testicle.
3. **This response recognizes Mr. Wilmot's concerns and offers a positive solution while still encouraging open dialogue.**
4. This response is not true.

CLASSIFICATION
Competency: **Foundations of Practice**
Taxonomy: **Application**

33.
1. This response dismisses Mr. Wilmot's concerns and offers false reassurance.
2. This response offers false reassurance.
3. **This response would be appropriate and indicates his concerns are being listened to.**
4. Although this response is true, it does not specifically address Mr. Wilmot's concerns.

CLASSIFICATION
Competency: **Professional Practice**
Taxonomy: **Application**

34.
1. Treatment is not an absolute guarantee of a cure, and other malignancies may occur.
2. This course of action is not required, as he will still have one functioning testicle.
3. **Even though the cure rate is positive for testicular cancer, all clients must have routine follow-ups to monitor for relapse.**
4. The incidence of relapse is not high.

CLASSIFICATION
Competency: **Foundations of Practice**
Taxonomy: **Application**

35.
1. **This is the correct procedure. The warmth of the water will allow the testis to be palpated more easily.**
2. This position will not aid in feeling the testis. Circular motions are not likely to detect abnormalities.
3. This procedure is used to examine a hydrocele.
4. The testis should feel like a hard-boiled egg, and the epididymis is rougher.

CLASSIFICATION
Competency: **Foundations of Practice**
Taxonomy: **Application**

CASE 8

36.
1. With the client's history of unstable and fluctuating blood pressure, the practical nurse needs to ensure that the blood pressure reading is accurate. Unregulated care providers (UCPs) do not have the same competencies as regulated health care workers, who have standardized education, knowledge, and skills.
2. The doctor has written the order and has nothing to do with assessing the blood pressure at this particular time.
3. This action will not ensure accuracy of the reading.

4. This action is the safest option. The practical nurse is accountable for her actions in administering/holding the nifedipine and thus would be accountable for the error should the blood pressure not be what the UCP recorded. Taking and interpreting vital signs is a nursing function.

CLASSIFICATION
Competency:
Professional Practice
Taxonomy:
Critical Thinking

---

37. **1. Consent must be obtained for all treatments and medications. Verbal consent is appropriate prior to the administration of each dose of ECASA.**

2. Enteric-coated tablets should not be crushed.
3. The practical nurse must ensure that the client takes all ordered medication. Leaving the ECASA at Ms. Bystriska's bedside is not a responsible nursing action unless this has been predetermined as appropriate for this particular client.
4. A written consent specifically for medication administration is not reasonable or indicated.

CLASSIFICATION
Competency:
Legal Practice
Taxonomy:
Application

---

38. 1. This site is an appropriate subcutaneous (SC) site.
2. This needle gauge is correct for SC injections.

3. Massaging the injected area is not recommended with insulin.

4. This technique is appropriate.

CLASSIFICATION
Competency:
Foundations of Practice
Taxonomy:
Application

---

39. 1. There is no indication that Ms. Banwait has been proven to be incapable of making decisions.
2. There is no indication that Ms. Banwait has been judged incapable and that her husband has been designated as the substitute decision maker.
3. The practical nurse would need to find out more concerning the upset stomach before withholding the medication.

4. Ms. Banwait has withdrawn consent; therefore, the nurse is not legally permitted to force treatment on her. There is no indication that she has been deemed incapable to make decisions regarding her health care.

CLASSIFICATION
Competency:
Legal Practice
Taxonomy:
Application

CASE 9

40. 1. Avoid vaginal lubricants or other oil-based products as these can weaken the rubber.
2. Requires inspection before each use for monitoring any defects in the diaphragm. It should be removed 6 to 8 hours after intercourse, and not used during menstruation.

3. Annual examinations are required to assess the fit of the diaphragm. The device should be inspected after each use, replaced every 2 years, and may have to be refitted for weight fluctuation, after each pregnancy, or after abdominal or pelvic surgery.

4. Effectiveness of the diaphragm is less when used without a spermicide.

CLASSIFICATION
Competency:
Foundations of Practice
Taxonomy:
Knowledge/Comprehension

---

41. 1. This response is judgemental.
2. This response is judgemental and implies that Sarah should feel guilty if she chooses to have an abortion.

3. This response is nonjudgemental and encourages Sarah to discuss her options.

4. The client is Sarah, not her parents. Sarah has the right to make her decision. However, if Sarah indicates that her parents are involved and supportive, they may be included in the discussion.

CLASSIFICATION
Competency:
Professional Practice
Taxonomy:
Application

42.
1. A diaphragm will not prevent sexually transmitted infections (STIs).
2. Some spermicides do provide protection against some STIs, but they are generally not effective against human immunodeficiency virus (HIV), chlamydia, or cervical gonorrhea.
3. Same as answer 1.
4. **A female condom is inserted by the woman prior to intercourse. If used correctly, it provides a barrier to sperm and STIs.**

CLASSIFICATION
Competency:
Foundations of Practice
Taxonomy:
Application

43.
1. **There is a strong link between human papilloma virus (HPV) and cervical cancer, and Papanicolaou (Pap) tests are required for diagnosis. Pap tests should be performed annually.**
2. Antibiotics are not effective against HPV.
3. This option is not realistic. The practical nurse should discuss with Ms. McLeod safe sexual practices, including the use of condoms.
4. Eradication of the virus is not considered conclusive, even after there is no visible evidence of HPV.

CLASSIFICATION
Competency:
Foundations of Practice
Taxonomy:
Application

44.
1. Oral birth control is very effective but not 100% effective. Ms. Ahmadi has complied with the recommendation that she use a method of birth control that is 100% effective. Also, oral contraceptives may have an effect on the cardiovascular system.
2. **All these methods are fairly effective; however, a tubal ligation (i.e., the tying of the fallopian tubes) is the most effective. A hysterectomy is the only method of birth control that is 100% effective, but surgery in someone with severe heart failure may not be recommended.**
3. While a vasectomy is close to 100% effective, it is Ms. Ahmadi who should not become pregnant. There is no information that Ms. Ahmadi is in a monogamous partnership.
4. This option is not 100% effective.

CLASSIFICATION
Competency:
Foundations of Practice
Taxonomy:
Critical Thinking

CASE 10

45.
1. This outcome may occur, but the practical nurse should obtain factual information about the vaccine prior to making a decision.
2. **This option is the best way for the practical nurse to become informed of the safety and efficacy of the new vaccine. To support safe practice, it is the practical nurse's responsibility to seek out current information from reliable resources.**
3. This outcome may occur, but the practical nurse should research information about the vaccine prior to making a decision.
4. While it is a good idea to consult with nursing colleagues, the practical nurse should recognize that their opinions may not be based on fact.

CLASSIFICATION
Competency:
Professional Practice
Taxonomy:
Critical Thinking

46.
1. **A dilemma is defined as a situation in which one must make an uneasy and difficult choice between two alternatives. In this situation, the most ethical course of action is not clear: the practical nurse has a strong moral reason to support both caring for her clients and keeping her family safe.**

CLASSIFICATION
Competency:
Ethical Practice
Taxonomy:
Knowledge/Comprehension

2. Ethical theory is a framework of assumptions and principles intended to guide decisions about morality.
3. Moral distress is stress caused by situations in which a person is convinced of what is morally right but is not able to act.
4. Nonmaleficence is a principle that obliges people to act so that harm to others is prevented.

47.
1. Based on guidelines by leaders in previous pandemic planning, the priority groups were health care workers and children and adults with underlying health conditions.
2. Same as answer 1.
3. The government does not legislate who receives priority care.
4. **Health care leaders and decision makers develop guidelines to help prioritize resources and identify vulnerable groups so that there is justifiable, reasonable, and fair allocation of resources and access to treatment.**

CLASSIFICATION
Competency:
Professional Practice
Taxonomy:
Application

48.
1. **The deltoid muscle is easily accessible and is the recommended IM site for small volume injections and routine immunizations.**
2. The ventrogluteal muscle is a safe site for IM injections for all clients; however, it is neither necessary nor practical for an immunization clinic.
3. The dorsogluteal muscle, although a traditional site for IM injections, has been associated with injury to the sciatic nerve and is not recommended.
4. The vastus lateralis is the preferred site for immunizations for infants.

CLASSIFICATION
Competency:
Foundations of Practice
Taxonomy:
Critical Thinking

49.
1. **Individuals who have developed an anaphylactic reaction to a previous dose of influenza vaccine should not receive a further dose.**
2. Sexual activity has no relation to the flu vaccine.
3. Antibodies from one type of influenza do not provide immunity from another type of influenza.
4. While childhood immunizations ideally should be current, it is not necessary prior to administration of the flu vaccine.

CLASSIFICATION
Competency:
Foundations of Practice
Taxonomy:
Knowledge/Comprehension

50.
1. While it is not easy to deny care to an ineligible person, the ethical use of available resources requires that the practical nurse refuse to give the vaccine to the adolescent at this time.
2. This statement may be true, but it does not provide a rationale for refusing the adolescent the vaccine and may cause the mother to become concerned and angry.
3. It is not necessarily true that the adolescent is not at risk for contracting this influenza; it is just that he, at present, is not in a priority group.
4. **The mother needs to be reassured that her adolescent son is not in a vulnerable group and that, with limited vaccine available, it must go to those people who are most at risk. The practical nurse also assures the mother that her son will most likely be able to receive the vaccine at a later date.**

CLASSIFICATION
Competency:
Ethical Practice
Taxonomy:
Critical Thinking

CASE 11

51.
1. This response dismisses Ms. Smith's concerns and shows no respect for her feelings.
2. Same as answer 1.

3. **This response indicates caring and provides Ms. Smith an opportunity for her to express her feelings.**
4. Ms. Smith may not be ready to socialize with other residents.

CLASSIFICATION
Competency: **Professional Practice**
Taxonomy: **Application**

52.
1. This action is neither professional nor caring and may be considered neglect.
2. Ms. Smith has stated she does not wish to participate in exercise.
3. There is no indication Ms. Smith requires a substitute decision maker (SDM). She has stated her rationale for her decision.
4. **The practical nurse must respect the decision of the client even if it is contrary to what the practical nurse believes is the "right" health care decision.**

CLASSIFICATION
Competency: **Ethical Practice**
Taxonomy: **Application**

53.
1. It is contrary to ethical nursing practice to accept valuable gifts from clients even if the client is cognitively intact.
2. Same as answer 1.
3. **This response is professional and complies with ethical guidelines for accepting gifts from clients.**
4. This is not true of all agencies, as some gifts, particularly if they are for the entire nursing team, are appropriate. It also places blame on the agency rather than showing the practical nurse practising ethical behaviour.

CLASSIFICATION
Competency: **Ethical Practice**
Taxonomy: **Critical Thinking**

CASE 12

54.
1. When presented early in the process, a list of "dos and don'ts" may cause resentment and impede compliance with a diet. This would be best offered later.
2. This information does need to be emphasized but may be presumptive and directive as an initial action.
3. This question presumes Mr. Hudson has behaviours that he needs to change and is not appropriate initially. In later conversations, it may be appropriate.
4. **This question is open ended, does not presume anything, involves Mr. Hudson in the nutrition plan, and puts the emphasis on his needs, not the practical nurse's.**

CLASSIFICATION
Competency: **Professional Practice**
Taxonomy: **Critical Thinking**

55.
1. **Smaller, more frequent meals help to maintain consistent blood glucose levels.**
2. Total carbohydrate intake should be 45 to 60% of the total diet. It is the type of carbohydrate that is more important.
3. There is no evidence that a diabetic diet does not provide adequate vitamins and minerals.
4. Total fat should remain approximately the same as for the general public. It is more important to restrict the amount of saturated and trans fats, not the total fat.

CLASSIFICATION
Competency: **Foundations of Practice**
Taxonomy: **Application**

56.
1. Simple carbohydrates include monosaccharides and disaccharides. Examples are sugars such as table sugar, honey, and fruit drinks.
2. **These foods are examples of complex carbohydrates that contain starch, glycogen, and fibre.**
3. *Monounsaturated* is a term used with fats.
4. Some of these foods have a moderate glycemic index.

CLASSIFICATION
Competency: **Foundations of Practice**
Taxonomy: **Knowledge/Comprehension**

57.
1. Most fish have a low fat content.
2. Canola oil contains unsaturated fat.
3. **Whole milk is high in saturated fat.**
4. Omega 3 is "heart healthy," and trans-fat-free margarine is low in saturated fat.

CLASSIFICATION
Competency:
Foundations of Practice
Taxonomy:
Knowledge/Comprehension

58.
1. The bran muffin is high in calories and may contain saturated fats, as may the margarine. For diabetics, fruits are best taken whole rather than as juice since the whole fruit contains fibre. This breakfast does not contain protein or dairy products.
2. **This menu is low in calories yet contains all the food groups, providing protein, complex carbohydrates, fibre, dairy, and fruits.**
3. This menu is high in protein but contains no fibre or fruits.
4. The raisins may be high in sugar, the lactose-free milk is not necessary in a diabetic or weight-loss diet, and whole fruit would be better than juice.

CLASSIFICATION
Competency:
Foundations of Practice
Taxonomy:
Critical Thinking

59.
1. Unless otherwise instructed by the physician, he should maintain his normal medication schedule.
2. **Monitoring of blood glucose will tell Mr. Hudson if he needs to adjust his diet. Unless otherwise instructed by a physician, he should maintain his normal medication schedule.**
3. It is not necessary to contact a physician for minor illnesses unless blood sugars become unstable.
4. Same as answer 2.

CLASSIFICATION
Competency:
Foundations of Practice
Taxonomy:
Critical Thinking

60.
1. A weight loss of 5 kg is good and will help the diabetes but does not particularly indicate how well blood glucose has been maintained.
2. A fasting blood-sugar reading will only tell the status of the blood sugar on that particular day.
3. **A glycosylated hemoglobin (HbA_{1c}) test provides an accurate long-term index of the client's average blood sugar. It is objective and reliable evidence of glucose control.**
4. This method of evaluation is important but not the best. Mr. Hudson may feel well even with high blood-glucose levels. If he is not managing the diabetes, he may not want to admit this to the practical nurse.

CLASSIFICATION
Competency:
Foundations of Practice
Taxonomy:
Critical Thinking

CASE 13

61.
1. People with anorexia tend to have cold intolerance rather than feeling hot.
2. **Women with anorexia often stop menstruating due to the loss of body fat.**
3. The skin of people with anorexia tends to be dry, not oily.
4. People with anorexia have constipation rather than diarrhea.

CLASSIFICATION
Competency:
Foundations of Practice
Taxonomy:
Application

62.
1. This test is important but monitors only one thing.
2. This test is very important for a client with anorexia, but a test for electrolytes would include potassium.
3. **An electrolytes test includes sodium, potassium, and chloride.**
4. Same as answer 1.

CLASSIFICATION
Competency:
Foundations of Practice
Taxonomy:
Critical Thinking

63.
1. Young women with anorexia tend to avoid intimacy and are generally not sexually active.
2. Clients with anorexia more frequently deny their illness.
3. Rather than acting out, the anorexic teen often strives to be the "model child."
4. **Clients with anorexia are often high achievers in school in their attempt to be perfect and have control.**

CLASSIFICATION
Competency:
Foundations of Practice
Taxonomy:
Application

64.
1. The physician should be notified but this is not the first action.
2. The apical rate should be monitored after fluids until it increases
3. **This is a very low apical rate and is due to low blood volume secondary to dehydration. The initial action is to increase the blood volume through the administration of fluids.**
4. A snack will not increase the blood volume, and Tiffany may not want to eat.

CLASSIFICATION
Competency:
Foundations of Practice
Taxonomy:
Critical Thinking

65.
1. **This statement is true of teens with anorexia, and Tiffany has a history of excessive exercising. With the forced increase in food, Tiffany will fear an increase in weight, which she may attempt to counter by exercising.**
2. Over-exercising may be harmful, but moderate exercise will be of no harm, particularly since her vital signs have stabilized.
3. Exercise is not an important part of the therapeutic plan for a teen with anorexia.
4. Exercise will not affect Tiffany's tolerance for food.

CLASSIFICATION
Competency:
Foundations of Practice
Taxonomy:
Critical Thinking

66.
1. This response may be true but is not likely to convince Tiffany to attend the sessions.
2. **This response focuses on Tiffany's feelings rather than the group therapy itself. The group would be effective only if Tiffany is able to discuss her feelings openly.**
3. Tiffany may never feel the need to talk with the other girls.
4. This response offers false reassurance; group therapy with other girls who have anorexia may help Tiffany develop insight but may not help her cope with the disease.

CLASSIFICATION
Competency:
Professional Practice
Taxonomy:
Application

67.
1. Rapid weight gain may cause cardiovascular overload and an overwhelming sense of loss of control.
2. **Gradual weight gain is metabolically safe and will prevent the feelings of loss of control that would occur with too rapid a weight gain.**
3. Hydration is important, but 3 L is too much. Tiffany would likely not be compliant with drinking this much fluid.
4. This weight gain would be too fast, particularly in a person who is underweight.

CLASSIFICATION
Competency:
Foundations of Practice
Taxonomy:
Application

CASE 14

68\. 1. This type of rash is common and usually benign in a new infant.
2. This behaviour is not necessarily a sign of illness unless the infant cannot be roused.
3. **Grunting and rapid respirations are abnormal behaviours in an infant. Grunting is a compensatory mechanism whereby an infant attempts to keep air in the alveoli to increase arterial oxygenation; increased respirations increase oxygen and carbon dioxide exchange.**
4. This behaviour is a normal sign of increasing fluid requirements with growth.

CLASSIFICATION
Competency:
Foundations of Practice
Taxonomy:
Application

69\. 1. Oral temperatures are not recommended for children under 3 years old.
2. This route is used only when no other route is possible because of the risk for rectal perforation and because it is intrusive.
3. **This is not invasive, and although it does not provide a core temperature, it is relatively accurate.**
4. Tympanic temperatures are not accurate with infants.

CLASSIFICATION
Competency:
Foundations of Practice
Taxonomy:
Application

70\. 1. Fluids will help decrease the temperature, but this is not the most important intervention.
2. **A temperature of 38.9°C in an infant is abnormal and indicates an infection, which could proceed rapidly to a life-threatening stage. The safest option is to seek medical attention.**
3. A temperature of 38.9°C is a concern, and the parent should not wait days for a physician's advice. The practical nurse has not given the parent any direction about what to do if the temperature increases.
4. Tempra will decrease the temperature, but it is more important to identify and treat the cause of the high temperature.

CLASSIFICATION
Competency:
Foundations of Practice
Taxonomy:
Critical Thinking

71\. 1. **This statement is true. Nurses must not share or reveal their password.**
2. Clients are allowed to view their health records as per agency policy, just as would occur with paper and pencil documentation.
3. If the person accessing the health record is a member of the circle of care, permission from the client is not required.
4. There is no research to prove this statement.

CLASSIFICATION
Competency:
Legal Practice
Taxonomy:
Application

CASE 15

72\. 1. Canada's health care system provides access to health care for all.
2. This statement is true but is not the most important factor.
3. **These clients may have to choose between food, rent, and transportation since they may not have enough money for all.**
4. There is no reason to assume these clients would not be compliant unless the treatment involved additional financial hardships.

CLASSIFICATION
Competency:
Professional Practice
Taxonomy:
Critical Thinking

73.
1. A wood-frame house is not necessarily of concern.
2. **Throw rugs are hazardous, particularly on bare floors. Older persons are most at risk for falls.**
3. Microwave ovens are generally safer for older adults to use than gas or electric stoves.
4. Electric baseboard heaters do not generally get hot enough to burn the skin, and this would not be the most common risk.

CLASSIFICATION
Competency:
Foundations of Practice
Taxonomy:
Critical Thinking

74.
1. **Fibre provides the stool with bulk and moves it through the intestine. Bran and fruits are good sources of fibre.**
2. Cellulose does help constipation, but corn on the cob may be difficult for an older adult to eat. Rice is not a good source of cellulose.
3. Bananas and milk are not natural laxatives.
4. Echinacea and feverfew are herbal remedies not indicated for constipation.

CLASSIFICATION
Competency:
Foundations of Practice
Taxonomy:
Application

75.
1. **Staying indoors protects Mr. Scanlon from inhaling pollutants and is the safest, easiest option.**
2. If ordinary activities include outdoor activities, the client will be at risk of inhaling airborne pollutants.
3. There is no need at this time for Mr. Scanlon to consult with a respiratory therapist.
4. This suggestion is a medical decision and may not necessarily be appropriate.

CLASSIFICATION
Competency:
Foundations of Practice
Taxonomy:
Application

CASE 16

76.
1. The practical nurse may not know what such treatment would involve. As well, the client has not stated that she wishes to be treated according to religious practices.
2. **This method is client-centred care.**
3. The client is the person who provides information about her own care. The family is consulted only if Ms. Merkel is not able to communicate her wishes.
4. Clients are to be cared for as individuals.

CLASSIFICATION
Competency:
Ethical Practice
Taxonomy:
Application

77.
1. **This action provides client-centred, culturally appropriate care.**
2. Ms. Merkel has already stated her reasons.
3. This situation is not about the nurse's rights but the client's rights.
4. This response is not culturally sensitive, client-centred care. The nurse, as a client advocate, must speak with the charge nurse about reassignment.

CLASSIFICATION
Competency:
Professional Practice
Taxonomy:
Application

78.
1. The practical nurse must first determine with the family which cultural practices should be followed. Viewing the body may not be desired or culturally appropriate.
2. Organ donation would likely have been discussed prior to Ms. Merkel's death. As she has already died, her organs will not be able to be harvested.
3. **This answer is the most inclusive one.**
4. There is no indication that this course of action is necessary. If it is, it would be included in information received about specific death rites in answer 3.

CLASSIFICATION
Competency:
Professional Practice
Taxonomy:
Critical Thinking

CASE 17

79. 1. Monilia, not herpes, causes thrush.

2. The infant may acquire the herpes infection from the vaginal birth, putting the infant at risk for systemic herpes, which has a very high mortality.

3. Chlamydia and gonorrhea, not herpes, are the most common causes of ophthalmia neonatorum.
4. Neurological complications may result from the infant's systemic herpes infection, but this is a late stage of the illness.

CLASSIFICATION
Competency:
Foundations of Practice
Taxonomy:
Knowledge/Comprehension

---

80. **1. This is a normal oxygen saturation level for a newborn infant; therefore, no action is required. If there were evidence of respiratory distress, the practical nurse should monitor the levels.**

2. This action is not necessary.
3. This action is not necessary or desirable.
4. This action will do nothing to affect blood levels of oxygen.

CLASSIFICATION
Competency:
Foundations of Practice
Taxonomy:
Critical Thinking

---

81. 1. Impaired reflex behaviour and a shrill cry indicate central nervous system damage.

2. Asymmetry of the gluteal dorsal surface of the thighs and inguinal folds indicates congenital dislocation of the hip; folds on the affected side appear higher than those on the unaffected side.

3. An inguinal hernia is evidenced by the protrusion of the intestine into the inguinal sac.
4. Peripheral nervous system damage would be manifested by limpness or flaccidity of the extremities.

CLASSIFICATION
Competency:
Foundations of Practice
Taxonomy:
Knowledge/Comprehension

---

82. 1. It is too soon to observe for signs of infection.

2. The surgical site is an extremely vascular area, and the infant must be closely observed for bleeding.

3. The infant is likely to cry during the procedure, but with an analgesic and comforting, the pain should be managed. A shrill, piercing cry is indicative of central nervous system difficulty.
4. Urinary output is assessed but is not the most essential nursing action in the initial postoperative period.

CLASSIFICATION
Competency:
Foundations of Practice
Taxonomy:
Critical Thinking

CASE 18

83. 1. Heart cells are damaged when a client experiences a myocardial infarction.
2. The pain of angina may be as severe as the pain of a myocardial infarction.
3. Sublingual nitroglycerin usually relieves pain within 5 minutes.

4. Rest and nitroglycerin relieve pain from angina. The hallmark symptom of a myocardial infarction is pain that persists despite rest and nitroglycerin administration.

CLASSIFICATION
Competency:
Foundations of Practice
Taxonomy:
Application

---

84. 1. Cholesterol is produced by the body, synthesized primarily in the liver.
2. Only animal-sourced foods furnish dietary cholesterol.

3. Cholesterol is an integral part of almost every cell in the body.
4. **Cholesterol is a sterol found in tissue and circulating in the blood. It can increase, in part, with diets high in saturated fats.**

CLASSIFICATION
Competency: **Foundations of Practice**
Taxonomy: **Application**

85.
1. **The patch should be removed for 10 to 12 hours each day to prevent a tolerance buildup to the medication.**
2. There are numerous adverse effects that the client may experience.
3. Patches should never be cut.
4. Neither of these options is a safe disposal method for medications. The best option is disposal in a biohazard container if available.

CLASSIFICATION
Competency: **Changes in Health**
Taxonomy: **Application**

CASE 19

86.
1. This response dismisses Mr. Bangay's feelings.
2. This response is a closed question that may obtain either "yes" or "no" as an answer.
3. Same as answer 1.
4. **This response is an open-ended question that will allow Mr. Bangay to discuss his feelings.**

CLASSIFICATION
Competency: **Professional Practice**
Taxonomy: **Application**

87.
1. This response is not appropriate. Mr. Bangay is grieving the absence of his wife, not looking for other female company.
2. This response presents a potential option for Mr. Bangay but does not respond to his statement.
3. **This response reaffirms Mr. Bangay's grief and allows him to speak about his wife and his feelings.**
4. This response dismisses Mr. Bangay's feelings.

CLASSIFICATION
Competency: **Professional Practice**
Taxonomy: **Application**

88.
1. This action follows the rules but does not employ nursing judgement.
2. **Mr. Bangay's temperature is above normal, especially considering he is an older adult. It is appropriate nursing judgement to monitor his temperature more frequently.**
3. The taking of vital signs does not require a physician order. It is within the scope of nursing practice.
4. This action is not necessary, and in an adult, the axillary route is not as reliable as an oral temperature.

CLASSIFICATION
Competency: **Professional Practice**
Taxonomy: **Critical Thinking**

89.
1. This action is not a specific resolution.
2. Collaborating rather than mandating action is likely to be more effective.
3. This action may have to occur if the issue cannot be solved.
4. **Collaboration is the most effective method of addressing conflict.**

CLASSIFICATION
Competency: **Collaborative Practice**
Taxonomy: **Critical Thinking**

CASE 20

90. 1. This documentation does not describe Olivia's behaviour.

2. Descriptions should be simple, objective, and easily interpreted. This documentation accurately describes Olivia's behaviour

3. "Well" is not an accurate description of behaviour.
4. This documentation is about the headaches, not Olivia's behaviour.

CLASSIFICATION
Competency:
Legal practice
Taxonomy:
Application

---

91. 1. This response describes electroencephalography.
2. This response describes echoencephalography.
3. This response is similar to a description of a positron emission tomography scan, but dye is not injected into the brain for either test.

4. This response is the definition of a computed tomography (CT) scan.

CLASSIFICATION
Competency:
Foundations of Practice
Taxonomy:
Knowledge/Comprehension

---

92. 1. This response may not be true.
2. This response does not answer Olivia's question.

3. After surgery, headaches may be aggravated rather than improved. It is better to be honest and not create false hope.

4. Same as answer 2.

CLASSIFICATION
Competency:
Foundations of Practice
Taxonomy:
Application

---

93. **1. The practical nurse should consult with the surgeon for the correct positioning since there must not be pressure on the operative site.**

2. This position is common after neurosurgery but is dependent on the operative site.
3. Trendelenburg's position may be contraindicated as with some types of surgery it may lead to increased intracranial pressure.
4. This position is incorrect as it may increase pressure on the operative site.

CLASSIFICATION
Competency:
Foundations of Practice
Taxonomy:
Critical Thinking

---

94. 1. If the drainage were sanguineous, this action would be appropriate.

2. Colourless drainage is a sign of cerebrospinal fluid leaking from the incision site and requires physician consultation.

3. The drainage needs to be documented, but this is not the initial action.
4. Dressings should be reinforced, not changed.

CLASSIFICATION
Competency:
Collaborative Practice
Taxonomy:
Critical Thinking

---

95. **1. Nurses have the authority to pronounce death.**

2. There is a legal requirement for physicians to certify death. Certifying death means determining the cause of death.
3. The physician does not need to be called to pronounce death.
4. The body should not be removed to the morgue until death has been pronounced and certified.

CLASSIFICATION
Competency:
Professional Practice
Taxonomy:
Knowledge/Comprehension

CASE 21

96. 1. Assistance with bathing may be important for the client but may take time and is not the priority action.

2. **This action can be accomplished fairly quickly. To delay the count prevents the day nurse from leaving the unit.**
3. Assisting the physician to reinsert the gastrostomy tube (G-tube) may take considerable time. It is not professional to ask the day practical nurse to wait until this is done. Reinsertion of a G-tube is not an emergency.
4. This client must be assessed, but there is no indication that it is urgent. Assessment will require more time than the narcotics count.

CLASSIFICATION
Competency: **Professional Practice**
Taxonomy: **Critical Thinking**

97.

1. This response is not logical. The unit staff has called in the family because Ms. David is about to die.
2. This response deflects the question. There is no need to refer this question to a physician as the practical nurse has the knowledge to reply.
3. The family has not expressed a need for the chaplain. This response does not answer the question.
4. **This response provides a truthful answer to the son's question.**

CLASSIFICATION
Competency: **Professional Practice**
Taxonomy: **Critical Thinking**

98.

1. Elevation of the extremities should be avoided because it increases venous return, placing an increased workload on the heart.
2. Excessive coughing and mucus production is characteristic of pulmonary edema and does not need to be encouraged.
3. **The orthopneic position allows maximum lung expansion because gravity reduces the pressure of the abdominal viscera on the diaphragm and lungs.**
4. Positioning for postural drainage does not relieve acute dyspnea; furthermore, it increases venous return to the heart.

CLASSIFICATION
Competency: **Foundations of Practice**
Taxonomy: **Application**

CASE 22

99.

1. This action is an appropriate method of assessment but is not as accurate as measuring.
2. Although assessing fluid balance by weighing a client is important, it does not determine the degree of edema in a specific extremity.
3. **Mr. Camponi's edema is likely to be most prevalent in his ankles. Measuring an area provides an objective assessment and is not subject to individual interpretation.**
4. Although monitoring intake and output helps in assessing fluid balance, it does not determine the degree of edema in a specific extremity.

CLASSIFICATION
Competency: **Foundations of Practice**
Taxonomy: **Critical Thinking**

100.

1. This action is taken cautiously and should be the decision of a physician.
2. **Elevation of an extremity promotes venous and lymphatic drainage by gravity.**
3. This action needs to be ordered by a physician.
4. This action will have little effect on edema.

CLASSIFICATION
Competency: **Foundations of Practice**
Taxonomy: **Critical Thinking**

INDEPENDENT QUESTIONS ANSWERS AND RATIONALES

101.

1. **Writing about clients, client care, and the organization would be contrary to ethical and legal principles. Even if the clients were not identified by name, other identifying characteristics, and knowledge of where the practical nurse works may breach confidentiality under the Personal Health Information Privacy Act (PHIPA).**
2. There is no reason a practical nurse may not participate in social networking sites as long as the practical nurse does not breach the confidentiality and privacy of clients, and the organization that she works for under the PHIPA.
3. Social networking sites are not professionally based and therefore may not be optimum for professional development.
4. Refer to answer 1. There is a great risk for breach of confidentiality because of the casual and unstructured nature of social networking sites. Misuse of technology can lead to potential breech of personal information. Refer to PHIPA.

CLASSIFICATION
Competency:
Ethical Practice
Taxonomy:
Application

102.

1. A family should not push the patient-controlled analgesia (PCA) device for an adolescent child unless directed to do so by the physician. Christopher is old enough to control the PCA himself.
2. The PCA provides consistent levels of medication.
3. The practical nurse does not need to be notified every time Christopher wants to push the button to relieve pain.
4. **Feelings of control, particularly in adolescents, are one of the documented advantages of PCAs.**

CLASSIFICATION
Competency:
Foundations of Practice
Taxonomy:
Application

103.

1. Legality is not the professional issue. If she is not able to communicate effectively in English, she is unable to provide safe client care.
2. **Professional responsibility includes having the ability to effectively communicate with clients. Until Ms. Levis is able to communicate effectively in English, care of clients would be compromised.**
3. This action may be a requirement from an agency but is not a requirement for registration. The professional and ethical issue is whether she is able to communicate effectively enough to provide safe client care, not whether she has passed a course.
4. This action is not professional, safe, or practical.

CLASSIFICATION
Competency:
Legal Practice
Taxonomy:
Critical Thinking

104.

1. Clients with advanced dementia would not be capable of using this pain scale.
2. This method of delivering an analgesic is inappropriate for a client with dementia since she will likely not be able to understand how to use the PCA.
3. This action does not provide for individualized care.
4. **Nonverbal client behaviour such as restlessness, facial grimaces, and crying may provide clues as to the effectiveness of the analgesic.**

CLASSIFICATION
Competency:
Foundations of Practice
Taxonomy:
Application

105.

1. This position would not help to prevent potential cerebral edema or increased intracranial pressure.

2. It is important to keep the head in the midline position and to prevent flexion of the neck.

3. **This position would facilitate drainage from the head region and thus help to prevent an increase in intracranial pressure.**

4. Lowering the head of the bed may increase intracranial pressure.

CLASSIFICATION
Competency:
Professional Practice
Taxonomy:
Critical Thinking

106.

1. **Ms. William has the right to make decisions regarding her disease and her life. The nurses may not agree with those decisions but must, without judgement, support the client's right to make her own informed decisions.**

2. There is no evidence that Ms. William is not mentally competent.
3. The choice of lifestyle is Ms. William's. A mediator is not indicated since there is no compromise to be achieved between Ms. William and the staff.
4. This action is abandonment of the client.

CLASSIFICATION
Competency:
Ethical Practice
Taxonomy:
Application

107.

1. This action will help to keep the secretions thin but is an ongoing action and not the most important.

2. **Hyperoxygenation will ensure that his oxygen level does not drop during suctioning. This action is the most important.**

3. Oral care needs to be provided, but it is not essential before suctioning.
4. Ties are not affected by suctioning.

CLASSIFICATION
Competency:
Foundations of Practice
Taxonomy:
Critical Thinking

108.

1. **A practical nurse is ethically not allowed to refuse to care for certain clients; however, she can ask if she can have her assignment modified. She will remain assigned to this client until a suitable replacement is found.**

2. This action is not ethical practice and could be considered abandonment of clients.
3. This action is not ethical and likely is not practical since she was needed on the palliative care unit.
4. This action is not ethical or professional. The practical nurse must ensure she does not advise or persuade the client in any way in the client's decision making.

CLASSIFICATION
Competency:
Ethical Practice
Taxonomy:
Application

109.

1. This client does not meet the criteria. The client must be mentally competent and capable of making decisions at the time of the request.
2. This client does not meet the criteria. The person must be at least 18 years of age and capable of making health care decisions.

3. **This client meets the criteria. Natural death is foreseeable in a period of time that is not too distant. The client is mentally competent and capable of making the decision at the time of his request and suffers from a serious and incurable illness.**

4. This client does not meet the criteria at this time. A comprehensive psychosocial assessment would be required to reveal any hidden problems or conflicts that may affect her rational decision making, a prerequisite to informed consent for any procedure. Her illness may be treatable with therapy and medications. More assessments would be required.

CLASSIFICATION
Competency:
Foundations of Practice
Taxonomy:
Knowledge and Comprehension

110.

1. **The scope of practice of a pharmacist includes comprehensive knowledge of medications and health teaching about medications to clients.**
2. This action may be appropriate; however, the pharmacist likely has more in-depth knowledge of the medications and may also be more available to the client.
3. While nurses have knowledge of drugs, the pharmacist is the more appropriate resource since a pharmacist's knowledge is more comprehensive.
4. This action is not the best method to educate the client unless there are no other resources available.

CLASSIFICATION
Competency: **Professional Practice**
Taxonomy: **Critical Thinking**

111.

1. This action is based on an assumption. The practical nurse does not know that continuing the teaching will improve understanding.
2. **This approach follows principles of teaching and learning. The practical nurse will be better able to observe and evaluate the clients understanding of the skill through visual demonstration and role playing.**
3. The practical nurse does not know what it is the client does not understand about the topic. Changing the topic does not address the issue and may cause the client to perceive that breathing exercises are not important.
4. This approach will not increase the understanding of the information. The practical nurse must determine the perceived learning needs of the client.

CLASSIFICATION
Competency: **Professional Practice**
Taxonomy: **Application**

112.

1. This action is a form of restraint. Canadian health care follows a philosophy of "least restraint." Clients must be individually and frequently assessed for the need for side rails.
2. The client might become more confused, a state that would be considered a chemical restraint.
3. **This would be the best choice for the client's safety. With the bed in the lowest position, it is likely a fall would not cause injury to the client. If the practical nurse checks on the client frequently, she may be able to assess for wakefulness and confusion.**
4. This action restricts the client's movement and is a restraint.

CLASSIFICATION
Competency: **Ethical Practice**
Taxonomy: **Application**

113.

1. **Fluctuations in mood are common in the early stages of Parkinson's disease as the client deals with the emotional stress of the diagnosis.**
2. This early manifestation is called a "resting tremor." It is evident when the extremity is at rest.
3. This manifestation occurs much later in the disease process.
4. There is no reason for an increase in appetite.

CLASSIFICATION
Competency: **Foundations of Practice**
Taxonomy: **Knowledge/Comprehension**

114.

1. **The primary health issue for the practical nurse and Mr. Mason is to assess the extent of the chemical dependence.**
2. This question addresses a legal issue and may break trust between Mr. Mason and the practical nurse.
3. Mr. Mason is likely to be aware of the legal and health issues related to his substance to use. This question serves no purpose.
4. This question can be explored at a further date. The initial assessment is to determine the extent of the dependency.

CLASSIFICATION
Competency: **Professional Practice**
Taxonomy: **Critical Thinking**

115.

1. Slowing the rate decreases the pressure but does not eliminate it.
2. Cramps are not a reason to discontinue the enema entirely; temporary clamping of the tubing usually relieves the cramps, and the procedure can be continued.
3. **Administration of additional fluid when a client complains of abdominal cramps adds to discomfort because of additional pressure. By clamping the tubing for a few minutes, the practical nurse generally allows the cramps to subside. Then the enema can be continued.**
4. This action will reduce the flow of the solution, in turn decreasing pressure, but may not reduce the cramping.

CLASSIFICATION
Competency:
Foundations of Practice
Taxonomy:
Critical Thinking

116.

1. **The practical nurse needs to have further assessment information prior to action. More data are required. He must find out if this is a new finding or if Mr. Nascad has had any previous tremors.**
2. The physician may need to be notified, but this is not the first step.
3. This statement is true, and the finding should be documented, but the practical nurse needs more data before assuming the tremor is benign.
4. This statement is not necessarily true. The cause of the tremor needs to be investigated.

CLASSIFICATION
Competency:
Foundations of Practice
Taxonomy:
Application

117.

1. This calculation is incorrect.
2. **To answer this question correctly, you must know Nägele's rule, which is to subtract 3 months and add 7 days to the first day of the last menstrual period. The information about spotting is a distracter, but the stem clearly states that June 11 was the date of the last normal menstrual period. With this calculation, the correct response is March 18.**
3. Same as answer 1.
4. Same as answer 1.

CLASSIFICATION
Competency:
Foundations of Practice
Taxonomy:
Application

118.

1. This may worsen her symptoms.
2. Same as 1.
3. Same as 1.
4. **Having the infant empty the affected breast will help to prevent worsening mastitis.**

CLASSIFICATION
Competency:
Foundations of Practice
Taxonomy:
Critical Thinking

119.

1. **The first action by the practical nurse must be to stop the abuse. This is achieved by intervening in the situation.**
2. This action will be done but is not the first action.
3. This action is possible but is not the first action.
4. Same as answer 2.

CLASSIFICATION
Competency:
Ethical Practice
Taxonomy:
Critical Thinking

120.

1. This statement is not accurate.
2. **Insulin assists the transport of glucose through the cell membrane.**
3. Same as answer 1.
4. Same as answer 1.

CLASSIFICATION
Competency:
Foundations of Practice
Taxonomy:
Knowledge/Comprehension

121.
1. This action is appropriate, but it is likely the teens already are aware of the health hazards of the snacks and make poor choices regardless.
2. This action is possible; however, the school administration may be reluctant to take this major step, particularly as schools sometimes receive monies from the snack companies.
3. It is a good idea to have a parent–teacher meeting, but there are many teens who may not be able to bring lunches, and bringing one may not prevent them from also purchasing snacks and drinks at school.
4. **This action is likely to be the most successful option. If the high-sugar snacks and pop are not in the machines, the students will not be able to purchase them.**

CLASSIFICATION
Competency:
Professional Practice
Taxonomy:
Critical Thinking

122.
1. The woman is hard of hearing so would not be able to hear what the practical nurse says.
2. **Provided the information on the paper was destroyed at the end of the shift, although not ideal, this is the most logical mechanism to ensure confidentiality.**
3. This action is not ethical practice.
4. It is not likely body language would be able to convey pertinent information about care.

CLASSIFICATION
Competency:
Professional Practice
Taxonomy:
Application

123.
1. It is not compassionate care to state that the mother does not need to have her children stay with her. The practical nurse does not know that the client will be fine.
2. While the practical nurse has the authority to enforce only one visitor, the family may view this action as only caring about rules, not the care of their mother.
3. Same answer as 2.
4. **This solution provides the family with an option of all being with their mother at some point during the night and allows the practical nurse to minimize noise and disruptions for other clients.**

CLASSIFICATION
Competency:
Professional Practice
Taxonomy:
Application

124.
1. **A client who has contracted one sexually transmitted infection (STI) will frequently have other STIs. Some are asymptomatic. Depending on reported symptoms, testing would be advised for gonorrhea, chlamydia, HIV, and syphilis. If other STIs are diagnosed, they will require treatment.**
2. Counselling implies there is a problem with the client's sexual activities, and this is not known. Transmission of genital herpes and other STIs needs to be discussed, but this is not the priority.
3. This needs to be discussed, as well as the fact the herpes cannot be cured, but is not the priority.
4. Although not necessarily common, it is possible to transfer herpes from the genital area of a partner during oral sexual activity. It is unlikely an exam would be warranted: Ms. Morrissey would be well aware of having oral herpes (cold sores), which would appear on her lips, not in her mouth.

CLASSIFICATION
Competency:
Foundations of Practice
Taxonomy:
Critical Thinking

125.

1. **To permit adequate visualization of the mucosa during the sigmoidoscopy, the bowel must be cleansed with a nonirritating enema before the exam.**
2. Stool will be eliminated from the colon by an enema before the exam. Collecting a stool specimen serves no purpose.
3. Because only the lower bowel is being visualized, it is unnecessary and debilitating to place these restrictions on the client; clear liquids and a laxative may be given the day before to limit fecal residue.
4. The client does not drink such a substance in preparation for a sigmoidoscopy.

CLASSIFICATION
Competency:
Foundations of Practice
Taxonomy:
Knowledge/Comprehension

126.

1. Compression bandages are used to mold and shape the limb for eventual prothesis not positioning on a pillow.
2. This will not reduce the development of phantom limb pain.
3. **Having the hip flexed will lead to flexion contractions. The client should not elevate the residual limb on a pillow postoperatively.**
4. This will not lead to incisional infection.

CLASSIFICATION
Competency:
Foundations of Practice
Taxonomy:
Knowledge/Comprehension

127.

1. The placenta is permeable to certain substances, which may include nicotine.
2. There is no evidence that the fetus becomes addicted to nicotine.
3. **Heavy cigarette smoking or continued exposure to a smoke-filled environment causes both maternal and fetal vasoconstriction, resulting in fetal growth retardation and increased fetal and infant mortality.**
4. The fetal circulation is separate from the maternal circulation; however, nicotine can cross the placental barrier.

CLASSIFICATION
Competency:
Foundations of Practice
Taxonomy:
Knowledge/Comprehension

128.

1. It is important to know a client's culture, but the country of origin does not necessary apply to culture. It is more important to assess for any risk factors, such as the use of herbal therapies.
2. **Herbal supplements and over-the-counter medicines may have adverse effects that interfere with clotting after surgery and may have interactions with other drugs.**
3. It is important that a client be adequately nourished before surgery, but the client's general health status should reflect this. This question is poorly worded for obtaining complete information about nutrition.
4. Sleep is important for healing after surgery but is not the most important factor at this time.

CLASSIFICATION
Competency:
Foundations of Practice
Taxonomy:
Critical Thinking

129.

1. While this statement may be true, it will shut down any communication between the practical nurse and the client.
2. This statement is true, but the client needs information about all types of treatment. This response by the practical nurse neglects the client's health and chances of survival.
3. This statement is not true.
4. **The client may be basing his decision on inadequate information. It is the practical nurse's responsibility to ensure the client has access to the knowledge he needs to make an informed decision.**

CLASSIFICATION
Competency:
Professional Practice
Taxonomy:
Application

130.
1. **This response provides a solution for Mr. Ciavello's complaint about flavourless food and is an appropriate referral to another health care provider.**
2. This response is inappropriate; Mr. Ciavello does not mention specific foods.
3. The practical nurse should first acknowledge Mr. Ciavello's feelings and then assess his level of knowledge before imparting such information.
4. This response suggests that adherence to the prescribed medical regimen is unnecessary.

CLASSIFICATION
Competency:
Collaborative Practice
Taxonomy:
Critical Thinking

131.
1. These symptoms do not indicate an electrolyte imbalance.
2. **Potassium, the major intracellular cation, functions with sodium and calcium to regulate neuromuscular activity and contraction of muscle fibres, particularly the heart muscle. In hypokalemia, these symptoms develop, and they may be life threatening.**
3. These symptoms would indicate hypocalcemia, which does not generally occur with colitis.
4. Nausea and vomiting might occur with a prolonged potassium deficit; however, this is not an early sign. Leg and abdominal cramps occur with potassium excess, not deficit.

CLASSIFICATION
Competency:
Foundations of Practice
Taxonomy:
Knowledge/Comprehension

132.
1. This result is a miscalculation.
2. Same as answer 1.
3. Same as answer 1.
4. **This calculation is correct and is outlined in the chart below.**

Intake (mL)	***Output (mL)***
IV fluid (350)	**Urine (290)**
G-tube feedings (600)	**Urine (320)**
Water (150)	**Emesis (25)**
TOTAL (1 100)	**(635)**

CLASSIFICATION
Competency:
Foundations of Practice
Taxonomy:
Application

133.
1. Elevation does not change the position of the IV cannula; the infusion must be discontinued.
2. **When an IV infusion is infiltrated, it should be removed to prevent swelling, possible damage of the tissues, and pain.**
3. This action would add to the infiltration of fluid.
4. Soaks may be applied, if ordered, after the IV is removed.

CLASSIFICATION
Competency:
Foundations of Practice
Taxonomy:
Application

134.
1. **The sequence for cardiopulmonary resuscitation should be maintained regardless of the setting or diagnosis. The practical nurse will need assistance in providing emergency care to the client; therefore, calling for help is the priority action.**
2. This action should be taken after the call for help.
3. Oxygen should be administered if Mr. Stephanopoulos is assessed to be breathing.
4. The assessment of a pulse is determined after the assessment of the airway.

CLASSIFICATION
Competency:
Collaborative Practice
Taxonomy:
Critical Thinking

135.

1. The physical craving for nicotine may last for months.
2. Increased vitamin intake may be beneficial but will not reduce withdrawal symptoms.
3. This suggestion will be helpful but will not reduce his withdrawal symptoms.
4. **This is practical advice that addresses Mr. Carter's concern.**

CLASSIFICATION
Competency:
Foundations of Practice
Taxonomy:
Application

136.

1. Generally, cardiac disease does not cause *abruptio placentae*.
2. Hyperthyroidism may cause endocrine disturbance in the infant but does not affect the blood supply to the uterus.
3. Cephalopelvic disproportion may affect the delivery of the fetus but does not affect the placenta.
4. **Pregnancy-induced hypertension leads to vasospasms; this, in turn, causes the placenta to tear away from the uterine wall (*abruptio placentae*).**

CLASSIFICATION
Competency:
Foundations of Practice
Taxonomy:
Knowledge/Comprehension

137.

1. Some jurisdictions may request annual official proof of compliance with quality assurance (QA) programs. However, ongoing and continuous quality assurance is essential to maintaining competency.
2. **Most quality assurance programs are based on the principle of lifelong learning, daily reflection, and continuous improvement in competency. Self-assessment, a common component of QA programs, is never static nor formally scheduled.**
3. While some employers do use a QA tool, its primary purpose is not employee evaluation.
4. While some jurisdictions require practical nurses to participate in QA programs to maintain registration, their primary purpose is not registration maintenance.

CLASSIFICATION
Competency:
Professional Practice
Taxonomy:
Critical Thinking

138.

1. This response is not necessarily true and negates Ms. Helena's feelings.
2. This response is not necessarily true and may alarm Ms. Helena unnecessarily.
3. **This response is a truthful and factual answer to Ms. Helena's question.**
4. This response implies that the practical nurse does not have the necessary knowledge to discuss the biopsy with Ms. Helena.

CLASSIFICATION
Competency:
Professional Practice
Taxonomy:
Application

139.

1. This action may be a solution but is not the first action the practical nurse should take.
2. **The practical nurse must first reflect on what is happening in her life and how it can be changed so she does not succumb to burnout. Implementing strategies without a complete understanding of what needs to be changed is not likely to be effective.**
3. The practical nurse must first assess the stressors in her life. She may not be able to afford to work part time.
4. This action is likely to happen, but the practical nurse must first assess her eating and sleeping habits to determine what changes need to be made.

CLASSIFICATION
Competency:
Professional Practice
Taxonomy:
Critical Thinking

140.

1. Caloric intake is increased to meet the demands of the growing fetus.
2. **As pregnancy progresses, there are usually alterations in glucose tolerance and in the metabolism and use of insulin. The result is an increased need for exogenous insulin.**

CLASSIFICATION
Competency:
Foundations of Practice
Taxonomy:
Knowledge/Comprehension

3. Pancreatic enzymes or hormones other than insulin are not taken by diabetics.
4. Same as answer 2.

141.

1. This statement is untrue; often the maternal instinct is nurtured by the sight of the infant.
2. **Almost all mothers, including multiparas, report some ambivalence and anxiety about their ability to be good mothers.**
3. This statement is untrue; it may take a much longer time.
4. This statement is untrue; ambivalent feelings are universal in response to mothering.

CLASSIFICATION
Competency:
Professional Practice
Taxonomy:
Knowledge/Comprehension

142.

1. This statement is untrue; excessive discipline leads to feelings of shame and self-doubt, the major crisis at this stage of development.
2. **The psychosocial need during the early toddler age is the development of autonomy. The toddler objects strongly to discipline.**
3. The sense of initiative is attained during the preschool age, not the toddler age.
4. It is frightening for a child to be left alone; it leaves the child with feelings of rejection, isolation, and insecurity.

CLASSIFICATION
Competency:
Foundations of Practice
Taxonomy:
Application

143.

1. This action is important, but maintenance of respiration has priority.
2. **Laryngeal spasms can occur abruptly; patency of the airway is determined by a constant assessment for symptoms of respiratory distress.**
3. Same as answer 1.
4. Same as answer 1.

CLASSIFICATION
Competency:
Foundations of Practice
Taxonomy:
Critical Thinking

144.

1. This action does not ensure movement but social interaction.
2. Although this statement may be true, it may not be motivating and may make the boy feel less masculine.
3. Limit setting meets the security needs of young children. Adolescents do not respond well to strict rules.
4. **Decision making fosters and supports independence, a developmental need of the adolescent. It also increases a sense of self-worth and control.**

CLASSIFICATION
Competency:
Professional Practice
Taxonomy:
Application

145.

1. Although this criterion is considered, the selection of drugs is based primarily on the ability of the drug to destroy the specific organism.
2. This criterion may be a factor if Ms. Sloane does not have a medical insurance plan, but it is not the most important factor.
3. **When the causative organism is isolated, it is tested for susceptibility (sensitivity) to various antimicrobial agents. When an organism is sensitive to a medication, the medication is capable of destroying the organism.**
4. Although the ordering practitioner's preference is considered, the selection of drugs is based primarily on the ability of the drug to destroy the specific organism.

CLASSIFICATION
Competency:
Professional Practice
Taxonomy:
Application

146.

1. He is not following his current diabetic diet and has been hyperglycemic. This action will not help. It does not promote independence in decision making and is not client centered.

2. This is the most appropriate action. It allows him to be part of the decision-making process in his health care. It helps the practical nurse to understand what types of food he enjoys whether it be cultural preference or not. It promotes his self-determination and is helping to build a trusting relationship with the client. The diabetic educator is a good resource to use for meal planning.

3. The practical nurse does not know if he follows an Indigenous diet. If he does, this may be helpful, but the practical nurse first needs to ask him his preference to promote self-determination and trust in relationship development.
4. This is not helpful. The practical nurse is closing down the therapeutic relationship by not empowering him as part of the decision-making process.

CLASSIFICATION
Competency:
Foundations of Practice
Taxonomy:
Critical Thinking

147.

1. These services are the ones covered under provincial health care plans and are transferable between provinces under the *Canada Health Act*.

2. Medications administered while in hospital are covered.
3. Specialists and intensive care services are covered under provincial plans.
4. Not all health services or health care providers are covered under provincial plans.

CLASSIFICATION
Competency:
Professional Practice
Taxonomy:
Knowledge/Comprehension

148.

1. This intervention is a tertiary intervention.
2. This intervention is a secondary intervention.
3. Same as answer 1.

4. Immunization programs prevent the occurrence of disease and are considered primary interventions.

CLASSIFICATION
Competency:
Professional Practice
Taxonomy:
Application

149.

1. This terminology is unclear; it does not indicate the specific stage of labour.
2. This stage lasts from the delivery of the fetus to the delivery of the placenta; the mother does not experience any physiological symptoms.
3. This stage lasts from full dilation to expulsion; a heavy bloody show and pushing are evident at this time.

4. The physiological intensification of labour occurring during transition is caused by a greater energy expenditure and increased pressure on the stomach; these result in feelings of fatigue, discouragement, and nausea.

CLASSIFICATION
Competency:
Foundations of Practice
Taxonomy:
Knowledge/Comprehension

150.

1. A client would have rapid, shallow respirations to compensate for poor gas exchange.
2. The distal lobes will have diminished sounds due to collapsed alveoli.
3. Atelectasis may cause a loose, productive cough.

4. Because atelectasis involves the collapsing of the alveoli distal to the bronchioles, breath sounds would be diminished in the lower lobes.

CLASSIFICATION
Competency:
Foundations of Practice
Taxonomy:
Knowledge/Comprehension

151.

1. This condition is caused by hypocalcemia. It is manifested by exaggerated muscular twitching.
2. This condition is an obvious defect of the spinal column; it is easily recognized.
3. Elevated potassium causes cardiac irregularities.

4. Intracranial bleeding may occur in the subdural, subarachnoid, or intraventricular spaces of the brain, causing pressure on vital centres; clinical signs are related to the area and degree of cerebral involvement.

CLASSIFICATION
Competency:
Foundations of Practice
Taxonomy:
Knowledge/Comprehension

---

152. **1. This statement adequately describes hemodialysis treatment.**

2. Fluids are restricted when on hemodialysis.
3. Clients with kidney failure who use hemodialysis require treatment 3 to 4 times a week for 3 to 4 hours each time.
4. This describes peritoneal dialysis not hemodialysis.

CLASSIFICATION
Competency:
Foundations of Practice
Taxonomy:
Knowledge/Comprehension

---

153. 1. This problem is unlikely to be life threatening.

2. Vomiting may result in aspiration of the vomitus because it cannot be expelled. This could cause pneumonia or asphyxia.

3. Same as answer 1.
4. Bronchospasm is not a common risk with wiring of the jaw.

CLASSIFICATION
Competency:
Foundations of Practice
Taxonomy:
Critical Thinking

---

154. 1. This is not ethical practice and is considered abandonment of the client.

2. The practical nurse has an ongoing legal duty to care for assigned clients, but she can ask to have her assignment changed.

3. This action is not ethical or professional. The practical nurse must ensure she does not advise or persuade the client in any way in the client's decision making.
4. Write an order to administer some other medication to treat the client's spasms.

CLASSIFICATION
Competency:
Ethical Practice
Taxonomy:
Application

---

155. 1. This approach may be perceived to be punitive and aggressive.
2. This approach is not supportive and implies that Wai is rude.
3. This approach may be inferred to be culturally insensitive and too forward.

4. Communicating directly may appear to be aggressive and insensitive to the foreign-trained nurse. This approach is supportive and culturally respectful.

CLASSIFICATION
Competency:
Professional Practice
Taxonomy:
Application

---

156. 1. This action is not necessary unless there is evidence that the mother is abusive or neglectful or if Lawrence's asthma is severe enough that his life is in danger if he is discharged.
2. This statement is not true.
3. The mother is his legal guardian; thus, agency policies would not prevent her from taking him home.

4. The mother is Lawrence's legal guardian and may discharge him. The important action is to ensure that she understands how to care for his asthma so that she can manage it at home. The practical nurse should ensure that the event is documented according to agency policies.

CLASSIFICATION
Competency:
Professional Practice
Taxonomy:
Critical Thinking

---

157. 1. This action is important but not the priority.
2. Same as answer 1.

3. All options could be correct, but respiratory assessment is the most crucial at this time.

4. Same as answer 1.

CLASSIFICATION
Competency:
Foundations of Practice
Taxonomy:
Critical Thinking

---

158. **1. Motor vehicle accidents are the most common cause of death among adolescents.**

2. Suicide is the second most prevalent cause of death.
3. Cancers are not the most common cause of death.
4. Sports injuries do occur but are not the most common cause of death.

CLASSIFICATION
Competency:
Foundations of Practice
Taxonomy:
Knowledge/Comprehension

---

159. 1. Sexual inhibitions are individual and not related to sexual orientation.
2. While companionship is important, it should not be assumed that it is any more important than sexual activity.
3. Sexual interest and activity do not cease in the older adult.

4. Sexual responses do not cease in the older adult. Older adults have an interest in sexual activities when a suitable partner and privacy are available.

CLASSIFICATION
Competency:
Foundations of Practice
Taxonomy:
Application

---

160. **1. Student practical nurses are responsible and accountable for their own actions. A second-year practical nursing student is fully prepared to take and interpret blood pressure readings.**

2. The nurse should reasonably expect a second-year practical nursing student to take and interpret a manual blood pressure reading.
3. The teacher is responsible only if she has given a client assignment that is beyond the expected knowledge and skills of the practical nursing student. Blood pressure reading is not beyond the skill of a second-year practical nursing student.
4. Same as answer 3.

CLASSIFICATION
Competency:
Professional Practice
Taxonomy:
Critical Thinking

---

161. 1. This teaching should come later in pregnancy but not before ascertaining the client's feelings about breastfeeding.
2. This teaching can be done in the latter part of pregnancy and reinforced during the postpartum period.
3. This teaching will have to be done, but it is not the priority intervention.

4. It is not uncommon for adolescents to avoid prenatal care; many do not recognize the deleterious effect that a lack of prenatal care can have on them and their babies.

CLASSIFICATION
Competency:
Foundations of Practice
Taxonomy:
Critical Thinking

---

162. 1. Paresis is a weakness or partial paralysis.

2. Hemiplegia is paralysis of one side of the body.

3. Paraplegia is the paralysis of both lower extremities and the lower trunk.
4. This statement describes quadriplegia.

CLASSIFICATION
Competency:
Foundations of Practice
Taxonomy:
Knowledge/Comprehension

---

163. 1. This complication would not result from long-term edema.
2. Same as answer 1.

3. **Oxygen perfusion is impaired during prolonged edema, leading to tissue ischemia.**
4. Same as answer 1.

CLASSIFICATION
Competency:
Foundations of Practice
Taxonomy:
Knowledge/Comprehension

164.
1. **The connective tissue degeneration of SLE leads to the involvement of the basal cell layer, producing a butterfly rash over the bridge of the nose and in the malar region.**
2. This manifestation occurs in scleroderma.
3. This manifestation occurs in muscular dystrophy, which is characterized by muscle wasting and weakness.
4. This manifestation occurs in polyarteritis nodosa, a collagen disease affecting the arteries and nervous system.

CLASSIFICATION
Competency:
Foundations of Practice
Taxonomy:
Knowledge/Comprehension

165.
1. **Radiation in controlled doses is therapeutic. When uncontrolled or in excessive amounts, it is carcinogenic.**
2. Therapeutic and controlled doses are used regardless.
3. Physical status does not affect the outcome of radiation therapy.
4. The nutritional status of the cells does not influence radiation's effect.

CLASSIFICATION
Competency:
Foundations of Practice
Taxonomy:
Knowledge/Comprehension

166.
1. Sperm do not move through the urine; they are found in semen.
2. Sperm are motile and achieve motility by motion of their flagella; they move from the epididymis to the vas deferens to the ejaculatory ducts to the urethra.
3. **Sperm cells are very fragile and can be destroyed by heat, resulting in sterility.**
4. During this period, the testes are not suspended.

CLASSIFICATION
Competency:
Foundations of Practice
Taxonomy:
Application

167.
1. Although it is considered a permanent form of sterilization, there has been some success reversing the procedure.
2. The procedure does not affect sexual functioning.
3. Precautions must be taken to prevent fertilization until absence of sperm in the semen has been verified.
4. **Some spermatozoa will remain viable in the vas deferens for a variable time after vasectomy.**

CLASSIFICATION
Competency:
Foundations of Practice
Taxonomy:
Application

168.
1. Although diversion is a method of altering pain perception and nausea, Ms. Angelo needs to see a physician for management of her dysmenorrhea.
2. **Ms. Angelo's symptoms may be serious and are compromising her lifestyle. She needs to consult a physician for treatment to correct the dysmenorrhea.**
3. Although ibuprofen may help with the pain, she initially needs to consult a physician.
4. Voluntary relaxation of the abdominal muscles does not cause cessation of uterine contractions.

CLASSIFICATION
Competency:
Professional Practice
Taxonomy:
Application

169.

1. This action is not required.
2. Same as answer 1.
3. **A full bladder is necessary so that the pelvic organs can be clearly visualized.**
4. Same as answer 1.

CLASSIFICATION
Competency: **Foundations of Practice**
Taxonomy: **Knowledge/Comprehension**

170.

1. Situational indicates a flexibility depending on the situation.
2. Laissez-faire is a relaxed and nondirective form of leadership.
3. **Autocratic indicates that the leader uses power and position to govern according to his or her own priorities.**
4. Positional is not a recognized form of leadership.

CLASSIFICATION
Competency: **Professional Practice**
Taxonomy: **Knowledge/Comprehension**

171.

1. The coronary blood flow is unconnected to the heart valves.
2. This statement is a description of electrocardiography.
3. **The catheter examines the condition of the coronary arteries. This statement provides a simple explanation of what a coronary artery is.**
4. The strength of contractions is not measured in angiography.

CLASSIFICATION
Competency: **Foundations of Practice**
Taxonomy: **Knowledge/Comprehension**

172.

1. This response creates a barrier to inclusive and appropriate care.
2. This is a form of discrimination. Heterosexism is the assumption that everyone is, or should be, heterosexual.
3. **This is a therapeutic response to help the adolescent practice safe sex. It demonstrates respect and shows the practical nurse is delivering care in an inclusive and appropriate manner.**
4. This response dismisses her health issues and is not supportive.

CLASSIFICATION
Competency: **Foundations of Practice**
Taxonomy: **Application**

173.

1. **Mr. Brendan is involved in high-risk behaviour that causes danger to his health. Safety topics would include, for example, safe sex, use of clean needles, physical safety, and signs of sexually transmitted infections.**
2. Mr. Brendan likely has poor nutrition, but this is not as important as safety.
3. Mr. Brendan likely has poor self-esteem, but this is not as important as safety.
4. Mr. Brendan likely is aware of the legal issues surrounding his work and heroin use.

CLASSIFICATION
Competency: **Professional Practice**
Taxonomy: **Critical Thinking**

174.

1. Although some herbal preparations may not have standardized dosages, this is not the most important aspect to discuss with Ms. Hoang.
2. This statement is presently true, although the government may move to regulate herbal preparations; however, it is not the most important aspect to discuss with Ms. Hoang.
3. **Some combinations of prescription drugs and herbal preparations interact. It is important that the health care provider be aware of all medications a client is taking, whether prescription or herbal. Ms. Hoang should be aware of the potential interactions.**
4. This statement is not necessarily true.

CLASSIFICATION
Competency: **Foundations of Practice**
Taxonomy: **Critical Thinking**

175.
1. Cannabis may relieve associated symptoms of tremors, spasticity, and inflammation in clients with multiple sclerosis.
2. Clients with inflammatory bowel diseases may find cannabis helpful for control of abdominal pain, diarrhea, and nausea.
3. Cannabis may be useful in alleviating nausea and vomiting associated with chemotherapy or radiation, anorexia, or severe intractable pain.
4. **Postoperative pain cannot be controlled well with cannabis use and may cause unacceptable side effects.**

CLASSIFICATION
Competency:
Foundations of Practice
Taxonomy:
Knowledge/Comprehension

176.
1. This notation means three pregnancies, one living child, and one abortion.
2. This notation means three pregnancies, no living children, and two abortions.
3. **This notation means four pregnancies, one living child, and two abortions, and is the correct notation.**
4. This notation means four pregnancies, one living child, and one abortion.

CLASSIFICATION
Competency:
Foundations of Practice
Taxonomy:
Application

177.
1. This statement shows little understanding or tolerance of the illness.
2. Ignoring the behaviour is a form of rejection; the client is not using the behaviour for attention.
3. **Recognizing the language as part of the illness makes it easier to tolerate, but limits must be set for the benefit of the staff and other clients. Setting limits also shows the client that the practical nurse cares enough to stop the behaviour.**
4. This statement demonstrates a rejection of the client and little understanding of the illness.

CLASSIFICATION
Competency:
Professional Practice
Taxonomy:
Application

178.
1. **A child learns to trust others by having his needs met in infancy. A child who has been maternally deprived is unlikely to have developed trust.**
2. Studies do not address this issue.
3. Some cognitive delay may be expected with prolonged hospitalization, but with appropriate care in hospital, cognitive milestones should ultimately be met.
4. These children frequently develop relationships with primary caregivers in place of the mother and father.

CLASSIFICATION
Competency:
Foundations of Practice
Taxonomy:
Knowledge/Comprehension

179.
1. This symptom is not related to methadone hydrochloride reduction.
2. **When methadone is reduced, a craving for narcotics may occur. Without narcotics, anxiety will increase, agitation will occur, and the client may try to leave the hospital to get drugs.**
3. Same as answer 1.
4. This symptom may occur with a methadone hydrochloride overdose.

CLASSIFICATION
Competency:
Professional Practice
Taxonomy:
Application

180.
1. A person must learn to cope with unpleasant objects and events.
2. Exposure to fearful situations without a plan of coping mechanisms may increase anxiety.
3. **Learning a variety of coping mechanisms helps reduce anxiety in stressful situations.**
4. Fearful situations can never be viewed as pleasurable.

CLASSIFICATION
Competency:
Foundations of Practice
Taxonomy:
Application

181.
1. This calculation is incorrect.
2. Same as answer 1.
3. **Correct calculation: 225 lb. – 180 lb. = 45 lb. 1 lb. = 2.2 kg 45 lb. ÷ 2.2 = x kg = 20.45 kg, which rounds down to 20 kg**
4. Same as answer 1.

CLASSIFICATION
Competency: **Professional Practice**
Taxonomy: **Application**

182.
1. An anomaly at birth would not likely produce the clinical signs listed and would be evident before the toddler years.
2. Acute respiratory infection usually has a gradual onset.
3. In view of the sudden onset of clinical signs and the age of the child, a hereditary condition is unlikely.
4. **All of the questions could be correct, but this question is the first the practical nurse should ask as it is the most likely. Respiratory tract obstructions generally occur in the larynx, trachea, or major bronchi (usually right). Hoarseness may indicate a vocal cord injury. Unintelligible speech may indicate interference in the flow of air out of the respiratory tract or obstruction or injury to the larynx. It is common for toddlers to choke on small objects.**

CLASSIFICATION
Competency: **Foundations of Practice**
Taxonomy: **Critical Thinking**

183.
1. This is not a culturally sensitive response. It is important that efforts be made to ensure that Mrs. George can practice her spirituality as completely as possible while in the hospital.
2. **For many Indigenous patients, being able to hold ceremonies where sweet grass or other medicines are burned is an important part of their spiritual wellbeing. The practical nurse should find out where ceremonies can be held at the hospital.**
3. Same as 1.
4. Same as 1.

CLASSIFICATION
Competency: **Professional Practice**
Taxonomy: **Critical Thinking**

184.
1. Vigorous scrubbing irritates the skin and increases the likelihood of an outbreak.
2. There may be no link between food and acne. Each individual should assess if any particular food causes an outbreak.
3. Sunscreen should be used, but oil-based sunscreens block the pores.
4. **Only mild soap and water are necessary; washing should be gentle in order not to irritate the skin tissues.**

CLASSIFICATION
Competency: **Foundations of Practice**
Taxonomy: **Application**

185.
1. Bending at the waist should be avoided because it strains the lower back muscles; the power for lifting should be supplied by the muscles of the thighs and buttocks.
2. **Placing the feet shoulder-width apart creates a wider base of support and brings the centre of gravity closer to the ground. This improves stability.**
3. Pressure on the abdomen is prevented by tightening the abdominal and gluteal muscles to form an internal girdle; keeping the body straight does not reduce strain on the abdominal musculature.
4. Relaxing the abdominal muscles with physical activity increases strain on the abdomen.

CLASSIFICATION
Competency: **Professional Practice**
Taxonomy: **Application**

186\. **1. A walker requires only partial weight bearing of the affected limb and gives the most overall support to the individual.**

2. A cane requires full weight bearing of the affected limb.
3. Crutches are used only when there should be no weight bearing.
4. A wheelchair is not appropriate because it does not promote the regaining of strength in the affected limb.

CLASSIFICATION
Competency:
Foundations of Practice
Taxonomy:
Critical Thinking

187\. 1. There are no data to support this. The amount of medication was probably inadequate for the client's pain tolerance level.
2. The practical nurse should not ignore the client's need for pain relief.

3. The practical nurse made the assessment that the medication was ineffective in relieving Mr. Ferguson's pain for the duration ordered. This information should be communicated to the physician for evaluation.

4. The physician's order is for administration q4hr prn. It should be given only within these guidelines.

CLASSIFICATION
Competency:
Collaborative Practice
Taxonomy:
Application

188\. 1. This calculation is incorrect.
2. Same as answer 1.
3. Same as answer 1.

4. Correct calculation:

$$x\,g = \frac{\frac{200\,\text{mg}}{\text{kg}}}{\text{day}} \times \frac{45\,\text{kg}}{1} \times \frac{6}{24/\text{day}}$$

$$x\,g = \frac{9000\,\text{mg}}{4}$$

$$x\,g = 2250\,\text{mg} = 2.25\,\text{g} = 2.3\,\text{g}$$

CLASSIFICATION
Competency:
Foundations of Practice
Taxonomy:
Application

189\. **1. In most cases, administration of pharmacological agents at regular intervals rather than as needed is preferable. Pain is easier to prevent than to treat. The round-the-clock approach alleviates pain before it becomes severe and can facilitate an earlier recovery.**

2. Same as answer 1.
3. Many clients are reluctant, for many reasons, to request pain medication and thus would not receive optimum pain management.
4. While nurses should be the expert at evaluating client pain, it is better to prevent pain from occurring rather than treating the pain.

CLASSIFICATION
Competency:
Foundations of Practice
Taxonomy:
Critical Thinking

190\. 1. This statement refers to a personal choice and is not indicative of gender identity.
2. How a person considers his or her own sexual orientation is not related to gender identity.

3. This statement offers the correct interpretation of gender identity. It is how a person identifies as being male, female, or a combination. It begins as soon as a person is aware of the difference in the sexes.

4. Same as answer 1.

CLASSIFICATION
Competency:
Professional Practice
Taxonomy:
Critical Thinking

191.

1. **The practical nurse needs to perform an initial thorough assessment. Based on this assessment, the practical nurse will be able to arrange suitable physical aids or the services of a foot care specialist.**
2. An assessment needs to be performed prior to arranging nursing care.
3. The assessment is the initial action.
4. Although regular physician's appointments are important, they do not address Mr. Akland's immediate concern.

CLASSIFICATION
Competency:
Foundations of Practice
Taxonomy:
Critical Thinking

192.

1. A fact sheet is not the most appropriate teaching tool at this time. The practical nurse needs to know why he is not taking his drugs.
2. There is no reason to suppose his noncompliance is due to confusion about doses or times.
3. There is no reason to suppose lifestyle interferes with the regimen.
4. **The practical nurse must first find out from Mr. James if there is a specific reason for his noncompliance. Initially, with HIV medication regimens, the adverse effects are unpleasant. Supporting Mr. James until the adverse effects are reduced is very important and will help him be compliant.**

CLASSIFICATION
Competency:
Professional Practice
Taxonomy:
Critical Thinking

193.

1. **The social worker is the correct health care provider to advise and arrange for community services. It is part of social workers' scope of practice.**
2. The physician may be able to assist, but the social worker is the best choice.
3. This action takes time for the practical nurse if he is not well acquainted with the community services. It is more appropriately within the scope of the social worker's practice.
4. This action may help the family, but if they are feeling overwhelmed, then the best action is to provide the personal assistance of a social worker who can best facilitate support.

CLASSIFICATION
Competency:
Collaborative Practice
Taxonomy:
Critical Thinking

194.

1. **This procedure is correct for obtaining the culture.**
2. This method will obtain only mucus, not a culture of the pharynx.
3. The client is much more likely to gag in a supine position.
4. It would be difficult to insert the swab with the client's head forward.

CLASSIFICATION
Competency:
Foundations of Practice
Taxonomy:
Application

195.

1. **The practical nurse must first gather all possible information (nursing process) about the new product prior to taking action.**
2. A physician does not necessarily have to be involved nor give permission for the ordering of an incontinence product.
3. This action is premature. The information must be compiled first and then discussed with the nurse manager.
4. The practical nurse may not independently conduct an action such as this without permission from hospital leaders.

CLASSIFICATION
Competency:
Professional Practice
Taxonomy:
Critical Thinking

196.

1. It may not be necessary for the practical nurse to accompany the client to the magnetic resonance imaging (MRI) scan, and doing so just to change an IV bag is not appropriate use of personnel.

2. Only if the practical nurse has previously consulted with the personnel in the MRI department and has been assured the bag can be changed would this action be appropriate.
3. It may not be appropriate to reduce the rate of the IV.
4. **This action is the safest and most logical.**

CLASSIFICATION
Competency:
Foundations of Practice
Taxonomy:
Critical Thinking

197.
1. **Once a client has been identified as being incompetent to make decisions, the identified SDM becomes the decision maker based on what the client would have wished had he been capable of making an informed decision.**
2. There is no need for the next of kin to be contacted unless he or she is the SDM.
3. The physician is not responsible to make the care decisions unless it is an emergency.
4. Mr. Balasingham has been identified as incompetent, thus this action is not appropriate.

CLASSIFICATION
Competency:
Legal Practice
Taxonomy:
Application

198.
1. **Ms. Lewis requires isolation as she likely has a communicable disease. The dialysis client must be moved to free up the room for isolation.**
2. Ms. Lewis requires isolation and should not share a room with another client.
3. This would be particularly hazardous as the cancer client may be immune suppressed, thus more likely to contract a communicable disease.
4. This action is not professional. Ms. Lewis has been admitted and requires care.

CLASSIFICATION
Competency:
Foundations of Practice
Taxonomy:
Application

199.
1. This approach is not professional. While the information may assist the mother with breastfeeding, it does not solve the problem of the preceptor advocating an outdated practice. In addition, the mother may be confused by receiving different advice from the two nurses.
2. **This approach is the professional choice. Even though the preceptor is an experienced postpartum practical nurse, she may not be aware of best practice regarding breastfeeding and supplementing with bottles of formula. It is in the best interest of the preceptor and the mother for the student to question and discuss the issue.**
3. This is adversarial and not professional.
4. The student practical nurse has a professional responsibility to question outdated or inaccurate practice, even if the practical nurse preceptor has more experience.

CLASSIFICATION
Competency:
Professional Practice
Taxonomy:
Critical Thinking

200.
1. This action must be done but is not the first action.
2. Same as answer 1.
3. **If the practical nurse is performing the action, he is responsible for ensuring that it has been ordered by the physician.**
4. Same as answer 1.

CLASSIFICATION
Competency:
Professional Practice
Taxonomy:
Critical Thinking

END OF ANSWERS AND RATIONALES TO PRACTICE EXAM 1

6 Practice Exam 2

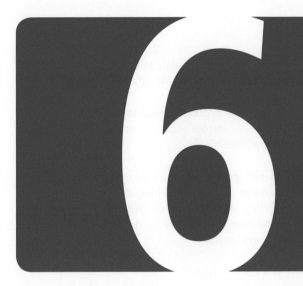

INSTRUCTIONS FOR PRACTICE EXAM 2

You will have 4 hours to complete the exam. The questions are presented as nursing cases or as independent questions. Read each question carefully, and then choose the answer that you think is the best of the four options presented. If you cannot decide on an answer to a question, proceed to the next question and return to this question later if you have time. Try to answer all the questions. Marks are not subtracted for wrong answers. If you are unsure of an answer, it will be to your advantage to guess.

Answers to Practice Exam 2 appear on page 110

CASE-BASED QUESTIONS

CASE 1

A practical nurse is facilitating a cardiac rehabilitation group for 10 men who have recently been discharged from the hospital post myocardial infarction (MI). The practical nurse will provide teaching and guidance about heart-healthy living.

QUESTIONS 1 to 5 refer to this case.

1. An important topic to be covered during the first class is the pathophysiology of a heart attack. What would be the most appropriate teaching technique to start the teaching session?

1. Ask each group member what he knows about myocardial infarctions.
2. Conduct a brief overview, with visual aids, about what happens during a heart attack.
3. Distribute pamphlets that provide complete information about MIs.
4. Organize a role-playing activity for group members to demonstrate what happens during a heart attack.

2. The practical nurse performs a health assessment on each of the men, many of whom are obese. Which of the following assessments is most indicative of a diagnosis of obesity?

1. Waist-to-hip ratio
2. Ratio of total body weight to height
3. Weight over the 85th percentile on standard adult growth charts
4. Hydrostatic weight

3. The practical nurse teaches a client about a heart-healthy diet. What recommendation should the nurse include in the teaching?

1. "Fruit juice may be consumed as an alternative to fruits."
2. "Portion your dinner plate to one-half vegetables and fruits, one-quarter whole grains, and one-quarter protein."
3. "Choose ultra processed foods more often."
4. "Replace complex carbohydrates with simple carbohydrates."

4. Many of the group members have hypertension. The practical nurse provides nutrition counselling regarding reducing their dietary sodium. Which of the following recommendations would offer the most effective advice for controlling salt intake?

1. "Use a salt substitute."
2. "Read nutrition labels on all purchased foods."
3. "Avoid adding salt when cooking."
4. "Purchase only foods advertised as having reduced sodium."

5. The practical nurse engages the men in active learning by having them evaluate various menus. Which of the following should they choose as the best low-sodium, low-calorie meal?

1. Salmon steak with lemon, baked sweet potato, green salad with vinegar dressing
2. 250 g of pasta with tomato sauce, whole-wheat roll, salad with low-calorie dressing
3. Breaded fish on a multi-grain bun with tartar sauce and baked beans
4. Ham and cheese omelette, avocado salad, and chicken broth

END OF CASE 1

CASE 2

Mr. Poulos, age 80, has periorbital cellulitis of his left eye and requires intravenous (IV) antibiotics. A saline lock was inserted in the emergency department, and Discharge Services has arranged for him to have home nursing care twice a day to infuse the medication and monitor the cellulitis.

QUESTIONS 6 to 12 refer to this case.

6. The home care practical nurse visits Mr. Poulos. After introducing himself, which of the following actions should he next perform?

1. Wash his hands
2. Examine the saline lock
3. Check the medications
4. Assess the cellulitis

7. The pharmacy has prepared preloaded syringes of the antibiotics. Which of the following actions is the correct nursing responsibility for the administration of the preloaded syringes?

1. The practical nurse must call the pharmacist to confirm the drug and dosage.
2. The practical nurse is not permitted to administer syringes that another health care provider has prepared.
3. The practical nurse must perform the rights of medication administration.
4. The practical nurse must confirm the labelling on the syringe against the physician order.

8. Mr. Poulos's eye is swollen and irritated and has an exudate that causes crusting. He asks the practical nurse what he should do as a comfort measure. Which of the following measures would be the most effective?

1. Apply a cold compress every 4 hours
2. Apply a warm compress as necessary
3. Wear sunglasses to protect his eye from light
4. Keep the eye patched at all times

9. Mr. Poulos lives alone in his own home. The cellulitis has affected his vision, and he finds it difficult to see. What question should the practical nurse ask him?

1. "Do you have family to help you?"
2. "Would you like a visiting homemaker to help with your daily activities?"
3. "Are you able to cook your meals and clean the house?"
4. "How are you managing with making meals and household chores?"

10. One of the antibiotics administered to Mr. Poulos is vancomycin. The practical nurse is aware that vancomycin requires therapeutic serum levels, which have not been ordered by the physician. In this situation, what is the practical nurse's responsibility?

1. Contact the physician to discuss an order for vancomycin levels
2. Draw blood from Mr. Poulos for vancomycin levels
3. Instruct Mr. Poulos to go to a community laboratory to have blood drawn for the levels
4. Consult with the nursing team leader concerning the most appropriate action

11. On the practical nurse's subsequent visit, Mr. Poulos states that his arm feels itchy close to the insertion site of the saline lock. Which of the following actions would be the practical nurse's first priority?

1. Stop the infusion
2. Check a medication reference for adverse effects of the antibiotics
3. Check the labelling on the syringes to ensure the correct drug and correct dose
4. Assess the insertion site

12. Mr. Poulos has completed 7 days of antibiotics and is now asymptomatic. The physician determines that he will not require a 10-day course. Six preloaded syringes remain. Which of the following statements would be the best advice from the practical nurse on how Mr. Poulos should dispose of them?

1. "You should throw the syringes in the garbage."
2. "You should empty the syringes into a sink."
3. "You should return the syringes to the pharmacy."
4. "I will take them and dispose of them for you."

END OF CASE 2

CASE 3

Several clients on a surgical floor begin to have frequent and uncontrollable watery stools. The hospital infection control specialist believes that this may be an outbreak of Clostridium difficile. Ms. Patel, who is day 1 post–major surgery, is among the affected clients.

QUESTIONS 13 to 15 refer to this case.

13. The practical nurse must collect a stool sample from Ms. Patel for *Clostridium* toxin assay. How should the practical nurse properly collect the specimen?

1. Have Ms. Patel defecate into a specimen container
2. Collect the stool from a clean bedpan or incontinence pad
3. Obtain a stool sample after Ms. Patel has defecated in the toilet
4. Apply an adult incontinence diaper to Ms. Patel

14. Ms. Patel is very weak and continues to have episodes of watery diarrhea occurring every 1 to 2 hours. Which of the following concerns is the most important for the practical nurse to assess for first?

1. Fluid and electrolyte imbalance
2. Potential for systemic infection
3. Perianal excoriation
4. Cardiovascular decompensation

15. Ms. Patel observes specific hygiene practices. In her culture, the left hand is used to perform unclean procedures. How would the practical nurse provide culturally competent care to Ms. Patel?

1. Allow Ms. Patel to guide the practical nurse in hygiene practice
2. Have Ms. Patel perform self-care hygiene after each bowel movement
3. Use her right hand to hold the bedpan and the left to clean the perineal area
4. Wash her hands before touching Ms. Patel

END OF CASE 3

CASE 4

A practical nurse works on a postpartum unit and provides breastfeeding support to mothers and families.

QUESTIONS 16 to 19 refer to this case.

16. Ms. Bunik asks the practical nurse if her small breasts will affect her ability to breastfeed. What would be the practical nurse's best response?

1. "Everybody can be successful at breastfeeding."
2. "You seem to have some issues with breastfeeding."
3. "The size of your breasts will not affect your milk production."
4. "The amount of fat and glandular tissue in the breasts determines the amount of milk produced."

17. Mrs. Akan says to the practical nurse, "I will wait for my milk to come in to begin breastfeeding." What is the priority action for the practical nurse?

1. Assess for cultural factors that influence breastfeeding practices.
2. Ask Mr. Akan to bring in formula and bottles for the baby.
3. Educate Mrs. Akan on the benefits of exclusive breastfeeding.
4. Make a referral to the lactation consultant.

18. Ms. Clarke complains of severe afterpains when breastfeeding her newborn infant. To increase her comfort, what would be the most appropriate nursing action?

1. Apply an ice pack to her back
2. Place her in the supine position
3. Instruct her to flex her knees
4. Apply a heating pad to the lower abdomen

19. The practical nurse is educating Mr. and Mrs. Corrigan on breastfeeding. Which of the following statements by Mrs. Corrigan indicates an understanding of the teaching?

1. "My baby should breastfeed on demand, at least eight times in a 24-hour period."
2. "I should consume an extra 1 000 calories per day while I am breastfeeding."
3. "I should combine breastfeeding with formula feeding during the first week."
4. "My baby will not require any vitamin D supplementation as long as my baby is breastfeeding."

END OF CASE 4

CASE 5

A practical nurse who works at a community pediatric clinic is responsible for performing health assessments and teaching parents.

QUESTIONS 20 to 24 refer to this case.

20. A father asks why his 14-month-old daughter must receive a rubella vaccination. Which of the following responses by the practical nurse provides accurate information?

1. "Because rubella is a severe disease in childhood."
2. "To prevent pregnant women from contracting rubella."
3. "Because it is the law in Canada."
4. "To prevent your daughter from having serious side effects, such as encephalitis, which may occur with rubella."

21. One of the routine immunizations administered to infants is the *Haemophilus influenzae* type B (Hib) vaccine. Why is the Hib vaccine given to infants?

1. It reduces the incidence of meningitis.
2. It eliminates the risk of influenza.
3. It prevents the contraction of hepatitis.
4. It increases the general immune system of the infant.

22. The practical nurse performs a health assessment on a 1-year-old boy. She takes his vital signs, including blood pressure. Which of the following readings would reflect a normal blood pressure for a 1-year-old child?

1. 65/40 mm Hg
2. 90/52 mm Hg

3. 109/64 mm Hg
4. 120/70 mm Hg

23. The parents of 19-month-old Ravi ask the practical nurse what they should do if he develops a fever. What would be the best advice for the nurse to give to the parents?

1. "If his temperature is over 38°C, you should take him to the doctor."
2. "If his temperature is over 39°C, you should administer liquid ibuprofen and sponge his skin with alcohol."
3. "The fever does not necessarily have to be treated, but if Ravi is not feeling well, you may give him liquid acetaminophen according to the directions on the box."
4. "If the fever lasts more than 24 hours, you should consult your physician."

24. The practical nurse counsels the parents of Yuri, age 12 months, about diet and nutrition. Which of the following foods would be the best source of iron for Yuri?

1. Milk
2. Lamb
3. Orange juice
4. Mineral-fortified cereal

END OF CASE 5

CASE 6

Ms. Blackhawk, a 27-year-old mother of two young children, requires investigation of weakness in her arms and legs, blurred vision, tinnitus, and increased emotional lability. She has been transported from her small northern community to a regional health centre.

QUESTIONS 25 to 27 refer to this case.

25. Ms. Blackhawk is scheduled for a number of tests to determine a diagnosis. She begins to cry, telling the practical nurse that she misses her family and is worried about how her husband and children will cope without her. Which of the following responses by the practical nurse would be most therapeutic?

1. "I'm sure your husband will manage. Sometimes we don't give dads the credit we should."
2. "I can see you are upset; perhaps you would like to speak with a chaplain about your concerns."
3. "Perhaps we could ask your husband to give you a call every evening before the children go to bed so you can talk to them."
4. "I understand how hard this must be for you, but right now you must concentrate on getting well yourself."

26. Ms. Blackhawk is diagnosed with primary relapsing multiple sclerosis (MS). Depressed about her diagnosis, she asks the practical nurse if she thinks she will live to see her children become adults. Which of the following responses by the practical nurse would be both honest and therapeutic?

1. "There is a possibility you will live to see them as teenagers."
2. "Progression of the disease is individual, and with new medications and therapies, you may be healthy for many years."
3. "I am not comfortable giving you any guess about how long you may live."
4. "Don't worry about that. I am sure you will be around for a long time to come."

27. Ms. Blackhawk tells the practical nurse that because of her illness, she has often felt too tired to prepare dinner for her family. They have been eating fast foods, and she is concerned about the effects this is having on her and her family's health. Which of the following nursing responses would be the most therapeutic?

1. "It is important that your diet include fibre to avoid constipation."
2. "Perhaps your husband and your children could help prepare meals."
3. "With children, as long as they have milk and eat some protein, they will be fine."
4. "You must stop eating fast foods because they are low in nutritive value."

END OF CASE 6

CASE 7

Mr. Bricker, aged 79, has been admitted to the medical unit with weakness. He has recently finished a course of chemotherapy for leukemia.

QUESTIONS 28 to 31 refer to this case.

28. The laboratory results indicate that Mr. Bricker is neutropenic. This state would place him at greater risk of developing which of the following conditions?

1. Infection
2. Internal bleeding
3. Anemia
4. Anorexia

29. Mr. Bricker has developed stomatitis. Which of the following interventions would his practical nurse implement?

1. Frequent rinsing of his mouth with mouthwash
2. Using foam-tipped applicators for mouth care

3. Having him brush three times a day with a toothbrush
4. "Swish and spit" mouth rinsing with hydrogen peroxide

30. The practical nurse assesses Mr. Bricker and discovers a stage 2 pressure injury on his right heel. What is a priority nursing intervention?

1. Reposition every 4 hours
2. Maintain on bedrest
3. Change the dressing frequently
4. Arrange for a nutritional assessment from a dietitian

31. Mr. Bricker has decided he does not wish any further medical treatments. He asks the practical nurse to help him arrange for medical assistance in dying (MAID). Which of the following responses by the nurse would be most therapeutic?

1. "Why don't I ask your wife to come in and you can talk this over with her."
2. "You have a lot on your mind, I will refer you to the social worker."
3. "I will let your physician know you would like to discuss MAID. Is there anything else that might be helpful to you right now?"
4. "I know chemotherapy has been difficult, but there are other treatment options to discuss with your oncologist."

END OF CASE 7

CASE 8

A practical nurse working in a facility that provides electroconvulsive therapy (ECT) is preparing Mr. Ahmed for his first treatment.

QUESTIONS 32 to 34 refer to this case.

32. The practical nurse should ensure Mr. Ahmed is provided with what information prior to the ECT?

1. "Sleep will be induced, so you will not feel the ECT."
2. "There will be some permanent memory loss as a result of the treatment."
3. "ECT can be frightening, so it is best not to ask any questions."
4. "With new methods of administration, the treatment is totally safe."

33. Which of the following statements by the practical nurse about the ECT may help to decrease Mr. Ahmed's anxiety?

1. "The treatments will make you feel better."
2. "You will not be alone during the treatment."
3. "A period of amnesia will follow the ECT."
4. "There is no need to be afraid."

34. Which nursing intervention would be most appropriate after Mr. Ahmed has awakened from his first ECT?

1. Bring him a lunch tray
2. Orient him to time and place and tell him that he has just had an ECT treatment
3. Get him up and out of bed as soon as possible and back into the unit's routine
4. Take his blood pressure and pulse rate every 5 minutes until he is fully awake

END OF CASE 8

CASE 9

Ms. Da Costa, age 64 years, has been admitted to a respiratory unit with manifestations of dyspnea and chest tightness. She has a tentative diagnosis of chronic obstructive pulmonary disease (COPD).

QUESTIONS 35 to 37 refer to this case.

35. Ms. Da Costa is scheduled for a number of diagnostic tests. Which of the following tests would be most conclusive in diagnosing COPD?

1. Pulmonary function tests
2. Arterial blood gases
3. Electrocardiography
4. Chest radiography

36. Ms. Da Costa has been a cigarette smoker for more than 30 years. Her oxygen saturation registers 89%. How should the practical nurse interpret this reading?

1. This reading is slightly low, but considering the client's age, it is acceptable.
2. This reading may be normal for a client with COPD.
3. This reading indicates that oxygen therapy should be started immediately.
4. This reading is normal for a client with dyspnea.

37. Ms. Da Costa is very anxious about exercising. Which of the following actions by the practical nurse would be the most effective in decreasing her anxiety level?

1. Thoroughly explaining the reasons for, and the scope of, the exercise program
2. Ensuring that Ms. Da Costa has portable oxygen and practical footwear
3. Walking with Ms. Da Costa to help maintain an appropriate pace and increase her confidence
4. Asking the physician to prescribe a mild antianxiety medication

END OF CASE 9

CASE 10

Ms. Jansen is admitted to hospital due to an acute, severe attack of ulcerative colitis.

QUESTIONS 38 to 41 refer to this case.

38. Which of the following is a common clinical manifestation of ulcerative colitis?

1. Constipation
2. Bloody diarrhea
3. Weight loss
4. Coffee-ground emesis

39. Ms. Jansen's condition deteriorates. She becomes restless, with pale skin and unstable vital signs. Which of the following actions would be most important for the practical nurse to implement?

1. Consult with the RN
2. Establish a secondary IV line
3. Assess urine output
4. Insert an oral airway

40. Ms. Jansen spends several days in the intensive care and requires surgery due to a perforated colon. She returns to the unit with an ileostomy. Which of the following manifestations of the stoma would be of greatest concern to the practical nurse?

1. Moderate edema
2. Scant bleeding when touched
3. Draining liquid stool
4. Dusky purple colour

41. Ms. Jansen has many questions about how the ileostomy will affect her day-to-day activities, how to manage odours, and what type of clothing will best conceal the outer appliance. Which of the following actions of the practical nurse would be most appropriate?

1. Recommend frequent appliance changes and loose clothing
2. Consult the enterostomal therapist (ET) and provide information for a local ostomy support group
3. Document the concerns and report to the physician
4. Reassure her and explain that she will learn to deal with the issues over time

END OF CASE 10

CASE 11

Mr. Donny, age 21, is admitted to hospital with a gunshot wound to his right femur. Because the injury occurred during an armed robbery, he is handcuffed to the bed and is guarded by two police officers. Mr. Donny does not speak English.

QUESTIONS 42 to 44 refer to this case.

42. Mr. Donny requires cleansing of his wound. His practical nurse speaks the same language as Mr. Donny but has been told by one of the police officers that she must not speak this language with Mr. Donny. What is the most appropriate action by the practical nurse?

1. Comply with police direction and not speak with Mr. Donny
2. Inform the police she will explain the wound cleansing to Mr. Donny in his language
3. Consult agency policies for directions
4. Explain the treatment of the wound to Mr. Donny in English

43. There is a great deal of media attention about the armed robbery and the condition of Mr. Donny. Many phone calls are coming to the unit, and the practical nurse needs to know how to respond to these calls. What is the priority consideration for the practical nurse in this situation?

1. Nurses are not permitted to speak with the media about a client.
2. The client must be consulted about his wishes for release of information to the media.
3. Agency spokespeople are permitted only to confirm that the client has been admitted to their facility.
4. The police control what information may be released to the media.

44. Both of Mr. Donny's hands are handcuffed to the bed rail. The practical nurse notices that the skin under the handcuffs is broken and bleeding. What should the practical nurse do?

1. Ask the police to remove both handcuffs so that skin care may be given
2. Provide skin care while the handcuffs are in place
3. Have the police officer remove one handcuff at a time and provide care
4. Do not provide skin care unless the area becomes infected

END OF CASE 11

CASE 12

Neville, age 11 years, has type 1 diabetes. Recently his blood sugars have been unstable, so he is admitted to hospital.

QUESTIONS 45 to 48 refer to this case.

45. Neville is placed in a two-bed room. Which of the following children would be the best roommate for him?

1. A 12-year-old girl with colitis
2. An 8-year-old boy with asthma
3. An 11-year-old girl with a fractured femur
4. A 10-year-old boy with rheumatoid arthritis

46. Which of the following topics should be included when teaching Neville about his type 1 diabetes?

1. "Always carry a concentrated form of glucose."
2. "Weigh all food on an accurate gram scale."
3. "Candies, sweets, and fast foods are not allowed in your diet."
4. "Eat crackers, cheese, or an apple if you feel dizzy and confused."

47. As part of the teaching plan, the practical nurse will review with Neville his need for insulin. During which of the following times will the dose of insulin likely decrease?

1. At the onset of puberty
2. When an infection is present
3. When there is emotional stress
4. When active exercise is performed

48. The practical nurse is teaching Neville and his parents the correct use of a prefilled insulin pen. Which of the following statements by his mother indicates a need for further teaching?

1. "I will ensure the insulin pen type matches the insulin brand ordered."
2. "I will shake the insulin cartridge to ensure appropriate mixing."
3. "I will prime the pen with a priming shot."
4. "I will hold the injection for 10 seconds."

END OF CASE 12

CASE 13

Mr. Gordon, age 36, has been diagnosed with a schizophrenia disorder. He has been admitted to hospital because he is experiencing an acute psychotic episode.

QUESTIONS 49 to 51 refer to this case.

49. Mr. Gordon states that he knows the police are out to kill him. Which of the following medical terms would best describe what Mr. Gordon is experiencing?

1. An illusion
2. A delusion
3. Autistic thinking
4. A hallucination

50. Mr. Gordon is refusing all food because he believes that it is being poisoned. Which of the following nursing interventions would be most appropriate to implement?

1. Taste the food in Mr. Gordon's presence
2. Suggest that food be brought in from home
3. Tell Mr. Gordon that the food is not poisoned
4. Tell Mr. Gordon that tube feedings will be started if he does not begin to eat

51. The practical nurse explores with Mr. Gordon his fear that his food is being poisoned. Which of the following statements would be the most appropriate?

1. "You really know the food is not poisoned, don't you?"
2. "You feel someone wants to poison you?"
3. "Your fear is a symptom of your illness."
4. "You'll be safe with me. I won't let anyone poison you."

END OF CASE 13

CASE 14

A practical nurse works in a rehabilitation hospital. On her days off, she operates a private business providing specialized foot care for people in their homes.

QUESTIONS 52 to 56 refer to this case.

52. The practical nurse visits Mr. and Mrs. Marsh, a couple in their 80s who live independently in their home. At the first visit, she completes a health history. What information would be most important for the practical nurse to determine prior to cutting the toenails of Mr. and Mrs. Marsh?

1. Any history of peripheral vascular disease
2. Any recent respiratory infections
3. Nutritional status
4. Signs of dementia or memory impairment

53. The practical nurse begins by soaking the feet of Mr. and Mrs. Marsh in basins of warm water. What is the primary reason to soak feet prior to care?

1. It is a comfort measure for the client.
2. The water softens nails and thickened epidermal cells.
3. Soaking will enable the nurse to assess blood flow to the extremities.
4. It will decrease the odour associated with the feet of older adults.

54. The practical nurse shortens the couple's toenails. Which of the following is the correct technique for shortening toenails?

1. Cut the nails straight across with nail clippers
2. File the nails with an emery board
3. Clip the nails in an arc around the toe
4. Cut the nails with sharpened pedicure scissors

55. Mr. Marsh asks the practical nurse why she changes gloves after completing his feet and before starting with his wife's. Which of the following statements would be the best response by the practical nurse?

1. "It is a best practice guideline for foot care."
2. "I need to use separate gloves for you and your wife."
3. "I feel more comfortable using a clean pair of gloves with every client."
4. "Gloves prevent transmission of possible fungal infections."

56. The practical nurse realizes that many of her clients in the rehabilitation hospital could use her foot-care services when they are discharged home. What would be an appropriate and professional way to inform them of her business?

1. Ask the director of care at her facility if she might post information on the unit bulletin board
2. Provide the clients with her business card
3. Tell the clients that they will require foot care when they get home and give them her business number
4. Provide foot care to clients who are about to be discharged and inform them that they could receive the same care from her when they are at home

END OF CASE 14

CASE 15

Mr. Morton, age 69 years, has a history of chronic kidney disease (CKD). He has been admitted to hospital with worsening symptoms and is now in end-stage renal disease.

QUESTIONS 57 to 60 refer to this case.

57. What is the leading cause of CKD in Canada?

1. Diabetes mellitus
2. Benign prostatic hypertrophy
3. Nonsteroidal anti-inflammatory drug allergy
4. Cardiovascular disease

58. The laboratory results indicate that Mr. Morton has hyperkalemia. What is a clinical manifestation of hyperkalemia the practical nurse will monitor for?

1. Polyuria
2. Irregular pulse
3. Seizures
4. Pulmonary edema

59. The practical nurse is evaluating the effectiveness of health teaching about drug therapy to Mr. Morton. Which statement demonstrates that Mr. Morton has increased health literacy?

1. He teaches back his medication regimen and describes where to find information and when he should contact a health care provider with concerns.
2. He listens to the practical nurse describe his medication regimen and thanks the practical nurse for sharing this knowledge.
3. He teaches back his medication regimen and is actively engaged in learning about the prescribed medications.
4. He listens to the practical nurse and describes his medication regimen and reports that he does not understand what the nurse has taught him.

60. Mr. Morton has chosen to begin peritoneal dialysis. What is a major disadvantage of peritoneal dialysis?

1. Severe fluctuations in blood pressure
2. Frequent electrolyte imbalances
3. Risk of peritonitis
4. Risk of hepatitis

END OF CASE 15

CASE 16

Mr. Stein, age 26 years, has a history of bipolar disorder and is experiencing a manic episode. He has been admitted to hospital because of increasing hyperactivity and erratic behaviour.

QUESTIONS 61 to 64 refer to this case.

61. Mr. Stein becomes loud, noisy, and disruptive in the client lounge. The practical nurse tells him to be quiet or he will be put in isolation. What are the legal implications of this situation?

1. The statement by the practical nurse constitutes a threat.
2. Isolation is justified for Mr. Stein's own protection.
3. Mr. Stein's behaviour is to be expected and should be ignored.
4. Because of his disease, Mr. Stein cannot be held responsible for not understanding instructions.

62. While the practical nurse is talking with Mr. Stein in the client lounge, he continues his disruptive behaviour and starts to use profane and vulgar language. How should the practical nurse respond?

1. Have him leave the lounge so that he does not upset the other clients

2. Tactfully include other clients in providing group censure for his behaviour
3. Refuse to talk to Mr. Stein when he is speaking in this manner
4. Ask Mr. Stein to limit the use of vulgarity but continue the conversation

63. That evening, Mr. Stein physically assaults another client on the unit. What precautions by the nursing staff would have been most appropriate to prevent this situation?

1. Mr. Stein should have been sedated with tranquilizers because he was known to have erratic behaviour.
2. Mr. Stein should have been placed in restraints because of his history of hyperactivity.
3. Mr. Stein should have been put in a secure, segregated unit, rather than an open ward, because of his disruptive behaviour.
4. The nursing staff should have provided close observation because they knew Mr. Stein's behaviour was volatile.

64. Two days later, Mr. Stein demands to be allowed to go downtown to shop. Because he is an involuntary admission who is legally not allowed to leave the facility, which of the following statements by the practical nurse would be the best response?

1. "You are not stable enough to leave the unit."
2. "You'll have to ask your doctor."
3. "Not right now. I don't have a staff member to go with you."
4. "You are not permitted to leave the unit. What do you need?"

END OF CASE 16

CASE 17

Mr. Atkinson comes to the health clinic because he has been having episodes of epigastric pain and back discomfort after meals. He smokes 10 cigarettes daily and drinks 2 alcoholic beverages most days.

QUESTIONS 65 to 70 refer to this case.

65. Mr. Atkinson is scheduled for an upper gastrointestinal series with a barium swallow. Which of the following post-test teaching points is most important for the practical nurse to review with Mr. Atkinson?

1. He should immediately report any nausea after the test.
2. His stool may be colourless for up to 72 hours after the procedure.
3. There are no restrictions on diet or fluid intake after the test.
4. He will be encouraged to increase his fluid intake after the test.

66. Mr. Atkinson is diagnosed with peptic ulcer disease (PUD). What information would be important for the practical nurse to include when teaching him and his family about PUD.

1. Cigarette smoking promotes ulcer development and delays ulcer healing
2. Avoid taking ASA (Aspirin) or NSAIDS with acidic juices
3. Elevate the head of the bed on 10- to 15-cm blocks
4. Read all over-the-counter (OTC) drug labels to avoid those containing lactic acid and calcium

67. Mr. Atkinson develops severe anemia related to PUD and is admitted to the hospital. What is an important nursing intervention?

1. Monitor stools for occult blood
2. Take vital signs every 8 hours
3. Administer cobalamin (vitamin B_{12}) injections
4. Administer all medications 1 hour before mealtime to prevent further bleeding

68. Mr. Atkinson receives a transfusion of packed red blood cells (PRBC). Which of the following is an important nursing action?

1. Stay with him for the first 15 minutes of the transfusion
2. Monitor his vital signs every 2 hours during the transfusion
3. Ensure the transfusion takes no more than 6 hours to administer
4. Slow the rate of infusion if he develops pruritus

69. Fifteen minutes after the second unit of blood is transfused, Mr. Atkinson develops dyspnea, a cough, and a rapid heart rate. This is likely to be caused by which of the following conditions?

1. Acute lung injury
2. Hemolysis
3. Allergic reaction
4. Circulatory overload

70. Mr. Atkinson tells the practical nurse that he does not believe he will be able to cope with all the lifestyle changes once he leaves the hospital. How should the practical nurse respond?

1. Help Mr. Atkinson identify previous coping methods
2. Provide him with the phone number for community resources

3. Reassure Mr. Atkinson that his family will help him
4. Consult with the physician about anxiolytic medications

END OF CASE 17

CASE 18

Ms. Connor returned from a holiday in Central America 2 weeks ago. She visits a local health clinic because she feels nauseated and very tired. She has a temperature of 37.9°C.

QUESTIONS 71 to 75 refer to this case.

71. The assessment by the practical nurse indicates that Ms. Connor may have contracted hepatitis A. Which of the following manifestations are indicative of hepatitis A?

1. Nausea and right upper quadrant pain
2. Right flank pain and hunger
3. Hypotension and bradycardia
4. Confusion and hypothermia

72. It is confirmed that Ms. Connor has a hepatitis A infection. She asks the practical nurse if this means that she will have to be hospitalized. Which of the following responses would answer this question most completely?

1. "Hospitalization and isolation will be required until the contagious period is over."
2. "Hospitalization will not be required, but quarantine in your home will be necessary."
3. "Hospitalization is not required unless you are unable to look after yourself or are incontinent of stool."
4. "There are no special restrictions other than enteric precautions, which I will explain."

73. Ms. Connor asks the practical nurse if this infection will cause permanent liver damage. Which of the following responses from the practical nurse would be most appropriate?

1. "With hepatitis A, normal liver function should return with no complications."
2. "As with all forms of hepatitis, long-term liver damage will occur."
3. "You will not have liver damage provided you comply with the special diet and drink alcohol only in moderation."
4. "The medication you will be prescribed will prevent damage to the liver."

74. Clients with hepatitis often have anorexia. Which of the following dietary recommendations would the practical nurse suggest to Ms. Connor?

1. "Eat a high-carbohydrate diet and limit protein intake."
2. "You will require supplemental nutrition for a number of weeks."
3. "Have several small meals a day that include foods you like."
4. "Eat the most nutrient-rich meal in the morning, when you are not as nauseated."

75. Which of the following measures would have been most effective in preventing Ms. Connor from contracting viral hepatitis A or B?

1. Hand hygiene
2. Proper personal hygiene
3. Prophylactic immunization
4. Environmental sanitation

END OF CASE 18

CASE 19

Seven-year-old Kofi has sickle cell anemia and has been admitted to hospital during a vaso-occlusive crisis.

QUESTIONS 76 to 79 refer to this case.

76. Kofi is to receive 3 000 mL of IV fluid over a 12-hour shift. Using a minidrip IV set, with a drop rate of 60 drops/mL, at what rate should the IV infuse?

1. 25 drops/hr
2. 36 mL/min
3. 250 mL/hr
4. 360 drops/hr

77. When the practical nurse checks Kofi during the night, he finds that Kofi has wet the bed. What should the practical nurse do?

1. Have Kofi help him remake the bed
2. Gently tell Kofi that he is too old to be having "accidents"
3. Put incontinence pants on Kofi
4. Change Kofi's clothes and bedding and help him back to bed

78. Kofi's parents are upset and say to the practical nurse, "We should never have had Kofi. We have given him this disease." What is the most therapeutic response by the practical nurse?

1. "It must be very hard to see your son in pain."
2. "It is not your fault Kofi has sickle cell disease."
3. "I know how you feel."
4. "Do your other children have sickle cell disease?"

79. Several days later, Kofi is well enough to visit the hospital playroom. During a game of tag with another client, Kofi complains of feeling dizzy. What should the practical nurse's initial response be?

1. Check his pulse and blood pressure
2. Have him sit down
3. Call for help
4. Assist him to his room

END OF CASE 19

CASE 20

Mr. Wogan, age 62, has been treated for depression for the past 10 years. He has recently shared with his friends and family that he has been thinking more and more about suicide. Mr. Wogan is admitted to the psychiatric unit of a hospital.

QUESTIONS 80 to 83 refer to this case.

80. Which of the following questions would the practical nurse find most beneficial to evaluate Mr. Wogan's potential for suicide?

1. Ask him about his plans for the future
2. Ask other clients if Mr. Wogan has discussed suicide
3. Ask the family if Mr. Wogan has ever attempted suicide
4. Ask Mr. Wogan if he has thoughts about suicide or a plan for harming himself

81. Mr. Wogan confides to the practical nurse that he has a plan to kill himself. What has likely motivated him to confide in the practical nurse?

1. He wishes to frighten the practical nurse.
2. He wants attention from the staff.
3. He feels safe and can share his feelings with the practical nurse.
4. He is fearful of his own impulses and is seeking protection from them.

82. Mr. Wogan is placed on suicide precautions. Which of the following measures would be the most therapeutic way to provide for his safety?

1. Not allow him to leave his room
2. Remove all sharp or cutting objects
3. Give him the opportunity to vent his feelings
4. Assign a staff member to be with him at all times

83. Mr. Wogan asks the practical nurse, "Why am I being watched round the clock, and why am I not allowed to move around the unit as I like?" Which of the following would be the practical nurse's best response?

1. "Why do you think we are observing you?"
2. "What makes you think that we are observing you?"
3. "We are concerned that you might try to harm yourself."
4. "Your doctor has ordered it, and she is the one you should ask about it."

END OF CASE 20

CASE 21

Mr. Patterson, age 72 years, has his eyes examined at the eye clinic. He reports that he occasionally has a dull headache in the morning and a mild pain in his left eye and that his peripheral vision is not as good as it used to be.

QUESTIONS 84 to 86 refer to this case.

84. It is determined that Mr. Patterson has open-angle glaucoma. He says that he thinks his father also had trouble with his eyes, and he eventually went blind. He asks the practical nurse if this will happen to him. Which of the following responses by the practical nurse would be accurate regarding glaucoma?

1. "With treatment, it is unlikely that you will lose your vision."
2. "Your vision will decrease over time, especially at night, but you will not lose it altogether."
3. "With this type of glaucoma, it is impossible to say what the outcome for your vision will be."
4. "People with this type of glaucoma generally lose most of their sight over time."

85. The practical nurse discusses glaucoma with Mr. Patterson. Which of the following topics is most important?

1. Modification of his environment for safety
2. Knowledge of signs and symptoms that require medical attention
3. The need for strict compliance with his prescribed therapy
4. Information on the relationship between increased eye pressures and vision

86. The practical nurse explains to Mr. Patterson that open-angle glaucoma is a chronic condition that will require lifelong treatment. Which of the following nursing interventions would best help Mr. Patterson to accept his condition?

1. Schedule several appointments for follow-up health teaching
2. Encourage him to express his feelings and concerns about the glaucoma

3. Provide Internet resources for glaucoma information and support groups
4. Involve his family in discussions about how he will manage his condition

END OF CASE 21

CASE 22

A practical nurse and a registered nurse are co-facilitators for a group of clients in a psychiatric facility. The purpose of the therapeutic group is to share experiences, gain peer support, and find effective stress-reduction strategies.

QUESTIONS 87 to 90 refer to this case.

87. The nurses meet with the group for the first time. What is the most appropriate initial statement by the practical nurse?

1. "My name is Gabriel. I am a practical nurse, and I will be one of your group leaders."
2. "Welcome to the group. Our purpose is to help you find stress-reduction strategies."
3. "Hello. I hope you will be able to attend these meetings every morning from 9:00 to 10:00."
4. "Let's start by sharing with each other a bit about ourselves."

88. The nurses would like the group members to begin to share their experiences. Which of the following statements would best help members to begin the dialogue?

1. "Mr. Pao, tell the group about your problems."
2. "Ms. Brankston, I believe you are here because you are addicted to heroin."
3. "Ms. Halsey, could you start us off by describing what led you to being admitted to hospital?"
4. "Who would like to start the conversation?"

89. After several meetings, the group becomes difficult for the nurses to manage. Clients arrive late, speak out of turn, and interrupt each other. What would be the best approach for the practical nurse to help the group to become functional?

1. "Let's make some group rules for how we are going to show respect for each other."
2. "I don't think the group is working well, and we need to do something about it."
3. "For the group to function, we need to stop interrupting each other."
4. "I am disappointed that we are not supporting each other in this group."

90. After group one day, a client with depression tells the practical nurse that she does not like the idea of taking medications for her depression and thinks she will start to take St. John's wort. What would be the best response by the practical nurse?

1. "Your depression is chronic and serious and requires prescription medications."
2. "I will certainly support you in your decision to use a herbal preparation."
3. "I have heard St. John's wort is very effective in treating depression."
4. "What have you heard about St. John's wort for the treatment of depression?"

END OF CASE 22

CASE 23

Mr. Desjardins, age 78, has been hospitalized for confirmation of a possible diagnosis of gastric cancer.

QUESTIONS 91 to 95 refer to this case.

91. Mr. Desjardins asks the practical nurse if his condition is "something like cancer." Which of the following responses by the practical nurse would be the most appropriate?

1. "Do you think you have cancer?"
2. "You are having tests to find out if you have cancer. Would you like to talk about it?"
3. "This is really a discussion you should have with your doctor."
4. "We are still waiting for a number of test results to come back, so don't worry about it now."

92. Mr. Desjardins has a surgical resection of his stomach. Because of his age, he may be at risk for which of the following postoperative complications?

1. Hemorrhage
2. Fluctuating blood glucose levels
3. Renal failure
4. Delayed wound healing

93. After Mr. Desjardins has surgery, which of the following factors would most influence his perception of pain?

1. Age and sex
2. Overall physical status
3. Intelligence and economic status
4. Previous experience and cultural values

94. Mr. Desjardins is to begin ambulating the morning after his surgery. His medications include morphine sulphate. When assisting him out of bed, the practical nurse initially has him sit on the edge of the bed, dangling his feet. Why is this action considered necessary?

1. Because movement may temporarily increase his abdominal pain
2. To restore adequate circulation to his legs and feet
3. Because he may have some respiratory distress due to the abdominal incision
4. Because he may have postural hypotension from lying in bed

95. Two days after surgery, Mr. Desjardins tells the practical nurse that while walking he has pain in his right calf. What initial action should the practical nurse take?

1. Put Mr. Desjardins back in bed
2. Notify the physician
3. Apply warm soaks to the leg
4. Elevate his right leg

END OF CASE 23

CASE 24

Ms. Kovacs, age 84 years, has degenerative osteoarthritis. She lives by herself in a two-storey home. She is admitted to hospital for a total right hip replacement.

QUESTIONS 96 to 100 refer to this case.

96. Which of the following statements is true regarding degenerative osteoarthritis?

1. It primarily affects weight-bearing joints and can be asymmetrical.
2. It primarily affects small joints and is symmetrical.
3. The rheumatoid factor is positive.
4. Joint effusion is common.

97. The practical nurse turns Ms. Kovacs on her side, placing several pillows between her legs so that the entire length of the upper leg is supported. Which of the following is the nurse's reason for this pillow placement?

1. To prevent prosthesis dislocation
2. To prevent thrombus formation of the leg
3. To prevent flexion contractures of the hip joint
4. To prevent skin surfaces rubbing together

98. The practical nurse plans nursing interventions to prevent circulatory complications postsurgery. Which of the following actions would best achieve this goal?

1. Turn from side to side every 3 hours
2. Exercise the ankles and other uninvolved joints
3. Ambulate as soon as the effects of anaesthesia are gone
4. Sit up in a low chair as soon as the effects of anaesthesia are gone

99. The practical nurse discusses with Ms. Kovacs her discharge from the hospital. Which statement by Ms. Kovacs indicates a need for further education?

1. "I will use a raised toilet seat"
2. "Crossing my legs at the ankle is preferred when sitting"
3. "Bending forward at the waist could dislocate my hip"
4. "Chairs with arms are needed to assist me when I stand"

100. Which would be the most appropriate plan for Ms. Kovacs to ensure appropriate postsurgical care and recuperation?

1. Home with biweekly community supports
2. Transfer to a long-term care facility
3. Remain an inpatient in the acute care hospital until she is able to walk
4. Discharge to a rehabilitation facility

END OF CASE 24

INDEPENDENT QUESTIONS

QUESTIONS 101 to 200 do not refer to a particular case.

101. Mr. Megadichan has five newly developed pressure injuries that the wound care specialist has ordered to be cleansed and dressed daily. The dressings take over an hour to complete. Mr. Megadichan's practical nurse has a busy assignment and does not have the time to do the dressings. What would be the most appropriate action by the practical nurse?

1. Leave the dressings to be done by the night-shift staff
2. Delegate the dressing changes to the unregulated care provider (UCP)
3. Document in Mr. Megadichan's health record the reason the dressings have not been done
4. Consult with nursing colleagues to obtain assistance with the dressings

102. A student practical nurse taking Mr. Camponi's blood pressure wraps the cuff very loosely around his arm because she does not want to hurt him. Which of the following consequences may result from this action?

1. A falsely low reading
2. A falsely high reading

3. An accurate systolic reading but inaccurate diastolic reading
4. Only the first and last Korotkoff sounds will be heard

103. Which of the following statements about informed consent is true?

1. The physician is responsible for obtaining written consent for procedures.
2. Practical nurses must co-sign all consent for treatment forms.
3. The person who is performing the procedure is responsible for obtaining verbal or written consent.
4. Consent is always in a written form and signed by the client.

104. Ms. Karmally has poorly controlled type 1 diabetes. The practical nurse teaches her about the possible complications of diabetes. Which of the following statements indicates that Ms. Karmally has fully understood the teaching about possible diabetic complications?

1. "I will book an appointment with an ophthalmologist."
2. "I will test my blood with a glucose meter once a week."
3. "I will test my urine for ketones every day."
4. "I will cut back from full-time work to part-time work."

105. Ms. Walters, age 25 years, has just received a prognosis of terminal cancer. That evening, a practical nurse observes a female colleague holding Ms. Walters's hand in the client lounge. The practical nurse is aware that her colleague is a lesbian. What is the practical nurse's responsibility in this situation?

1. Report her colleague's behaviour to the unit manager
2. Discuss with her colleague her possible inappropriate behaviour
3. Discuss the hand holding with Ms. Walters
4. Accept this as therapeutic touch and take no action

106. A practical nurse who works full time in an acute care hospital and part time as a community nurse sustained a back injury. The practical nurse claimed sick benefits from her full-time employer but continued to work part time at the community nursing agency. Evaluate this professional behaviour.

1. Professional misconduct
2. Professional incompetence
3. Malpractice
4. Lack of accountability

107. Cassandra, age 14 years, is to have surgical excision of a mole. Her parents did not accompany her to the appointment. Cassandra tells the practical nurse she will sign her own permission form for treatment. Which of the following statements is true?

1. Cassandra is able to give independent consent as long as she understands the treatment, and its risks and benefits.
2. Cassandra is not able to make a mature or informed choice.
3. Cassandra is able to give voluntary consent when her parents are not available.
4. Cassandra will most likely be unable to choose between alternatives when asked to consent.

108. Which of the following infections, caused by the yeast *Candida albicans*, occurs often in infants and immunosuppressed persons?

1. Thrush
2. Dysentery
3. Impetigo
4. Scabies

109. A practical nurse who has been assigned to care for a client with acquired immune deficiency syndrome (AIDS) requests a change in assignment. She tells the charge nurse that she does not wish to care for clients with HIV (human immunodeficiency virus) or AIDS because they "bring the problem on themselves." Which of the following statements would be true in this situation?

1. Practical nurses may not discriminate in the provision of nursing care.
2. Because of the practical nurse's ethics, she should be assigned to another client.
3. Practical nurses may refuse to care for clients whose lifestyle choices have caused illness and resulting expense to the health care system.
4. The practical nurse should choose to work in an area where her personal ethics are not compromised.

110. Which of the following statements represents a major influence on the eating habits of the early-school-aged child?

1. The availability of food selections
2. The smell and appearance of food
3. The example set by parents at mealtime
4. Food preferences of the peer group

111. A 10-month-old infant has a gastrostomy tube and is receiving 240 mL of formula every 4 hours.

Which of the following actions is a primary nursing responsibility?

1. Open the tube 1 hour before feeding
2. Position the infant on the right side after feeding
3. Give 10 mL of normal saline before and after feeding
4. Warm the formula in a microwave

112. A practical nurse in a pediatrician's office is reviewing the birth record of an infant brought into the office for a newborn assessment at 2 weeks of age. Which of the following data indicate that the infant may require special attention?

1. A birth weight of 3 000 g
2. An Apgar score of 3 at birth
3. A positive Babinski reflex
4. A pulsating fontanelle

113. Samantha is a 10-year-old girl admitted to hospital for orthopedic surgery. Samantha's mother hands the practical nurse a bottle of capsules and says, "These are for Samantha's allergies. Would you make sure she takes one at 9 o'clock?" Which of the following responses would be the most appropriate by the practical nurse?

1. "One capsule at 9 p.m.? Of course, I will give it to her."
2. "Did you ask the doctor if she should have this tonight?"
3. "Samantha should not have this medication before her surgery."
4. "I will speak with your daughter's doctor about the allergies and ask for an order to give her pills."

114. A client is ordered atropine 0.3 mg subcutaneously preoperatively. The vial reads, "atropine 0.4 mg/mL." What is the correct dosage to administer to the client?

1. 0.12 mL
2. 0.3 mL
3. 0.75 mL
4. 1.2 mL

115. Which of the following precautions should the practical nurse take when administering a parenteral iron preparation?

1. Apply ice packs to the site after the injection
2. Rotate injections among the four extremities
3. Firmly massage the site after withdrawal of the needle
4. Change needles after drawing the drug into the syringe

116. One evening while making rounds in a long-term care facility for older people, a practical nurse opens the door of a client's room and finds him engaged in sexual intercourse with a female resident. Which of the following actions would be the most appropriate by the practical nurse?

1. Quietly leave the room and close the door
2. Discuss this with the nursing team
3. Ask the two residents if they would like privacy
4. Counsel the residents about sexuality in the older person

117. Which of the following steps is involved in making an occupied bed?

1. Ensure both side rails are in the raised position prior to turning the client.
2. Adjust the bed height to a comfortable working position.
3. Assemble equipment and place it on the bottom of the bed.
4. Remove soiled top sheets, then cover the client with a bath blanket.

118. Following a spontaneous abortion, the practical nurse notes that the client and her partner are visibly upset. The partner has tears in his eyes, and the woman has her face turned toward the wall and is sobbing quietly. Which of the following statements by the practical nurse would be the most therapeutic?

1. "I know that you are upset now, but hopefully you will become pregnant again very soon."
2. "I see that both of you are very upset. I brought you a cup of coffee and will be here if you want to talk."
3. "I know how you feel, but you should not be so upset now. It will make it more difficult for you to get well quickly."
4. "I can understand that you are upset, but be glad it happened early in your pregnancy and not after you carried the baby for the full term."

119. A woman experiencing perimenopause asks the practical nurse about the use of herbal supplements and soy products to decrease her symptoms. How should the practical nurse respond?

1. "These are not proven to work."
2. "You are better to take prescribed medications."
3. "I recommend that you take these natural supplements rather than medicines."
4. "Talk this over with your physician, and try the ones you find helpful."

120. Ms. Samuels has just returned to the surgical unit following extensive liposuction surgery. What observation would indicate to the practical nurse that Ms. Samuels is starting to experience acute respiratory insufficiency?

1. Restlessness and confusion
2. Anxiety and constricted pupils
3. Decreased pulse and respirations
4. Cyanosis and dyspnea

121. Which of the following vitamins is not stored in the body and must be included in the daily diet?

1. A
2. C
3. D
4. K

122. A practical nurse working in a long-term care facility smells smoke as he makes his rounds. He opens the door to Mrs. Cummings's room and finds it full of smoke. What should be the practical nurse's first priority action?

1. Dial the agency fire code number
2. Call out "Fire" to alert the residents and staff
3. Shut all the doors and windows
4. Get Mrs. Cummings to a safe place

123. A practical nurse receives a panicked phone call from her neighbour. She is screaming and crying that her 2-year-old daughter has just had a "fit." The practical nurse determines that the child has had a febrile seizure. What would be the best advice the practical nurse could give to her neighbour?

1. To call 9-1-1
2. To take the child to the emergency department or family physician immediately
3. To make an appointment with a neurologist as this is likely the start of epilepsy
4. To give the child liquid acetaminophen for the fever and monitor for any further seizures

124. A practical nurse working in a long-term care facility develops nausea and a headache within hours after the installation of a new carpet throughout the facility. Several clients in the facility voice similar complaints. The practical nurse believes that these manifestations are related to the new carpet and that he and the residents are exposed to a toxic environment. What would be the most appropriate initial action for the practical nurse to take?

1. Move the clients away from the new carpet
2. Research the toxic effects of environmental chemical exposure
3. Communicate his safety concerns to management
4. Document his concerns on the agency risk-management report

125. A young couple have just learned from the pediatric neurologist that their 2-year-old son, Charlie, has autism spectrum disorder (ASD). They tearfully ask the practical nurse what will happen to Charlie for the rest of his life. What response by the practical nurse would be most appropriate?

1. "There is a wide range of severity and disability with ASD, and at this stage, a prediction is not possible."
2. "Charlie will be mildly delayed but will be able to function within a normal school environment."
3. "Charlie will likely be severely cognitively impaired."
4. "This is a degenerative disorder, and Charlie's condition will likely deteriorate by about age 6 years."

126. The practical nurse is unable to read the physician's handwriting for the postoperative orders for a client. The physician has returned to his office. What should the practical nurse do?

1. Ask the client what his doctor ordered
2. Contact the doctor for clarification of the orders
3. Ask another nurse for clarification of the handwriting
4. Consult with another available physician regarding what the ordering physician likely wanted

127. A medical student has requested a practical nurse's computer password to access a client's chart. What should the practical nurse do?

1. Share the password; the medical student is part of the health care team
2. Ask the supervising doctor for permission to share the password
3. Not share the password; have the medical student obtain access to the client chart via the medical team
4. Share the password; it is not confidential

128. A physician is admitted to the psychiatric unit of a hospital as a client. He is restless, loud, and aggressive during the admission procedure and states, "I will take my own blood pressure." What is the most therapeutic response by the practical nurse?

1. "I am sorry, Doctor, but right now you are not capable of taking blood pressure."
2. "It is my responsibility to take your blood pressure."
3. "Certainly, Doctor. I'm sure you will do it okay."
4. "You must cooperate, or I will need assistance to take your blood pressure."

129. Majid, age 5 years, has a history of being physically and sexually abused. Which of the following therapies would be most appropriate for him?

1. Play therapy
2. Group therapy
3. Individual counselling
4. Role play

130. A female client tells the practical nurse that she takes one "coated baby aspirin" every day. Which of the following adverse effects would be of greatest concern to the practical nurse?

1. Urinary calculi
2. Atrophy of the liver
3. Prolonged bleeding time
4. Premature erythrocyte destruction

131. Ms. Buchwold has type 2 diabetes. Recently her blood sugars have been unstable. She tells the practical nurse, "I know I can tell you, but I don't want to tell the doctor. I have been drinking a fair bit of gin every evening." Which of the following responses by the practical nurse would be most appropriate?

1. "I won't mention this to the doctor, but I want you to assure me you will not continue with the drinking because we must get your blood sugars more stable."
2. "Your drinking is affecting your health, and you must tell the doctor about it."
3. "We must let the doctor know because this is affecting your health. I will be with you while you explain it to him."
4. "I am not allowed to keep important information from the doctor."

132. Tom, age 11, has had surgery. He sees the pulse oximeter on his finger and asks the practical nurse why he has it. Which of the following responses by the practical nurse would provide the best answer?

1. "It is a noninvasive method of measuring the percentage of oxygen in your circulating blood."
2. "It measures how well your blood is carrying oxygen to all of your body. Anything over 95% is good."
3. "It measures how red your blood is."
4. "It tells us how well you are breathing."

133. Mr. Clements, age 82, tells the practical nurse that he does not feel like eating because nothing tastes as good as the food he remembers eating when he was young. Which of the following explanations by the practical nurse would provide the most accurate response?

1. "As we age, our taste buds do lose their sensitivity."
2. "These days foods are sometimes not cooked the way you remember."
3. "Much of our food is processed, and we lose some taste in the process."
4. "Your appetite decreases as you age, and that affects the way you perceive the taste of the food."

134. Ms. Saunders, a client with a history of endometriosis, has just delivered a healthy baby boy. She tells the practical nurse that now that the pregnancy is over, she is concerned that the endometriosis will return. Which of the following responses by the practical nurse would be most accurate and appropriate?

1. "Pregnancy almost always cures endometriosis."
2. "Endometriosis will usually cause an early menopause."
3. "A hysterectomy will be necessary if the symptoms recur."
4. "Breastfeeding your baby may delay the return of symptoms."

135. Kayla Gibson is awake and alert following a bronchoscopy and biopsy for suspected esophageal cancer. Which of the following nursing interventions is the most appropriate initial action?

1. Provide ice chips to reduce swelling
2. Advise her to cough frequently
3. Evaluate for the presence of a gag reflex
4. Advise her to stay flat for 2 hours

136. Cannabis was legalized in Canada in 2018. What is the main substance that is most responsible for the "high" associated with cannabis use?

1. CBD (cannabidiol)
2. THC (delta-9-tetrahydrocannabinol)
3. PCP (phencyclidine)
4. MDA (methylenedioxyamphetamine)

137. Mr. Kovicki has had a transurethral prostatectomy. Immediately after the surgery, his urinary catheter drainage is light pink with several clots. How long after prostate surgery are blood clots expected?

1. 1 to 12 hours
2. 12 to 24 hours
3. 24 to 36 hours
4. 36 to 48 hours

138. A practical nurse is obtaining a health history from a client who has peptic ulcer disease. Which of the following statements by the client might indicate a possible contributing factor for the peptic ulcer?

1. "My blood sugars are a little high."
2. "I smoke two packs of cigarettes a day."
3. "I have been overweight most of my life."
4. "My blood pressure has been high lately."

139. Mr. Peterkin has heart failure. He admits to the practical nurse that he has not followed a salt-restricted diet. He is now experiencing ankle edema, orthopnea, and dyspnea on exertion. What additional signs of fluid retention may be manifested by Mr. Peterkin?

1. Dizziness on rising
2. Rhinitis
3. A weak and thready pulse
4. A decreased hemoglobin and hematocrit

140. Which of the following components is the most important aspect of hand hygiene?

1. Time
2. Soap
3. Water
4. Friction

141. A practical nurse takes a picture of a sleeping Ms. Tang with his cellphone camera. What may the practical nurse do with this picture?

1. Show it to Ms. Tang, and then save it
2. Show it to Ms. Tang's family, and then delete it
3. Show it to his colleagues, and then save it
4. Show it to no one, and then delete it

142. A practical nurse is a manager of a home health care company. Mr. Eigo contracts with the company to provide a companion for his wife, who has Alzheimer's disease. Mrs. Eigo is physically well but is forgetful and sometimes wanders out of the house. What would be the most appropriate category of caregiver for the practical nurse to assign to Mrs. Eigo?

1. A registered nurse (RN)
2. A registered or licensed practical nurse (RPN or LPN)
3. A geriatric activation therapist
4. A personal support worker or unregulated care provider (PSW or UCP)

143. Maude Grant has been on prolonged antibiotic therapy for a persistent abdominal infection. Which of the following diseases can arise from normal microbial flora, especially after prolonged antibiotic therapy?

1. Q fever
2. Candidiasis
3. Scarlet fever
4. Herpes zoster

144. Following a total hysterectomy, Ms. Mengal asks the practical nurse if it would be wise for her to take hormone replacement therapy (HRT) right away to prevent symptoms of menopause. Which of the following responses by the nurse would be most appropriate?

1. "It is best to wait; you may not have any symptoms at all."
2. "You should wait until symptoms are severe, as the hormones are dangerous."
3. "It would be best for you to take herbal supplements rather than hormones."
4. "You should discuss with your physician since there are risks associated with taking HRT."

145. Which of the following is a complication following a transurethral prostatectomy (TURP)?

1. Abdominal wound infection
2. Retrograde ejaculation
3. Bladder spasms
4. Cystocele

146. Which of the following nursing actions is correct when caring for a client with continuous bladder irrigation?

1. Monitor urinary-specific gravity
2. Record urinary output every hour
3. Subtract irrigating fluid volume from total output to determine the urine volume
4. Include irrigating solution in any 24-hour urine tests ordered

147. Following abdominal surgery, Ms. Roark is encouraged to ambulate. Her wound is still draining a moderate amount of serosanguineous fluid. What type of dressing should the practical nurse use for Ms. Roark prior to ambulation?

1. A dressing with gauze reinforcing the suture line
2. A dressing with additional gauze at the base
3. A dressing with additional gauze over the site of drainage
4. A pressure dressing covering the abdomen

148. Which of the following is true concerning the use of evidence-informed practice in nursing?

1. It was recommended by physicians who were using evidence-informed medicine.
2. It was designed by hospitals to reduce client care delivery costs.

3. It grew out of the demand for high-quality, cost-effective care and the availability of rapidly expanding knowledge.
4. It developed as a result of nurses' sharing information on the Internet.

149. A practical nurse must perform perineal care on a male client. Which of the following actions is the correct procedure for cleansing his penis?

1. Using a circular motion, first cleanse the tip of the penis at the urethral meatus.
2. With gentle but firm downward strokes, cleanse the shaft of the penis first.
3. Initially, retract the foreskin and then cleanse around the base of the glans penis.
4. First, grasp the shaft of the penis and cleanse in upward strokes toward the meatus.

150. The mother of a preschool child asks the practical nurse how she can best ensure that her child always wears his bicycle helmet. Which of the following suggestions from the practical nurse would be the most effective?

1. She should buy him one that he chooses.
2. She should tell him the importance of wearing a helmet.
3. She should reward him each time he puts the helmet on.
4. She should role-model by always wearing a helmet when she rides her bicycle.

151. A practical nurse is caring for a client who has chosen to die in his home. The practical nurse assesses he is experiencing significant pain and requires an increase in his narcotic analgesic. What should the practical nurse do?

1. Administer the increased dose and have the physician sign the order at a later date
2. Contact the physician to obtain a telephone order for the increased dose of narcotic
3. Advise the family to administer the increased dose of narcotic
4. Provide non-narcotic pain relief therapies

152. Parents of 12-month-old Ava take her to a clinic for her scheduled immunizations. What vaccine will Ava receive?

1. Diphtheria, tetanus, pertussis (DTaP)
2. Measles, mumps, rubella (MMR)
3. Rota (Rotavirus)
4. None because she does not require any immunizations at 12 months

153. Three-month-old baby Jason has Down syndrome. His parents ask the practical nurse if the soft spot on his head is related to this disorder. What might the practical nurse respond?

1. "This is called the fontanelle and is normal in all infants."
2. "The soft spot is bigger in Jason because with Down syndrome he needs more room for his brain to grow."
3. "Children with Down syndrome have incomplete closure of the bones in their head, and this is the soft spot."
4. "One of the defects in Down syndrome is a premature closure of the fontanelle, so his soft spot is smaller than normal."

154. The practical nurse is caring for an Asian client after abdominal surgery. When performing a pain assessment, which of the following statements reflects a correct inference?

1. All Asian clients are stoic about pain.
2. Asian clients have a high pain threshold.
3. Asian clients prefer herbal therapies for pain control.
4. All clients are individual in their response to pain.

155. A practical nurse realizes on his day off that he forgot to sign off administration of ampicillin from the previous evening. There are no agency policies concerning this type of situation. Which of the following actions by the practical nurse would be most appropriate?

1. Sign the medication record on his next shift, in two days' time
2. Return to the unit to sign the medication record
3. Call the nursing supervisor to report the incident and consult regarding the appropriate action
4. Call the charge nurse and ask her to document that he administered the medication

156. A young female, Ms. Holly, has a blood pressure of 160/90 mm Hg. She tells the practical nurse that she would prefer to take an herbal preparation rather than the prescribed antihypertensive. What would be the practical nurse's best action?

1. Discuss with Ms. Holly the health risks and benefits of the herbal therapy
2. Tell Ms. Holly that she must not use herbal therapy
3. Advise Ms. Holly that her prescribed antihypertensive is the necessary treatment
4. Support Ms. Holly in her choice of the herbal preparation

157. Which of the following clients should be referred to a physician for further assessment?

1. A 45-year-old woman with tenderness in both breasts 3 days prior to her menstrual period
2. A 31-year-old woman in her third trimester of pregnancy with increased breast size and a yellow fluid discharge from her nipples
3. A 26-year-old male with a fixed mass that is 2 cm × 2 cm in the upper outer quadrant of his left breast
4. A 4-day-old male child with bilateral enlargement of the breasts and a white discharge from both nipples

158. Mr. MacDonald, age 32 years, returned from the Middle East several months ago. As part of a military operation engaging in counterterrorism, he witnessed many atrocities, including the death of a comrade. Mr. MacDonald has been diagnosed by physicians as having post-traumatic stress disorder and has been admitted to a psychiatric unit. What is the priority consideration for his treatment?

1. Provide a positive, nonjudgemental attitude toward Mr. MacDonald
2. Encourage Mr. MacDonald to express his grief and guilt
3. Provide for group therapy with other soldiers with similar experiences
4. Maintain observation for suicidal thoughts or violent behaviour

159. A practical nurse working in a long-term care facility includes a spiritual assessment as a regular part of the admission process for new clients. Which of the following questions would be most appropriate when initiating a spiritual assessment?

1. "What is your religion?"
2. "Would you like to have the chaplain visit you?"
3. "What is your source of strength when you face challenging situations?"
4. "Do you participate in any spiritual practices we should know about?"

160. Candace, age 21 years, tells the practical nurse at the health clinic that her boyfriend punched her last evening. There is a bruise under Candace's eye. Which of the following actions should be the practical nurse's first priority?

1. Contact the police
2. Ask if Candace would like an ice pack
3. Ask Candace for a brief history of the event
4. Perform a complete head-to-toe exam

161. A prenatal client voices apprehension to the practical nurse about the coming delivery of her baby. Which of the following responses is the most therapeutic?

1. "If you have had an uneventful pregnancy, there will be no problem."
2. "What in particular are you worried about?"
3. "Your prenatal classes should have reviewed the stages of labour."
4. "Do you feel your partner will not be here to support you during labour?"

162. The practical nurse notes that the premature newborn's core temperature is 35.0°C. What would be the most appropriate nursing action?

1. Place a stockinette cap on the baby's head
2. Take the infant to the mother for transfer of body heat
3. Place the infant under a radiant heater or in a warmed Isolette
4. Give the baby a bath in warm water

163. Which of the following parents might be at most risk for abusing their child?

1. Mr. Couture, who is unemployed and living in subsidized housing with his family
2. Ms. Patrick, who was abused as a child
3. Ms. Steele, a high school dropout who is depressed with her factory job
4. Mr. Miyagi, a socially isolated recent immigrant from South America

164. Mrs. Cooke, age 87 years, has mild dementia related to Alzheimer's disease. Her husband assists her with activities of daily living as necessary. A practical nurse working in the community performs a home assessment. What would be the most important safety assessment related to bathing?

1. Need for bathing devices, such as a hand-held shower
2. Solutions used by Mr. Cooke for his wife's bathing and skin care
3. Need for devices such as grab bars in the tub and shower area
4. Cognitive and musculoskeletal function of Mrs. Cooke

165. A child who receives the varicella vaccine has a greatly reduced risk of contracting which of the following childhood illnesses?

1. Mumps
2. Chicken pox
3. Whooping cough
4. Rubella

166. Mr. and Mrs. Pappandreaou bring their 1-week-old infant son into the clinic. The infant is receiving formula, and they are concerned because he regurgitates with each feeding. What should the practical nurse instruct them to do?

1. Keep him prone following feedings
2. Prevent him from crying for prolonged periods
3. Administer a minimum of 240 mL of formula at each feeding
4. Keep him in a semi-sitting position, particularly after feedings

167. Which of the following statements is most accurate when describing depression during pregnancy?

1. Estrogen and progesterone levels associated with pregnancy protect against depression.
2. Signs and symptoms of antenatal depression are different from those in depression at other stages of life.
3. Depression in pregnancy is most frequent during the first trimester.
4. Antenatal depression is a risk factor for postpartum depression.

168. A newly graduated practical nurse is employed in an adult medical–surgical setting. Most of her previous clinical experience has been in mental health and pediatrics, so she is not familiar with adult medications. She asks her preceptor many questions about the medications. The preceptor is surprised at her knowledge gap and is not receptive to the new practical nurse's questions. What should the new practical nurse do to practise safely?

1. Change her employment to a pediatric setting
2. Continue to ask the preceptor for support and teaching
3. Tell the preceptor that if she makes a mistake, it will be the preceptor's responsibility
4. Study a medications text so that she can learn everything about the unfamiliar adult medications

169. A 4-month-old infant is brought to the health centre. The mother indicates that the infant has been refusing his pacifier, so she has been dipping it in honey. The practical nurse recognizes that the infant is at risk for the development of which of the following?

1. Dental caries
2. Infant botulism
3. Sudden infant death syndrome
4. Toxic shock syndrome

170. The physician orders morphine 2 mg SC for a 9-year-old child. The container reads, "5 mg/mL." What dose should the practical nurse administer?

1. 0.2 mL
2. 0.4 mL
3. 0.6 mL
4. 0.8 mL

171. A practical nurse is returning to work on a medical unit since being on a short bereavement leave after the death of his father. He has been assigned to care for a client receiving palliative care and does not feel emotionally prepared for this assignment. Which of the following actions by the practical nurse would be most appropriate?

1. Continue with the current assignment.
2. Assign the client to the unregulated care provider.
3. Tell the client he is unable to provide care for him.
4. Consult with his supervisor to arrange withdrawal from the assignment.

172. Mr. Parsons tells the practical nurse at the health clinic that he is tired all day and that his snoring keeps his wife awake at night. What should the practical nurse recommend?

1. That he try to have naps during the day at work
2. That his wife sleep in another room so that he does not wake her
3. That he discuss this with the physician as he may have sleep apnea
4. That he take a herbal sleep aid, such as melatonin

173. A blood test has revealed that Ms. Clarisse has iron-deficiency anemia. Which of the following menus would be best to treat her anemia?

1. Salmon steak, rice, and asparagus
2. Liver, spinach salad, and lima beans
3. Pork chops, cauliflower, and raw carrots
4. Cheeseburger, French fries, and a milkshake

174. Mr. Firth has told his practical nurse that he wishes to try acupuncture for his chronic pain. What would be the best response by the practical nurse?

1. "Acupuncture is not recommended for pain."
2. "Acupuncture is not an approved therapy in Canada."
3. "I will help you find an acupuncture practitioner."
4. "You probably need some help taking your pain medication."

175. An agency practical nurse is working his first shift in a long-term care facility where he must administer digoxin (Toloxin) to Mr. Masters. What is the safest action?

1. Check Mr. Masters's recent photo identification on the health record
2. Ask Mr. Masters his name

3. Ask the roommate if this is Mr. Masters
4. Ask the other nurses which client is Mr. Masters

176. The father of a child who is dying of cancer asks the practical nurse if he should tell his 7-year-old son that his sister is dying. Which of the following answers would be the practical nurse's best response?

1. "A child his age cannot comprehend the real meaning of death, so don't tell him until the last moment."
2. "Your son probably fears separation most and wants to know that you will care for him, rather than what will happen to his sister."
3. "Why don't you talk this over with your doctor, who probably knows best what is happening in terms of your daughter's prognosis."
4. "Your son probably doesn't understand death as we do but fears it just the same. He should be told the truth to let him prepare for his sister's death."

177. A client in her fourth month of pregnancy tells the practical nurse that her husband just admitted he has genital herpes. What should the practical nurse teach this client regarding sexual activity?

1. "It will be necessary to refrain from all sexual contact with him during pregnancy."
2. "You will need to use spermicides during sexual activity."
3. "You and your husband should use a condom for sexual activity."
4. "Meticulous cleaning of the vaginal area after intercourse is essential."

178. Ms. Gentile, a frail 86-year-old woman, begins to fall while she is ambulating with her practical nurse. What should be the initial action by the practical nurse?

1. Call for assistance
2. Assume a wide stance, bend the knees, and gently lower Ms. Gentile to the floor
3. Prevent her from falling to the floor by supporting her under her arms
4. Support Ms. Gentile against her body as she regains her strength

179. A practical nurse hears an unregulated care provider (UCP) introduce herself as a nurse to a client. Which of the following actions by the practical nurse would be most appropriate?

1. Tell the UCP that she is not allowed to call herself a nurse and she will be reported to the manager
2. Take the UCP aside and explain the title "nurse" is protected and may be used only by registered and practical nurses.
3. Tell the client that she is the nurse and the UCP is employed just to provide non-nursing care
4. Ask the nurse educator to hold an in-service for the staff to explain various levels of nursing care

180. Which of the following statements regarding substance misuse and older persons is correct?

1. Nurses are less likely to recognize substance misuse in older persons than in younger adults.
2. It involves a small percentage of older persons, and the misuse is primarily limited to over-the-counter medications.
3. Alcohol is the most common substance abused and is abused by over 50% of people over 60 years of age.
4. Older persons are more likely to be willing to discuss the issue than are younger people.

181. Ms. Marie, age 26 years, is scheduled for surgical removal of a small, benign cyst on her neck. She is concerned that she will form an "ugly" keloid scar since keloids run in her family. Which of the following statements by the practical nurse would be most therapeutic?

1. "It is unlikely that you will form a keloid just because your mother and sister did."
2. "This surgery is necessary. The scar will be very small, and I am sure no one will notice it."
3. "I understand your concern. Would you like to talk to the surgeon about the possibility of scar formation?"
4. "I know you are concerned, but the doctor will make sure that a keloid will not form."

182. Which of the following facts about the use of the female condom is correct?

1. Because the female condom is a polyurethane sheath, it may be washed and reused.
2. Only water-soluble lubricants should be used with these condoms.
3. A male condom should always be used at the same time as a female condom.
4. The condom may not be used for anal intercourse.

183. Ms. Evelyn Grant is scheduled to have a tracheotomy. The tracheotomy tube will have an inflated cuff. She asks her practical nurse if she will be able to talk with the tube in place. Which of the following would be the practical nurse's best response?

1. "The tube does not allow for speech, but we will be able to communicate in other ways."
2. "We will remove the tube when you wish to say something."

3. “Sometimes you can make yourself understood, but your speech will be slurred.”
4. “Your throat will be too sore for you to want to talk, so it will not be a concern.”

184. Sally lives in a youth shelter. She has come to a street health clinic with a persistent, productive cough. She asks the practical nurse if she has contracted tuberculosis (TB). Which of the following responses would be most therapeutic?

1. “TB has been pretty well eradicated in Canada, so I imagine it is just a cold.”
2. “There is a risk you have contracted TB. If that is the diagnosis, you can be treated.”
3. “Most cases of TB in Canada are among people who have come from another country.”
4. “You seem to have a good immune system, so it is unlikely.”

185. Ms. Pargeter, age 29, has hypertension. Ms. Pargeter has a history of poor compliance with her prescribed antihypertensive medication, having stated that the medications make her tired. The practical nurse determines Ms. Pargeter’s blood pressure to be 165/100 mm Hg. What is the nurse’s best approach to this situation?

1. Tell Ms. Pargeter her blood pressure is too high and that she must take her medications as prescribed
2. Suggest to Ms. Pargeter she make an appointment with the physician to discuss possible modifications to her medication plan
3. Tell Ms. Pargeter if she is not going to be compliant with her medication regime, then there is nothing to be done for her
4. Discuss with Ms. Pargeter what she can do to rest and reduce the stress in her life

186. A practical nurse has made an entry in the hard copy of the wrong client’s health record. What should be the corrective action?

1. Remove the entry from the wrong chart
2. Draw a line through the entry, write “wrong chart,” and date and sign it
3. Use whiteout to eliminate the entry
4. Complete an incident report and place a copy in both client charts

187. Ms. Leonard calls the telephone nursing consultation service. She tells the practical nurse that her husband has suddenly experienced dizziness, headache, and weakness in his left side and is having difficulty speaking. What is the most important directive the practical nurse should give to Ms. Leonard?

1. “Call 9-1-1.”
2. “Take your husband to the family physician immediately.”
3. “Give your husband an aspirin.”
4. “Place him in a head-down position and call the doctor.”

188. Jeanine, age 6 years, has a severe allergy to peanuts and is attending summer camp. She carries a commercial preloaded epinephrine injection kit (EpiPen) as she has experienced previous anaphylactic reactions. One day, the practical nurse is called to the dining hall because Jeanine has collapsed after accidentally eating some peanut butter. Which is the most important initial action of the practical nurse in the emergency care of Jeanine?

1. Call Jeanine’s parents
2. Administer the epinephrine injection
3. Take Jeanine’s vital signs
4. Administer diphenhydramine hydrochloride (Benadryl) after ensuring a patent airway

189. Ms. Cameron has a history of urinary tract infections (UTIs). What would the practical nurse recommend to help prevent the incidence of her infections?

1. Drink cranberry juice regularly
2. Use commercially available perineal wipes
3. Limit her fluid intake to reduce urine production
4. Take a urinary antiseptic prophylactically

190. Mrs. Gingras is experiencing anorexia and cachexia as a result of severe COPD. Which of the following measures would the practical nurse recommend to help her increase her protein and calories?

1. Eat more food at each meal
2. Plan menus that include her favourite foods
3. Add high-calorie sauces and condiments to foods
4. Consume nutritional supplement drinks such as Ensure between meals

191. Mr. Michener died at 1830 hours. His family is at the bedside. It is now 1845 hours, and the practical nurse feels she should prepare the body before the night-shift staff arrives at 1915 hours. What should the practical nurse do?

1. Begin to prepare the body but encourage the family to stay at the bedside
2. Ask the family if they would leave because she has to prepare the body
3. Allow the family to stay as long as they need but request overtime pay for staying to prepare the body
4. Provide support to the family and offer the night staff assistance in preparing the body

192. Mr. Spinosa is to receive prednisone (Apo Prednisone) for treatment of an acute exacerbation of chronic obstructive pulmonary disease (COPD). Which of the following adverse effects might he experience?

1. Alopecia
2. Anorexia
3. Weight loss
4. Mood changes

193. A practical nurse is working for the second day in a first aid clinic at a charity marathon race. What is the practical nurse's priority action when he arrives to work his shift at the event?

1. Check the equipment and supplies
2. Read the communication report about clients discharged on the previous shift
3. Perform a head-to-toe assessment on any clients awaiting care
4. Ensure medical directives (standing orders) are in place

194. Mr. Frost is recovering from an acute exacerbation of colitis. For what reason would he be placed on a high-protein diet?

1. To repair tissue
2. To slow peristalsis
3. To correct anemia
4. To improve smooth muscle tone in the colon

195. Mr. Sanderson, age 18 years, sustained a severance of the spinal cord during a gymnastics competition. The physician explained to him that he is now a paraplegic. Three weeks later, Kyle asks when he can leave hospital to practise for an upcoming tournament. Which of the following defence mechanisms is Mr. Sanderson using?

1. Denial
2. Verbalization of a fantasy
3. Inability to adapt
4. Extreme motivation to get well

196. Ms. Mills, age 54 years, is starting an estrogen–progestin hormone therapy. What potential adverse effect would the practical nurse advise her to report?

1. Nausea
2. Weight gain
3. Calf tenderness
4. Breast tenderness

197. Ms. Kirk has had a thrombotic cerebrovascular accident in the left hemisphere of her brain. She is conscious. What manifestations would the practical nurse expect Ms. Kirk to exhibit?

1. Left-sided paralysis and increased diaphoresis
2. Increased deep-tendon reflexes and rigidity
3. Urinary retention with dribbling
4. Anxiety, communication, and mobility difficulties

198. A practical nurse is visited in her home by her neighbour, who tearfully confesses to the practical nurse that she has been beating her children for many months. She begs the practical nurse to help her but not to tell anyone. What action must the practical nurse take?

1. Examine the neighbour's children to assess the seriousness of their injuries
2. Discuss with the neighbour community services that are available to help her
3. Ask the neighbour what she can do to help her
4. Tell the neighbour she will have to contact the local child welfare authorities

199. Ms. Carlyle, a 91-year-old client in a long-term care facility, is dehydrated. The physician orders hypodermoclysis with normal saline to run over 12 hours during the night. Where would be the best place for the practical nurse to insert a butterfly catheter?

1. Into a vein on the dorsal surface of the hand
2. Into the abdomen or upper thigh
3. Into the brachial vein in the antecubital fossa
4. Into a vein in Ms. Carlyle's pedal circulation

200. Which of the following is the greatest risk factor for a woman to develop peripheral arterial disease?

1. Her sex
2. Smoking a pack of cigarettes a day
3. An intake of 180 mL of wine daily
4. A diet high in saturated fats

END OF PRACTICE EXAM 2

7

Answers and Rationales for Practice Exam 2

ANSWERS EXAM 2

CASE–BASED QUESTIONS ANSWERS AND RATIONALES

CASE 1

1.

1. This teaching technique may be more effective with a group that is cohesive and familiar with one another. As part of a newly formed group, many members might be reluctant to volunteer answers because of fear of others viewing them as lacking in knowledge.
2. **This teaching technique, particularly when paired with visuals, is an efficient and effective method to impart knowledge.**
3. Pamphlets would provide an effective follow-up to the presentation as they would help the group members to recall the information at home.
4. Role-playing allows participants to actively apply knowledge in a controlled situation, but the participants must first have the knowledge of the pathophysiology of MIs. Role-playing may not be the best strategy to teach pathophysiology.

CLASSIFICATION
Competency:
Foundations of Practice
Taxonomy:
Critical Thinking

2.

1. **All of these methods can be used to evaluate for obesity; however, waist-to-hip ratio is recommended, particularly with cardiac clients.**
2. This measurement will be taken and used to compute the body mass index (BMI).
3. Although there are standard weight and height charts for adults, they are not generally used to determine adult obesity. Pediatric growth charts may be used to determine obesity in children.
4. Hydrostatic weight provides the most accurate measure of lean body weight; however, it is not considered to be practical in most clinical settings.

CLASSIFICATION
Competency:
Foundations of Practice
Taxonomy:
Critical Thinking

3.

1. *Canada's Food Guide* recommends choosing whole fruits instead of juice.
2. **These portions help promote a heart-healthy diet that is well balanced with protein and complex carbohydrates in the form of vegetables and that is also low in fat.**
3. *Canada's Food Guide* recommends limiting intake of ultra processed foods.
4. Complex carbohydrates are healthier than simple carbohydrates.

CLASSIFICATION
Competency:
Foundations of Practice
Taxonomy:
Application

4.

1. This option will reduce sodium intake, but the group members may still eat foods that have high sodium content.
2. **Many foods, especially purchased fast foods, have high sodium content. The men will be best able to monitor their sodium intake if they are aware of the actual amount of salt in the foods. Reading labels will also help educate them about high-sodium and low-sodium foods.**
3. This option will reduce salt intake but will not help the men avoid the high sodium content in many prepared foods.
4. This option may reduce salt intake, but "reduced sodium" does not necessarily mean low sodium.

CLASSIFICATION
Competency:
Foundations of Practice
Taxonomy:
Critical Thinking

---

5. **1. Salmon is a low-calorie and -sodium fish with omega 6 and omega 3 fats; a baked sweet potato contains carbohydrates and vitamins; a green salad is low-calorie vegetables containing fibre; vinegar dressing is low in calories and sodium.**

2. 250 g is far too large a quantity of pasta. Also, a low-calorie dressing may not be low in sodium.
3. Breaded fish may be high in calories. Baked beans may be high in sodium and calories.
4. Eggs, ham, and cheese are high in calories. Avocados, although a good fat, are also high in calories. Chicken broth is high in sodium.

CLASSIFICATION
Competency: **Foundations of Practice**
Taxonomy: **Application**

CASE 2

6. **1. All of the options must be performed by the practical nurse; however, he must wash his hands first to prevent transmission of microorganisms.**

2. Same as answer 1.
3. Same as answer 1.
4. Same as answer 1.

CLASSIFICATION
Competency: **Foundations of Practice**
Taxonomy: **Application**

---

7. 1. This action is not necessary. The pharmacist would have prepared the medications according to the physician order. The scope of practice for pharmacists allows them to prepare and dispense medications.
2. Nurses may administer medications that pharmacists have prepared provided they have performed the rights of medication administration. Nurses may not administer medications another nurse has prepared.

3. Nurses must perform the rights of medication administration (variably documented as 5, 6, 7, 8, or 10) before administering any medication.

4. This step is included in the rights.

CLASSIFICATION
Competency: **Professional Practice**
Taxonomy: **Application**

---

8. 1. Cold compresses will not provide comfort although they may help to reduce the swelling. If used, they should be cool rather than cold.

2. Moist heat provides comfort, increases circulation to the area, and cleanses the exudates.

3. This measure will not help with the swelling and exudate.
4. Patching may provide some comfort, but the patch should be removed at intervals to cleanse the area and assess the eye.

CLASSIFICATION
Competency: **Foundations of Practice**
Taxonomy: **Application**

---

9. 1. This question may receive a yes or no answer, which will not provide the nurse with sufficient information to assess how he is managing.
2. Same as answer 1.
3. Same as answer 1.

4. This question is open ended and will be more likely to elicit information about how Mr. Poulos is managing with his daily activities and meal preparation.

CLASSIFICATION
Competency: **Professional Practice**
Taxonomy: **Critical Thinking**

---

10. 1. **The vancomycin levels must be ordered by a physician. It is the practical nurse's responsibility to ensure client safety and advocate for the client, so the practical nurse must ensure that the physician orders the levels.**
2. The practical nurse cannot draw blood for vancomycin levels without an order unless a medical directive is in place.
3. Mr. Poulos needs a requisition signed by a physician in order to have his blood drawn for the levels.
4. The practical nurse has a professional responsibility and accountability for the client, Mr. Poulos. Consultation with another nurse is not required.

CLASSIFICATION
Competency:
Collaborative Practice
Taxonomy:
Application

---

11. 1. This action may be necessary depending on the observations after the site is assessed.
2. The practical nurse should research drug references after assessing the site.
3. This action should have occurred prior to the infusion of the antibiotics.
4. **All options could be correct and may occur but remember the nursing process: the first action needs to be an assessment of the insertion site to look for signs of infiltration or tissue irritation.**

CLASSIFICATION
Competency:
Foundations of Practice
Taxonomy:
Critical Thinking

---

12. 1. This option is not safe because it could lead to a needle-stick injury by anyone handling the garbage.
2. Medications should not be disposed of into the public water supply.
3. **The appropriate method of disposal is through the pharmacy. Pharmacies encourage the public to bring in unused medications for safe disposal.**
4. The medication is the property of Mr. Poulos, and it is his responsibility to dispose of it. If the client asks the practical nurse to take the drugs because he is not able to dispose of them, the practical nurse can document this request and take the medication to the pharmacy.

CLASSIFICATION
Competency:
Professional Practice
Taxonomy:
Application

CASE 3

13. 1. Ms. Patel would not be able to pass stool into a specimen container.
2. **Ms. Patel may have limited mobility due to being day 1 postsurgery, and with this type of diarrhea, she would be unable to get to a bathroom quickly enough. If there are sufficient warning signs, the stool may be collected in a bedpan. If not, the stool may be scraped from an incontinence pad.**
3. It is not likely that a nurse would be able to collect a specimen from a toilet.
4. This action may embarrass Ms. Patel and be disrespectful.

CLASSIFICATION
Competency:
Foundations of Practice
Taxonomy:
Application

---

14. 1. **All options are a concern. Ms. Patel is losing fluid and necessary electrolytes in the diarrhea, and these losses must be closely monitored and corrected to prevent dehydration and circulatory collapse.**
2. This situation is a possibility, but the fluids are the first concern.
3. This situation may occur but is not the initial concern.
4. This situation may occur if Ms. Patel becomes dehydrated.

CLASSIFICATION
Competency:
Foundations of Practice
Taxonomy:
Critical Thinking

---

15. **1. The practical nurse respects Ms. Patel's cultural preferences by consulting with her about appropriate practice for personal hygiene.**
2. Ms. Patel is day 1 postoperative and weak. She may not be able to cleanse herself adequately.
3. The right hand is considered to be clean and would become unclean by touching the bedpan. The left hand should be used for both the bedpan and the cleansing.
4. This action is expected of all nurses with all clients regardless of cultural practices.

CLASSIFICATION
Competency: **Professional Practice**
Taxonomy: **Application**

CASE 4

16. 1. This response is untrue: successful breastfeeding requires mastery, and some women have difficulty.
2. This response presumes Ms. Bunik has issues with breastfeeding and may be interpreted negatively by Ms. Bunik.
3. This response offers correct information and would be reassuring to Ms. Bunik.
4. The baby's sucking and emptying of the breasts, not the amount of fat and glandular tissue, determine the amount of milk produced.

CLASSIFICATION
Competency: **Foundations of Practice**
Taxonomy: **Application**

---

17. **1. It is important for the practical nurse to assess cultural factors that may influence Mrs. Akan's beliefs about the best time to initiate breastfeeding.**
2. The infant may require formula if Mrs. Akan will not breastfeed the infant but the practical nurse needs to assess her first.
3. This may be necessary, but the practical nurse needs to assess Mrs. Akan first.
4. Same as 3.

CLASSIFICATION
Competency: **Foundations of Practice**
Taxonomy: **Application**

---

18. 1. Application of warmth to the lower abdomen may be helpful in relieving the discomfort.
2. Lying prone, not supine, may be helpful in relieving the discomfort.
3. Same as 1.
4. This is the correct nursing action. Application of warmth (e.g., heating pad) or lying prone may relieve discomfort associated with uterine contractions (afterpains).

CLASSIFICATION
Competency: **Foundations of Practice**
Taxonomy: **Application**

---

19. **1. Newborns need to breastfeed at least eight times in a 24-hour period.**
2. Most women require an additional 450 to 500 calories per day.
3. Formula feeding is not required if the infant is breastfeeding adequately.
4. Daily supplementation of vitamin D is recommended for all breastfed infants as breast milk may not have enough vitamin D to meet an infant's needs.

CLASSIFICATION
Competency: **Foundations of Practice**
Taxonomy: **Application**

CASE 5

20. 1. Rubella is not a severe disease in childhood.
2. Rubella in a pregnant woman may cause teratogenic effects in the fetus. Thus, children are immunized to prevent them from transmitting the disease to a pregnant woman.

CLASSIFICATION
Competency: **Foundations of Practice**
Taxonomy: **Application**

3. Canadian law does not require children to be vaccinated against rubella.
4. Rubeola and chicken pox may cause severe sequelae, but rubella generally does not.

21.
1. **The Hib, *Haemophilus influenzae* type B, vaccine has greatly reduced the incidence of infant meningitis, a disease with high mortality and morbidity.**
2. The Hib vaccine does not protect against various strains of influenza. It specifically protects against *H. influenzae* type B, which causes meningitis.
3. The Hib vaccine does not prevent hepatitis. Hepatitis is prevented by the hepatitis B vaccine.
4. The Hib vaccine does not increase general immunity.

CLASSIFICATION
Competency:
Foundations of Practice
Taxonomy:
Knowledge/Comprehension

22.
1. This blood pressure is normal for a newborn.
2. **This blood pressure is normal for a 1-year-old.**
3. This blood pressure is normal for a 12-year-old.
4. This blood pressure is normal for an adult.

CLASSIFICATION
Competency:
Foundations of Practice
Taxonomy:
Knowledge/Comprehension

23.
1. Fevers in children normally subside within several days. It is not necessary for the parents to take Ravi to the doctor with a temperature of 38°C.
2. No liquids other than room-temperature water should be sponged on a child.
3. **Because fever is not an illness, parents do not necessarily have to "fight" the fever. If the child is more than 3 months old and is feeling uncomfortable, the parents can administer acetaminophen in liquid form. It is important to follow the directions on the box for the correct dosage based on the child's weight.**
4. The parents should consult a physician if the fever lasts longer than 3 days.

CLASSIFICATION
Competency:
Foundations of Practice
Taxonomy:
Application

24.
1. Milk is a poor source of iron.
2. Lamb contains iron in small amounts and is not as easily digested as cereal.
3. Orange juice does not contain iron.
4. **Fortified cereal is a rich source of iron that is easily digested by children.**

CLASSIFICATION
Competency:
Foundations of Practice
Taxonomy:
Application

CASE 6

25.
1. This response dismisses the client's concerns.
2. The client has made no reference to wanting to speak to any member of the clergy.
3. **This response addresses the client's concern and also provides a practical solution.**
4. Same as answer 1.

CLASSIFICATION
Competency:
Professional Practice
Taxonomy:
Application

26.
1. Most people with this type of multiple sclerosis live for approximately 25 years after diagnosis.
2. **This response offers hope without false reassurance.**
3. This response is neither therapeutic nor professional.
4. This response is glib and does not answer the client's concerns.

CLASSIFICATION
Competency:
Professional Practice
Taxonomy:
Application

---

27. 1. This response does not address the issue of eating fast food because of Ms. Blackhawk's fatigue.

2. This response addresses the client's concerns and offers practical help.

3. This response is not helpful and trivializes the importance of a balanced diet.
4. It is true that fast foods offer little nutrition, but this does not mean they may not be occasionally enjoyed.

CLASSIFICATION
Competency:
Professional Practice
Taxonomy:
Critical Thinking

CASE 7

28. **1. The extensive growth of lymphoblasts suppresses the normal growth of red cells, white cells, and platelets. Neutropenia is a low level of white cells, specifically neutrophils, which are part of the immune system and are required to prevent infection.**

2. Internal bleeding would be the result of thrombocytopenia.
3. Anemia would be the result of decreased red blood cells and hemoglobin.
4. Anorexia may occur with leukemia and neutropenia but is not a specific risk.

CLASSIFICATION
Competency:
Foundations of Practice
Taxonomy:
Application

29. 1. This intervention may irritate the oral mucosa; mouthwash should always be diluted.

2. Foam is soft and will not damage the oral mucosa.

3. This intervention will injure the oral mucosa.
4. This intervention has an offensive taste and will irritate the mucosa.

CLASSIFICATION
Competency:
Foundations of Practice
Taxonomy:
Application

30. 1. Reposition him every 2 hours, not every 4 hours.
2. A heel pressure injury is not a reason to maintain him on bedrest.
3. Frequent dressing changes will increase risk of infection.

4. Adequate nutritional intake is essential for wound healing.

CLASSIFICATION
Competency:
Foundations of Practice
Taxonomy:
Knowledge/Comprehension

31. 1. This response dismisses Mr. Bricker's request.
2. Same as answer 1.

3. This response indicates acceptance and respect and provides Mr. Bricker an opportunity to continue the conversation.

4. Same as answer 1.

CLASSIFICATION
Competency:
Ethical Practice
Taxonomy:
Application

CASE 8

32. **1. Clients fear this therapy because of the expected pain. If they are reassured that they will be asleep and will feel no pain, there will be less anxiety and more cooperation.**

2. Permanent memory loss should not occur.
3. While electroconvulsive therapy (ECT) may be frightening to Mr. Ahmed, this statement cuts off future communication.
4. No treatment requiring anaesthesia is totally safe.

CLASSIFICATION
Competency:
Professional Practice
Taxonomy:
Application

33.

1. This statement may be false reassurance.
2. **The staff's presence will provide continued emotional support and help relieve anxiety.**
3. Not all clients experience amnesia, and the amnesia passes; placing emphasis on amnesia will increase fear.
4. The practical nurse should not place focus on Mr. Ahmed's fear. It is more reassuring for him to know that someone will be with him.

CLASSIFICATION
Competency:
Professional Practice
Taxonomy:
Application

34.

1. This intervention would come later if the client asked for food.
2. **Clients are confused when they awaken after ECT. They may experience temporary disorientation, so it is important to orient them to time, place, and situation.**
3. This intervention would not be appropriate for a client who has just awakened after a treatment.
4. This intervention is not necessary. Routine postoperative vital signs are adequate.

CLASSIFICATION
Competency:
Foundations of Practice
Taxonomy:
Application

CASE 9

35.

1. **These tests, which include tidal volume, airway resistance, peak expiratory volume, and others, would provide the most useful information.**
2. This test may be indicated but is not conclusive in diagnosing chronic obstructive pulmonary disorder (COPD).
3. This test would be done but is not diagnostic for COPD.
4. This test would be ordered but would not be conclusive.

CLASSIFICATION
Competency:
Foundations of Practice
Taxonomy:
Critical Thinking

36.

1. Oxygen saturations are lower in older persons. Ms. Da Costa, however, is only 64 years old.
2. **Hypoxemia is a common finding for clients with COPD.**
3. Oxygen therapy may or may not be indicated for clients with COPD and is sometimes contraindicated since it may suppress the respiratory centre.
4. Dyspnea is not always accompanied by low oxygen saturation.

CLASSIFICATION
Competency:
Foundations of Practice
Taxonomy:
Critical Thinking

37.

1. This action should be done but may not be the most effective way of decreasing anxiety.
2. This action is also recommended but, again, would not reduce anxiety.
3. **This action would give the nurse an opportunity to observe as well as to set an appropriate pace.**
4. This action would not generally be necessary at this time.

CLASSIFICATION
Competency:
Foundations of Practice
Taxonomy:
Critical Thinking

CASE 10

38.

1. Bloody diarrhea, not constipation, is a common clinical manifestation of ulcerative colitis.
2. **Bloody diarrhea and abdominal pain are common clinical manifestations of ulcerative colitis.**

CLASSIFICATION
Competency:
Foundations of Practice
Taxonomy:
Knowledge/Comprehension

3. Weight loss can occur but is less common.
4. Coffee-ground emesis would not be a common clinical manifestation.

39.
1. **This action is needed as Ms. Jansen's care needs are more complex and her condition has become unpredictable.**
2. A secondary IV line may be required for infusion of medications and fluid resuscitation; however, the most important action for the practical nurse is to consult with the RN.
3. This action will be done at some time but is not a priority.
4. It is possible that Ms. Jansen will need assistance maintaining a patent airway, but this is not yet indicated and is not the initial intervention.

CLASSIFICATION
Competency:
Collaborative Practice
Taxonomy:
Critical Thinking

40.
1. Moderate edema is a normal finding in the initial postoperative period.
2. Scant bleeding is normal when the stoma is touched or cleansed because of its vascularity.
3. Liquid to pasty is the normal stool consistency of an ileostomy.
4. **A stoma that is a dusky purple colour may indicate inadequate blood supply.**

CLASSIFICATION
Competency:
Foundations of Practice
Taxonomy:
Critical Thinking

41.
1. This does not address Ms. Jansen's concerns.
2. **Ms. Jansen will be able to receive practical advice from the ET and a support group.**
3. Documentation and reporting Ms. Jansen's concerns does not address her needs.
4. Same as 1.

CLASSIFICATION
Competency:
Foundations of Practice
Taxonomy:
Critical Thinking

CASE 11

42.
1. The practical nurse's priority responsibility is to the client. The police do not have authority in this case to prevent the practical nurse from obtaining informed consent and reassuring Mr. Donny about his condition.
2. **The priority responsibility is to the client. The practical nurse must ensure the therapeutic relationship is maintained and must ensure Mr. Donny understands his treatment plan.**
3. There is no reason to consult agency policies, as the duty to the client is clear.
4. This action is inappropriate as Mr. Donny does not understand English.

CLASSIFICATION
Competency:
Professional Practice
Taxonomy:
Critical Thinking

43.
1. In some situations, a nurse may be the spokesperson for the agency to the media.
2. **This consideration addresses confidentiality. A nurse is not allowed to share client information with others unless the client's consent is obtained.**
3. With the client's permission, agency spokespeople can confirm the client has been admitted to the facility. A status report may also be released with client permission.
4. In some situations, the police may legally restrict what is divulged to the media; however, the nurse's first priority is the confidentiality of the client.

CLASSIFICATION
Competency:
Legal Practice
Taxonomy:
Critical Thinking

44.
1. It may not be safe to remove both of Mr. Donny's handcuffs.
2. The practical nurse will not likely be able to provide complete skin care while the handcuffs are in place.

3. **This option provides safety for the practical nurse and enables the practical nurse to provide care for the skin.**
4. Mr. Donny has a right to appropriate care. Skin care must be provided to prevent further injury and infection.

CLASSIFICATION
Competency:
Professional Practice
Taxonomy:
Application

CASE 12

45. 1. Same-gender roommates at this age are desirable for companionship and to maintain privacy needs.
2. An 8-year-old boy would be too young to provide companionship for Neville.
3. Same as answer 1.
4. **A 10-year-old is closer in age to Neville. He will prefer the company of someone of the same gender and age group.**

CLASSIFICATION
Competency:
Professional Practice
Taxonomy:
Application

---

46. 1. **With type 1 diabetes, particularly in younger children, blood glucose levels may fluctuate. Neville is admitted to hospital because his blood sugar levels have been unstable. At the first sign of hypoglycemia, Neville needs to have a quick, concentrated source of glucose to immediately raise his blood sugar.**
2. This action may be advisable for some people with diabetes but is generally not necessary.
3. This statement is not completely true and telling Neville he is not allowed treats may cause him to rebel against his disease and the diet.
4. These items should be eaten once his blood sugar has been raised by quick-acting glucose.

CLASSIFICATION
Competency:
Foundations of Practice
Taxonomy:
Application

---

47. 1. With increased growth and the associated dietary intake, the need for insulin increases.
2. An infectious process, if severe enough, may require increased insulin.
3. An emotional upset is a stress that increases the need for insulin.
4. **Exercise reduces the body's need for insulin. Increased muscle activity accelerates the transport of glucose into the muscle cells, thus producing an insulinlike effect.**

CLASSIFICATION
Competency:
Foundations of Practice
Taxonomy:
Application

---

48. 1. This is a correct statement.
2. **This statement is incorrect. Shaking may cause the formation of bubbles that take up space in the cartridge and thereby alter the dose. Roll and tip NPH and premixed insulin.**
3. This statement is correct. Typically, it is recommended to use two units to prime the pen; however, refer to the pen instruction sheet from the manufacturer.
4. This statement is correct. It is necessary to hold the injection for 10 seconds to ensure full delivery of the dose.

CLASSIFICATION
Competency:
Foundations of Practice
Taxonomy:
Application

CASE 13

49. 1. An illusion would be a misinterpretation of a sensory stimulus.

2. A delusion is a fixed, false personal belief that is not founded in reality.

3. Autistic thinking is a distortion in the thought process associated with schizophrenic disorders.
4. A hallucination is a perceived experience that occurs in the absence of an actual sensory stimulus.

CLASSIFICATION
Competency:
Foundations of Practice
Taxonomy:
Knowledge/Comprehension

---

50. 1. This intervention would be a form of entering into the client's delusions. The client may feel that only a particular part of the food was free of poison.
2. This suggestion may reinforce the delusion that the hospital food is poisoned.

3. Clients cannot be argued out of delusions, so the best approach is a simple statement of reality.

4. Threats are always poor nursing interventions, no matter how exasperated the nurse feels.

CLASSIFICATION
Competency:
Foundations of Practice
Taxonomy:
Application

---

51. 1. This question is close ended and may not encourage Mr. Gordon to explore his fears.

2. This statement is the only one that helps Mr. Gordon to focus and explore his feelings.

3. Although this statement is true, it is not something Mr. Gordon is ready to understand; it is a closed statement.
4. This statement offers false reassurance and is not realistic; Mr. Gordon will still have concerns as to what will happen when the nurse is not there.

CLASSIFICATION
Competency:
Professional Practice
Taxonomy:
Application

CASE 14

52. **1. All history is potentially important. However, clients with peripheral vascular disease are at risk for infection, foot ulceration, and poor wound healing. They may require a physician order for nail cutting.**

2. This information may have significance but is not the most important information.
3. This information will have relevance to wound healing and maintenance of skin integrity but is not the most important information.
4. This information has significance for ability to perform foot care and respond to health teaching but is not the most important initial information.

CLASSIFICATION
Competency:
Foundations of Practice
Taxonomy:
Critical Thinking

---

53. 1. While it is a comfort measure, this is not the most important reason for the foot soaks.

2. Warm water softens nails and thickened epidermal cells and allows for easier removal of the nails and dead skin.

3. Soaking will increase circulation to the area, which is therapeutic. However, assessment of circulation to the feet is best done prior to the foot soaks.
4. While it will decrease odour, this is not the most important reason for the foot soaks.

CLASSIFICATION
Competency:
Foundations of Practice
Taxonomy:
Critical Thinking

---

54. **1. Cutting the nails straight across prevents splitting of nail margins and formation of sharp nail spikes that can irritate lateral nail margins.**

2. Filing the nails with an emery board is not an efficient method for shortening them; however, an emery board may be used to smooth rough nail edges after clipping.
3. Nails should be cut straight across.
4. Nail clippers are preferable since they are designed for the thickness of toenails. Using sharpened scissors presents more of a risk for accidentally injuring the toes and may not be safe.

CLASSIFICATION
Competency:
Foundations of Practice
Taxonomy:
Knowledge/Comprehension

---

55. 1. It is a best practice, but this does not adequately answer Mr. Marsh's question.
2. This response does not answer the question.
3. This response may be true, but the nurse should change gloves to prevent transmission of possible fungal infections, not because it makes her more comfortable to do so.

4. This response correctly answers Mr. Marsh's question, providing the reason for the change of gloves between clients.

CLASSIFICATION
Competency:
Professional Practice
Taxonomy:
Application

---

56. **1. The practical nurse must keep her salaried and private work completely separate. The only action that could not be perceived as a conflict of interest is receiving permission from the director of care.**

2. This action is a conflict of interest and would not be professional behaviour.
3. Same as answer 2.
4. Same as answer 2.

CLASSIFICATION
Competency:
Professional Practice
Taxonomy:
Application

CASE 15

57. **1. Diabetes mellitus is the leading cause of CKD in Canada.**

2. Benign prostatic hypertrophy is a common cause of acute, not chronic, kidney injury.
3. Nonsteroidal anti-inflammatory drug allergy is a common cause of acute, not chronic kidney injury.
4. Renal vascular disease, not cardiovascular disease, is a leading cause of CKD in Canada.

CLASSIFICATION
Competency:
Foundations of Practice
Taxonomy:
Critical Thinking

---

58. 1. Polyuria is not a clinical manifestation of hyperkalemia.

2. Irregular pulse is a clinical manifestation of hyperkalemia the practical nurse should monitor for.

3. Seizures are not a clinical manifestation of hyperkalemia.
4. Pulmonary edema is not a clinical manifestation of hyperkalemia.

CLASSIFICATION
Competency:
Foundations of Practice
Taxonomy:
Application

---

59. **1. When Mr. Morton teaches back what he has learned, describes how to access additional information, and reports when to contact health care providers, he is demonstrating that he has increased health literacy.**

2. This does not provide sufficient evidence that Mr. Morton has increased health literacy about his drug therapy.

CLASSIFICATION
Competency:
Professional Practice
Taxonomy:
Application

3. This meets some of the criteria, however, there is insufficient evidence that Mr. Morton is able to implement what he has learned.
4. In this case, Mr. Morton would need further teaching to increase health literacy.

---

60. 1. Because fluid shifts are gradual, blood pressure fluctuations are not severe.
2. Electrolyte imbalances are less likely to occur because fluid shifts are gradual.
3. Risk of developing peritonitis is the major disadvantage of peritoneal dialysis.
4. Risk of developing peritonitis, not hepatitis, is the major disadvantage of peritoneal dialysis.

CLASSIFICATION
Competency: **Foundations of Practice**
Taxonomy: **Application**

CASE 16

61. **1. These words constitute a threat. A threat is a type of assault that is an intentional tort.**
2. Isolation is considered to be a restraint. It may be ordered by a physician when the client is assessed to be a danger to others. It is unnecessary at this time.
3. Mr. Stein's behaviour may be expected but should be dealt with directly. Behaviour should never be ignored.
4. This generalization draws a conclusion that may not be true.

CLASSIFICATION
Competency: **Legal Practice**
Taxonomy: **Application**

---

62. 1. This response does not show acceptance of the client, nor does it help Mr. Stein control his behaviour.
2. It is not appropriate at this stage to involve the other clients. The practical nurse needs to take responsibility for actions to decrease Mr. Stein's inappropriate behaviour.
3. This response does not deal with the problem directly and may confuse Mr. Stein because he may not be aware of why the practical nurse is refusing to talk to him.
4. This response sets appropriate limits for Mr. Stein, who cannot set self-limits; it rejects the behaviour but accepts the client.

CLASSIFICATION
Competency: **Professional Practice**
Taxonomy: **Application**

---

63. 1. It would be unrealistic, not therapeutic, and not indicated to keep Mr. Stein sedated at all times.
2. This precaution is not necessary unless the client commits repeated acts of violence, in which case, a physician may order the client to be placed in four-point restraints.
3. There had been no previous history of violence that would warrant a secure, segregated unit.
4. The nursing staff, knowing the client was disruptive and volatile, was negligent in not providing close supervision. Mr. Stein should have been closely observed to protect him against self-imposed injury as well as to protect others.

CLASSIFICATION
Competency: **Professional Practice**
Taxonomy: **Critical Thinking**

---

64. 1. This response is true but shows no consideration of how Mr. Stein may feel.
2. It may be true that Mr. Stein must ask the physician for a change in his involuntary status, but this response implies that the practical nurse simply does not wish to deal with his request and is putting him off.
3. This response implies Mr. Stein may be able to go shopping later when there is a staff member available, yet this may not be the case.
4. This response clearly states that Mr. Stein is not allowed to leave and may decrease his anxiety by taking the time to find out what he thinks he needs.

CLASSIFICATION
Competency: **Professional Practice**
Taxonomy: **Critical Thinking**

CASE 17

65. 1. Nausea sometimes occurs with the swallowing of barium. It does not need to be reported.
2. This information is correct but does not pose any risk to the client. It is not as important as the need for increased fluids.
3. This information is correct but is not most important.
4. Increased fluid intake is required after the procedure to flush the barium out of the system and prevent impaction.

CLASSIFICATION
Competency:
Foundations of Practice
Taxonomy:
Critical Thinking

---

66. **1. This information is correct.**
2. ASA (Aspirin) and NSAIDs should not be taken unless approved by the health care provider.
3. This is not a recommended treatment for PUD.
4. The client should avoid all OTC drugs unless approved by the health care provider.

CLASSIFICATION
Competency:
Foundations of Practice
Taxonomy:
Application

---

67. **1. Blood in stools may indicate gastrointestinal bleeding.**
2. Vital signs should be taken more frequently.
3. Cobalamin (vitamin B_{12}) injections are often required after gastrectomy.
4. This action will not prevent further bleeding.

CLASSIFICATION
Competency:
Foundations of Practice
Taxonomy:
Critical Thinking

---

68. **1. This is the correct action.**
2. Mr. Atkinson's vital signs need to be retaken after the first 15 minutes and he needs to be observed every half hour.
3. The transfusion should take no more than 4 hours to administer.
4. The transfusion should be stopped if Mr. Atkinson develops pruritus.

CLASSIFICATION
Competency:
Foundations of Practice
Taxonomy:
Knowledge/Comprehension

---

69. 1. An acute lung injury would cause similar clinical manifestations but would not be caused by a blood transfusion.
2. The client may experience these symptoms; however, additional manifestations such as fever and low back or abdominal pain would occur.
3. Flushing, itching, pruritus, and urticaria (hives) would occur with a mild allergic reaction.
4. Symptoms of circulatory overload occur when fluid administration is faster than the circulation can accommodate.

CLASSIFICATION
Competency:
Foundations of Practice
Taxonomy:
Application

---

70. **1. Mr. Atkinson can become more confident in his ability to handle stressors by reflecting on his previous successful coping mechanisms.**
2. Community resources may be helpful, but the better response is to help Mr. Atkinson identify strategies he can use.
3. This may not be accurate.
4. Other strategies should be implemented prior to anxiolytic medications.

CLASSIFICATION
Competency:
Professional Practice
Taxonomy:
Critical Thinking

CASE 18

71. **1. These manifestations, along with malaise, are the most common manifestations of hepatitis A.**
2. Anorexia is more likely with these manifestations, and flank pain is associated with renal problems.
3. Hypertension is more usual than hypotension in the case of hepatitis A, and bradycardia is not a manifestation.
4. The client is more likely to have a fever than hypothermia, and no confusion.

CLASSIFICATION
Competency:
Foundations of Practice
Taxonomy:
Knowledge/Comprehension

---

72. 1. Hospitalization is not usually required for hepatitis A, and isolation is only for clients incontinent of stool.
2. There is no reason for quarantine.
3. Incontinence of stool is not an indication for hospitalization. It is not likely that Ms. Connor will be unable to care for herself because of the infection. If, however, this does occur, there are care options other than hospitalization.
4. Appropriate infection control and enteric precautions are sufficient.

CLASSIFICATION
Competency:
Foundations of Practice
Taxonomy:
Application

---

73. **1. Long-term damage is rare with hepatitis A.**
2. This statement is untrue.
3. The client should not consume alcohol until there is no remaining trace of infection.
4. No medication will protect the liver.

CLASSIFICATION
Competency:
Foundations of Practice
Taxonomy:
Application

---

74. 1. A high-carbohydrate diet may not be palatable, and protein will be required for healing.
2. There is no requirement for supplementation.
3. The most successful approach is to recommend eating appetizing foods in small quantities.
4. Ms. Connor will more likely be most nauseated in the morning.

CLASSIFICATION
Competency:
Foundations of Practice
Taxonomy:
Application

---

75. 1. This measure is necessary but not the most effective.
2. Same as answer 1.
3. Immunization is the most successful method since it provides complete protection.
4. Same as answer 1.

CLASSIFICATION
Competency:
Foundations of Practice
Taxonomy:
Critical Thinking

CASE 19

76. 1. This calculation is incorrect. Also, infusion pumps are not regulated in drops.
2. Same as answer 1.
3. This calculation is correct: Amount of fluid = 3 000 mL

÷ 12 hr
= 250 mL/hr

4. Same as answer 1.

CLASSIFICATION
Competency:
Foundations of Practice
Taxonomy:
Application

77\. 1. Kofi may feel he is being punished by having to make the bed. Also, he is likely in pain and likely has an IV line, which would make assisting with the bed making difficult.
2. This action would embarrass Kofi and make him feel worse.
3. This action would be demeaning to Kofi as he would view the incontinence pants as diapers.
4. **Kofi will have received a large amount of fluids to provide hemodilution. With the excess fluids and the expected regression that occurs with hospitalization of children, urinary incontinence happens frequently. The practical nurse can best help Kofi handle this embarrassment by helping him into dry clothing and back into a dry bed.**

CLASSIFICATION
Competency: **Professional Practice**
Taxonomy: **Application**

78\. 1. **This response validates the parents' feelings of distress.**
2. Sickle-cell disease is genetically transmitted, so the parents may legitimately feel it is their fault.
3. The practical nurse does not know how the parents feel.
4. This response changes the subject and does not provide support to the parents' feelings.

CLASSIFICATION
Competency: **Professional Practice**
Taxonomy: **Application**

79\. 1. Immediate physical safety takes priority over further assessment.
2. **The child's immediate physical safety takes priority. The child must sit down to avoid falling.**
3. The subjective symptom of dizziness alone does not warrant calling for help at this time.
4. Immediate physical safety takes priority; walking at this time would be unsafe.

CLASSIFICATION
Competency: **Foundations of Practice**
Taxonomy: **Critical Thinking**

CASE 20

80\. 1. At this point, Mr. Wogan is most likely unable to think beyond the present, much less deal with future plans; this question is too general.
2. This action is inappropriate and a violation of confidentiality.
3. The family would be one resource, but it is best to approach Mr. Wogan directly.
4. **Directness is the best approach at the first interview because the practical nurse can thereby set the focus and concern and also determine how serious Mr. Wogan is about suicide.**

CLASSIFICATION
Competency: **Foundations of Practice**
Taxonomy: **Application**

81\. 1. This statement could be true but is an unlikely motivation for the behaviour.
2. Same as answer 1.
3. This statement may be true, but more important, the client is seeking help and protection.
4. **Clients frequently report suicidal feelings so that staff will have the chance to stop them. They are really asking, "Do you care enough to stop me?"**

CLASSIFICATION
Competency: **Foundations of Practice**
Taxonomy: **Application**

82.
1. This measure would be punishment for the client, and he still may find a way to carry out a suicide attempt in the room.
2. This measure would be routinely taken. By itself, it is not necessarily therapeutic.
3. This measure is not a suicide precaution.
4. **Emotional support and close surveillance can demonstrate to Mr. Wogan that the staff cares and is attempting to prevent his acting out of suicidal ideation.**

CLASSIFICATION
Competency:
Foundations of Health
Taxonomy:
Critical Thinking

83.
1. This response would place the client on the defensive.
2. This response is inappropriate in a rather obvious situation.
3. **This response helps the client realize that staff members care and believe that the client is worthy of care.**
4. This response is an evasive tactic by the practical nurse.

CLASSIFICATION
Competency:
Professional Practice
Taxonomy:
Application

CASE 21

84.
1. **This response is accurate. This type of glaucoma does have a strong familial component, but with appropriate treatment, Mr. Patterson should experience no further deterioration in his vision.**
2. It is true that night vision can be affected, but this response is not therapeutic.
3. This response is untrue. With appropriate treatments, the prognosis may be determined.
4. This response is not therapeutic and is also untrue.

CLASSIFICATION
Competency:
Foundations of Practice
Taxonomy:
Application

85.
1. This action may be necessary, but if the intraocular pressure is controlled, there should be no deterioration in Mr. Patterson's vision.
2. This knowledge could be important; however, there are often no symptoms of increased pressure.
3. **The client must understand that strict compliance with his prescribed therapy is essential. Routine administration of eye drops can prevent further increases in intraocular pressure and prevent loss of vision.**
4. This information is important but not as necessary as information about the importance of compliance.

CLASSIFICATION
Competency:
Foundations of Practice
Taxonomy:
Critical Thinking

86.
1. Follow-up appointments will be scheduled and will help him to feel supported. They will likely help with compliance. However, they are not likely to be the most effective intervention for assisting Mr. Patterson to accept the glaucoma.
2. **Encouraging Mr. Patterson to discuss his condition and express his concerns will help to decrease his anxiety and help him to deal with the diagnosis of a chronic illness.**
3. This intervention will provide Mr. Patterson with additional information to assist him to manage his glaucoma but is not likely to be as effective as discussing his feelings and concerns.
4. The family may need to be involved with the treatment regimen and will provide support, but that will not help him to accept his condition as much as being able to verbalize his feelings.

CLASSIFICATION
Competency:
Professional Practice
Taxonomy:
Critical Thinking

CASE 22

87.
1. **In the initial stage of group process, the leader's responsibility is to create an atmosphere of respect and trust. He can demonstrate respect through common manners of introducing himself and his role.**
2. This statement may be the next most important one as it states the purpose of the group (i.e., what goals the group aims to accomplish).
3. Although it is important to provide timing for the group, this initial statement may not be perceived as welcoming.
4. While a group task is to get to know each other, this is best left until after the initial "housekeeping" activities have occurred.

CLASSIFICATION
Competency: **Professional Practice**
Taxonomy: **Critical Thinking**

88.
1. Mr. Pao may view this approach as an authoritative statement that does not demonstrate respect.
2. This statement is a breach of confidentiality.
3. **It is often helpful with a new group to start the dialogue with a specific person since many will not want to be the first to speak. This question invites Ms. Halsey to describe her experiences rather than label her with a diagnosis.**
4. This statement is not likely to elicit volunteers to begin the conversation.

CLASSIFICATION
Competency: **Professional Practice**
Taxonomy: **Critical Thinking**

89.
1. **This statement applies principles of effective group process by involving all members in establishing group norms.**
2. While this statement may be true, the practical nurse's saying the group is not working may make the clients anxious and may be perceived to be punitive.
3. While this statement may be true, the problem is not just that the group members are interrupting each other. This statement does not seek a solution.
4. While the practical nurse may be disappointed and may share this feeling with the group, it does not seek a solution to the dysfunction.

CLASSIFICATION
Competency: **Professional Practice**
Taxonomy: **Critical Thinking**

90.
1. This response does not respect the client's choice to use alternative therapies.
2. While the practical nurse should support the client's choice, the nurse needs to first find out if the client has made an informed choice.
3. While this response is supportive of the client's choice, there has been controversy about the effectiveness of St. John's wort. Also, the practical nurse needs to find out if the client has made an informed choice.
4. **This open-ended question enables the practical nurse to find out if the client is making an informed choice regarding St. John's wort.**

CLASSIFICATION
Competency: **Professional Practice**
Taxonomy: **Critical Thinking**

CASE 23

91.
1. This response may elicit only a "yes" or "no" from Mr. Desjardins, and it may make him feel defensive.
2. **The practical nurse should demonstrate to Mr. Desjardins recognition of his verbalized concern and a willingness to listen.**
3. Avoiding the question indicates that the practical nurse is unwilling to listen.
4. This response could increase anxiety rather than reduce worry; furthermore, it cuts off communication and denies Mr. Desjardins's feelings.

CLASSIFICATION
Competency: **Professional Practice**
Taxonomy: **Application**

92\.
1. Postoperative hemorrhage is a danger with liver disease and use of anticoagulants, not age.
2. Fluctuating blood glucose levels are a concern for people with diabetes, not people of advanced age.
3. Renal failure is associated with dehydration and an electrolyte imbalance, not age.
4. **Older persons are at increased risk for delayed wound healing and decreased tolerance to anaesthesia.**

CLASSIFICATION
Competency:
Foundations of Practice
Taxonomy:
Application

93\.
1. Age and sex affect pain perception only indirectly.
2. Overall physical condition may affect one's ability to cope with stress, but it would not greatly affect pain perception.
3. Intelligence is a factor in understanding pain, but it does not affect the perception of pain intensity; economic status has no effect on pain perception.
4. **Interpretation of pain sensations is highly individual and is based on past experiences, which include cultural values.**

CLASSIFICATION
Competency:
Foundations of Practice
Taxonomy:
Critical Thinking

94\.
1. Abdominal pain will not be prevented by sitting on the edge of the bed.
2. There should be no circulation problems with his legs and feet by the morning after surgery.
3. He may experience shallow breathing due to the abdominal incision, but this is not respiratory distress and is not prevented by sitting on the side of the bed.
4. **Following the administration of narcotics, the client's neurocirculatory reflexes may have some difficulty adjusting to the force of gravity when an upright position is assumed. Postural or orthostatic hypotension occurs, and the blood supply to the brain is temporarily decreased.**

CLASSIFICATION
Competency:
Foundations of Practice
Taxonomy:
Critical Thinking

95\.
1. **Pain in the calf may be a sign of thrombophlebitis, a possible postoperative complication. If the thrombus becomes dislodged, it may lead to pulmonary embolism. Any client with this complaint should immediately be confined to bed.**
2. The physician needs to be notified, but this is not the first action.
3. The application of heat may be contraindicated if a thrombus has developed.
4. The leg should not be elevated above heart level without a physician's order; gravity may dislodge the thrombus, creating an embolism.

CLASSIFICATION
Competency:
Foundations of Practice
Taxonomy:
Application

CASE 24

96\.
1. **Degenerative osteoarthritis affects the weight-bearing joints, such as knees, hips, and spine, and is not usually symmetrical.**
2. This finding is true of rheumatoid arthritis.
3. Same as answer 2.
4. Same as answer 2.

CLASSIFICATION
Competency:
Foundations of Practice
Taxonomy:
Knowledge/Comprehension

97.

1. This position supports the operative site; the involved leg must be maintained in alignment, avoiding adduction.

2. The pillow will not affect venous return, which relates to thrombus formation.
3. Adduction, not flexion contractures, are of most concern after surgery.
4. Although friwction is decreased when skin does not interface with skin, this is not the reason for separating the thighs and lower limbs.

CLASSIFICATION
Competency:
Foundations of Practice
Taxonomy:
Application

98.

1. The client must be turned at least every 2 hours to help prevent the complications of immobility. Three hours is too long to keep a client in one position.

2. Ankle movement, particularly dorsiflexion of the foot, allows muscle contraction, which compresses veins, reducing venous stasis and the risk of thrombus formation.

3. It is too soon for this action.
4. It is too soon for this action and sitting in a low chair is contraindicated because hip flexion can cause displacement of the prosthesis.

CLASSIFICATION
Competency:
Foundations of Practice
Taxonomy:
Application

99.

1. This statement is correct.

2. Crossing the legs at the knee and ankle increases the risk of dislocation of the prosthesis.

3. This statement is correct.
4. This statement is correct.

CLASSIFICATION
Competency:
Foundations of Practice
Taxonomy:
Application

100.

1. Ms. Kovacs will need initial intensive physiotherapy that would not be able to be provided at home with biweekly community supports. Her living arrangements, living alone in a two-storey house, are not appropriate for rehabilitation care.
2. Ms. Kovacs does not require this level of care.
3. This plan is not the best use of limited acute care facilities.

4. Ms. Kovacs will require intensive physiotherapy to enable her to regain mobility. This can best be achieved at a rehabilitation centre.

CLASSIFICATION
Competency:
Foundations of Practice
Taxonomy:
Critical Thinking

INDEPENDENT QUESTIONS ANSWERS AND RATIONALES

101.

1. The night shift may not have time to do the dressings either. Leaving the care to the night shift demonstrates a lack of accountability and will also cause a delay in Mr. Megadichan receiving care.
2. This delegation is inappropriate. The pressure injuries are new and require skills and knowledge beyond those of an unregulated care provider.
3. Documenting does not solve the problem of the wounds requiring care by the practical nurse.

4. This option is the only one that involves a possible solution to the need to complete the dressing changes and provide safe care to Mr. Megadichan.

CLASSIFICATION
Competency:
Collaborative Practice
Taxonomy:
Critical Thinking

102.

1. This consequence will result if the cuff is too wide.

2. This consequence will result from a loosely or unevenly wrapped cuff.

CLASSIFICATION
Competency:
Foundations of Practice
Taxonomy:
Application

3. This consequence will result if multiple caregivers use different interpretations of Korotkoff sounds.
4. This consequence will result from too rapid deflation of the cuff.

103.

1. The physician is responsible for obtaining consent for only those procedures that she is performing.
2. A practical nurse may sign a written consent as a witness to a client signature; however, the witness does not have to be a practical nurse.
3. **If a practical nurse is performing a procedure, it is she who must obtain consent.**
4. Consent may be written, verbal, or implied.

CLASSIFICATION
Competency:
Legal Practice
Taxonomy:
Knowledge/Comprehension

104.

1. **Diabetic retinopathy is a common complication of poorly controlled diabetes. People with diabetes need to have their eyes examined on a routine basis by an ophthalmologist or optometrist.**
2. It is important to test the blood, but it should be done at least three times a day rather than once a week.
3. This action is not necessary unless blood sugar levels are very high.
4. There is no need to reduce the number of hours worked unless Ms. Karmally's lifestyle is interfering with her management of the diabetes.

CLASSIFICATION
Competency:
Foundations of Practice
Taxonomy:
Application

105.

1. This action is not appropriate. There is no cause for a report.
2. There is no evidence of inappropriate behaviour.
3. It would be inappropriate to approach Ms. Walters; it would likely upset her and could lead to legal and professional sanctions against the practical nurse.
4. **There is no indication that the colleague's action was anything other than therapeutic touch. It is prejudicial to assume sexual behaviour just because the colleague is a lesbian.**

CLASSIFICATION
Competency:
Professional Practice
Taxonomy:
Application

106.

1. **Professional misconduct is behaviour that would be considered a fundamental breach of nursing ethics, conduct that discredits the profession. Falsely claiming sick benefits is professional misconduct.**
2. Incompetence relates to a lack of knowledge, skills, or judgement required to provide safe comprehensive care.
3. Malpractice is negligence performed in professional practice, an unreasonable lack of skill, or illegal or immoral conduct that results in the injury of a client.
4. Accountability is being responsible for one's actions and the consequences of those actions. There is no indication that the practical nurse accepts or does not accept responsibility for her actions.

CLASSIFICATION
Competency:
Professional Practice
Taxonomy:
Application

107.

1. **In all provinces and territories except Quebec, the maturity of the individual is the marker for giving consent. In Quebec, the age of consent is 14.**
2. An adolescent may be capable of mature and informed decisions.
3. Cassandra's ability to give consent does not depend on whether her parents are available.
4. Adolescents have the capacity to choose between alternatives.

CLASSIFICATION
Competency:
Legal Practice
Taxonomy:
Application

108.

1. Thrush, also called moniliasis and candidiasis, usually affects the mucous membranes of the oral cavity, causing painful white patches. Individuals with immunological deficiencies, those receiving prolonged antibiotic therapy, and infants are particularly susceptible to this organism.

2. Dysentery is usually caused by an amoeba or a bacterium; it is not common in infants.
3. Impetigo is a bacterial infection of the skin caused by streptococci or staphylococci.
4. This infectious condition of the skin is a result of infestation by mites.

CLASSIFICATION
Competency:
Foundations of Practice
Taxonomy:
Knowledge/Comprehension

109.

1. Practical nurses may not discriminate on cultural, socioeconomic, or health status grounds.

2. This action allows the practical nurse to choose clients based on her biases, not professional ethics.
3. This action is not ethically permitted in Canada.
4. This possible solution to the problem does not change this particular situation. As well, it is unlikely that the practical nurse will find an area of practice that meets the criteria for her personal ethics.

CLASSIFICATION
Competency:
Ethical Practice
Taxonomy:
Application

110.

1. Selection does not have a major influence on eating habits.
2. Food's smell and appearance certainly have some influence, though not major, on eating habits at this age.

3. The early-school-aged child has become a cooperative member of the family and will mimic parents' attitudes and food habits readily.

4. The peer group does not become highly influential until a later school age and adolescence.

CLASSIFICATION
Competency:
Foundations of Practice
Taxonomy:
Knowledge/Comprehension

111.

1. Feeding may proceed immediately after opening the tube.

2. Positioning the infant on the right side after feeding facilitates digestion because the pyloric sphincter is on this side and gravity aids in emptying the stomach.

3. It is standard procedure to flush the tube with water, not normal saline, after the feeding to ensure that all the formula gets into the stomach; it is not necessary before the feeding.
4. Place the formula in a lukewarm water bath to bring to room temperature, never use a microwave.

CLASSIFICATION
Competency:
Foundations of Practice
Taxonomy:
Application

112.

1. This weight is within the normal range. The average birth weight is about 3 200 g.

2. An Apgar score of 3 indicates neonatal distress and should signal to the practical nurse that the infant requires close supervision and support.

3. A positive Babinski reflex is normal through the age of 2 years.
4. It is normal to detect a mild pulsation in the fontanelle of an infant.

CLASSIFICATION
Competency:
Foundations of Practice
Taxonomy:
Application

113.

1. The practical nurse cannot administer medication without authorization from a registered prescriber.
2. The practical nurse must get a physician's order for the medication and cannot accept the parent's information alone.

3. The practical nurse does not know if Samantha should have the medication and must consult with the physician.
4. **A practical nurse should not administer these medications without a prescription. The practical nurse should also ensure that the doctor is aware of Samantha's allergies before the surgery.**

CLASSIFICATION
Competency:
Professional Practice
Taxonomy:
Knowledge/Comprehension

---

114. 1. This calculation is incorrect.
2. Same as answer 1.
3. **Correct calculation:**

$$x\ \text{mL} = \frac{1\ \text{mL}}{0.4\ \cancel{\text{mg}}} \times \frac{0.3\ \cancel{\text{mg}}}{1}$$

$$x\ \text{mL} = \frac{3}{4}\ \text{mL} = 0.75\ \text{mL}$$

4. Same as answer 1.

CLASSIFICATION
Competency:
Foundations of Practice
Taxonomy:
Application

---

115. 1. This action would constrict blood vessels and impair absorption.
2. Deep penetration is necessary; only the ventral gluteal muscles should be used because of their size and the decreased visibility of staining.
3. This action should be avoided. It might cause seepage of the drug into the muscle, with subsequent tissue irritation and staining.
4. **Residual medication on the needle may stain and irritate the tissues during penetration.**

CLASSIFICATION
Competency:
Professional Practice
Taxonomy:
Application

---

116. 1. **Humans are sexual from birth to death. Consenting older persons engaging in intercourse are no different from younger adults and must be afforded the same respect. Resident rooms in a long-term care facility are considered the clients' homes. The practical nurse should not have entered the room without knocking and asking permission to enter.**
2. This action is not appropriate. The practical nurse witnessed a private relationship and does not need to share what she saw with the nursing team.
3. To ask would be an interruption. The couple should already have privacy in his room. At another time, the practical nurse could discuss with the resident the possibility of changing rooms to one that may offer more privacy.
4. This action is not appropriate or, obviously, necessary.

CLASSIFICATION
Competency:
Professional Practice
Taxonomy:
Critical Thinking

---

117. 1. While side rails are considered a restraint, when making an occupied bed, the practical nurse may raise one rail at a time for safety, but not both.
2. **This action minimizes strain on the back. It is easier to remove and apply linen evenly when the bed is in a flat position, and a comfortable height provides easy access to the bed and linen.**
3. The equipment is assembled before starting the procedure, but it should be placed on a clean chair or overbed table. Placing it on the bottom of the bed puts it on the soiled linen and interferes with the making of the bed.
4. The client is covered with the bath blanket, and then the soiled top sheet is removed. This provides for client warmth and comfort.

CLASSIFICATION
Competency:
Professional Practice
Taxonomy:
Knowledge/Comprehension

118.

1. This statement assumes that another pregnancy will ensue; it also cuts off further communication.
2. **This statement allows both partners to comfort each other and lets them know the practical nurse is available; it also allows them to recognize and accept their feelings of loss.**
3. Telling clients not to be upset cuts off communication and wrongly implies that sadness prolongs recovery.
4. Grieving for the unborn child will and should occur during any period of pregnancy.

CLASSIFICATION
Competency: **Professional Practice**
Taxonomy: **Application**

119.

1. This response closes off discussion and is not necessarily true.
2. This response is not necessarily true, and there are some established risks in taking hormone replacement therapy.
3. The practical nurse should avoid recommendations based on personal beliefs. It is up to the client to decide.
4. **The woman is best to discuss treatment options with her physician to get full information. The physician should be aware of any herbal supplements the woman is taking. After the discussion, if the woman chooses, she can safely try alternative therapies for symptom relief.**

CLASSIFICATION
Competency: **Professional Practice**
Taxonomy: **Application**

120.

1. **Inadequate oxygenation of the brain may produce restlessness or behavioural changes. The pulse and respiration rates increase as a compensatory mechanism for hypoxia.**
2. The pupils dilate with cerebral hypoxia.
3. The pulse and respiration rates increase with hypoxia.
4. There will be cyanosis at a later stage. Dyspnea may or may not be present.

CLASSIFICATION
Competency: **Foundations of Practice**
Taxonomy: **Application**

121.

1. This vitamin is fat soluble and stored in the body.
2. **Vitamin C is water soluble and not stored in the body.**
3. Same as answer 1.
4. Same as answer 1.

CLASSIFICATION
Competency: **Foundations of Practice**
Taxonomy: **Knowledge/Comprehension**

122.

1. This action needs to be done but is not the first priority.
2. The practical nurse does need to immediately alert the other staff, but not by yelling, "Fire," which may cause residents to panic.
3. This action should be done as soon as possible, but removing Mrs. Cummings is the priority.
4. **Client safety is the practical nurse's first priority. Mrs. Cummings must be removed from danger.**

CLASSIFICATION
Competency: **Professional Practice**
Taxonomy: **Critical Thinking**

123.

1. This action is not necessary. Febrile seizures are generally not a medical emergency.
2. **Febrile seizures are frightening but generally harmless and usually stop by themselves. The child should be seen by a physician immediately to check on her condition, monitor for other seizures, and advise on temperature control.**

CLASSIFICATION
Competency: **Foundations of Practice**
Taxonomy: **Application**

3. Febrile seizures are not related to epilepsy.
4. The child should be examined by a physician.

124.

1. This action would be a wise initial action if there were a safe place to take the residents. However, the carpet has been installed throughout the facility.
2. This action is beneficial, but the most immediate concern is to inform management of the possible dangers of the chemical exposure.
3. **Management needs to be made aware of the situation so that corrective action may be taken, and staff and clients protected.**
4. This action will need to be done but is not the initial action.

CLASSIFICATION
Competency:
Professional Practice
Taxonomy:
Critical Thinking

125.

1. **Autism spectrum disorder has a wide range in severity of clinical manifestations and cognitive and behavioural outcomes. Early recognition and early interventions help to manage the disorder. It is not possible at the time of diagnosis to predict eventual functioning.**
2. It is not possible to predict this outcome when the child is 2 years old.
3. Same as answer 2.
4. ASD is not a degenerative disorder.

CLASSIFICATION
Competency:
Foundations of Practice
Taxonomy:
Knowledge/Comprehension

126.

1. It is not up to the client to determine the orders of the physician.
2. **The practical nurse is legally responsible for ensuring that he implements the physician orders correctly. The only way to do this is to speak directly with the physician.**
3. The physician, not another nurse, must clarify the physician's orders.
4. It is the responsibility of the ordering physician to clarify his orders.

CLASSIFICATION
Competency:
Collaborative Practice
Taxonomy:
Application

127.

1. Same as answer 3.
2. Same as answer 3.
3. **Passwords should never be shared. Passwords protect client confidentiality. The medical student should have her own password if allowed access to the chart.**
4. Same as answer 3.

CLASSIFICATION
Competency:
Legal Practice
Taxonomy:
Application

128.

1. Being a doctor may be a big part of this client's self-esteem, and this remark threatens that self-esteem.
2. **This response simply states facts without getting involved in role conflict.**
3. Firm, consistent limits need to be set so that the nurse–client role is established.
4. This response could be viewed as a threat and is more about the practical nurse's need than the client's behaviour.

CLASSIFICATION
Competency:
Professional Practice
Taxonomy:
Application

129.

1. **The most effective therapy method is for the child to play out his feelings; when feelings are allowed to surface, the child can then learn to face them by controlling, accepting, or abandoning them. Through this process, the child can experience growth.**

CLASSIFICATION
Competency:
Foundations of Practice
Taxonomy:
Application

2. This therapy is not child specific and, generally, is more suited for adolescents, young adults, and adults.
3. Same as answer 2.
4. Same as answer 2.

130.

1. Urate excretion is enhanced by high doses of Aspirin.
2. Aspirin is readily broken down in the gastrointestinal tract and liver.
3. **Aspirin interferes with platelet aggregation, thereby lengthening bleeding time.**
4. Aspirin inhibits platelet aggregation; it does not destroy erythrocytes.

CLASSIFICATION
Competency: **Foundations of Practice**
Taxonomy: **Application**

131.

1. This response does not present a therapeutic solution to the situation. The practical nurse is aiding the client.
2. This response places the responsibility on the client, but she may not be compliant with the practical nurse's advice.
3. **This response supports the client and also ensures that the physician will be informed of the client's drinking.**
4. This response implies the practical nurse is functioning by rules, not by nursing standards.

CLASSIFICATION
Competency: **Professional Practice**
Taxonomy: **Critical Thinking**

132.

1. This response is too technical and would not be understood by an 11-year-old.
2. **This response provides accurate information in a manner easily understood.**
3. This response is partly true but is not a complete answer and is too simplistic for an 11-year-old.
4. Same as answer 3.

CLASSIFICATION
Competency: **Foundations of Practice**
Taxonomy: **Critical Thinking**

133.

1. **With aging, the taste buds become less sensitive.**
2. This response may be true but is not the most accurate explanation.
3. Same as answer 2.
4. Same as answer 2.

CLASSIFICATION
Competency: **Foundations of Practice**
Taxonomy: **Critical Thinking**

134.

1. Pregnancy temporarily suppresses ovarian function; the aberrant endometrial tissue is still present.
2. Endometriosis may lead to sterility; it does not cause menopause.
3. Conservative medical therapy will be used first; a hysterectomy is a last resort.
4. **Lactation may delay ovarian function after delivery. It also therefore may delay the symptoms of endometriosis.**

CLASSIFICATION
Competency: **Foundations of Practice**
Taxonomy: **Application**

135.

1. Ice chips must not be given until the gag reflex returns.
2. Coughing should not be encouraged; it might initiate bleeding from the site of the biopsy.
3. **After administration of a local anaesthetic during a bronchoscopy, fluids and food should be withheld until the gag reflex returns.**
4. To allow drainage and minimize the possibility of aspiration, the client should be kept in a semi-Fowler position.

CLASSIFICATION
Competency: **Foundations of Practice**
Taxonomy: **Application**

136.
1. CBD (cannabidiol) is not responsible for the 'high' associated with cannabis use. CBD counteracts some of the negative effects of THC.
2. **THC (delta-9-tetrahydrocannabinol) is the main substance most responsible for the "high" associated with cannabis use.**
3. PCP (phenycyclidine) is not a substance in cannabis.
4. MDA (methylenedioxyamphetamine) is not a substance in cannabis.

CLASSIFICATION
Competency:
Foundations of Practice
Taxonomy:
Knowledge/Comprehension

137.
1. The trauma of surgery will result in some bleeding from the prostate, which will continue until coagulation takes place; the clots that occur need to clear from the bladder. This time range is too short.
2. Same as answer 1.
3. **The trauma of surgery normally results in blood clots in the bladder for the first 24 to 36 hours after prostate surgery. Bladder irrigation is typically done to remove clotted blood from the bladder.**
4. It is abnormal for blood clots to still be occurring 36 to 48 hours after surgery; the physician should be notified.

CLASSIFICATION
Competency:
Foundations of Practice
Taxonomy:
Application

138.
1. There is no correlation between high blood sugars and peptic ulcers.
2. **Smoking increases the acidity of gastrointestinal secretions, which damages the mucosal barrier.**
3. Weight is unrelated to peptic ulcer disease.
4. High blood pressure is not directly related to peptic ulcer disease.

CLASSIFICATION
Competency:
Foundations of Practice
Taxonomy:
Knowledge/Comprehension

139.
1. This manifestation occurs when the pooling of blood in the peripheral vessels causes hypotension; it rarely occurs with hypervolemia.
2. Rhinitis would not be a manifestation of heart failure.
3. An increased fluid volume in the intravascular compartment (overhydration) will cause the pulse to feel full and bounding.
4. **An increase in the extracellular fluid volume can cause a relative decrease in the hemoglobin and hematocrit by dilution of the blood.**

CLASSIFICATION
Competency:
Foundations of Practice
Taxonomy:
Application

140.
1. Although this aspect of hand hygiene is important, without friction it has minimal value.
2. Although soap reduces surface tension, without friction it has minimal value.
3. Although water flushes some microorganisms from the skin, without friction it has minimal value.
4. **Friction is necessary for the removal of microorganisms.**

CLASSIFICATION
Competency:
Foundations of Practice
Taxonomy:
Critical Thinking

141.
1. Ms. Tang has not provided consent for the picture to be taken. For confidentiality reasons, the photo must not be saved.
2. Ms. Tang may not wish her family to see the photo. There is no indication Ms. Tang has provided consent for the photo to be shown.
3. Same as answer 1.
4. **Taking the picture in itself is a breach of confidentiality. The photo must be immediately deleted.**

CLASSIFICATION
Competency:
Legal Practice
Taxonomy:
Application

142.
1. For the level of care she needs, Mrs. Eigo does not require an RN.
2. For the level of care she needs, Mrs. Eigo does not require a registered or licensed practical nurse.
3. Mrs. Eigo does not require the services of a geriatric activation therapist.
4. **A personal support worker (PSW) or unregulated care provider (UCP) is most suitable for Mrs. Eigo. The PSW or UCP has the education and skills to assist a client with the activities of daily living.**

CLASSIFICATION
Competency: **Collaborative Practice**
Taxonomy: **Critical Thinking**

143.
1. *Coxiella burnetii*, the causal agent of Q fever a *Rickettsia*, is not part of the normal flora; it is spread by contact with infected animals, drinking of contaminated milk, or the bite of a vector tick.
2. **Candidiasis (a *Candida* infection) arises in certain individuals when local resistance is decreased through prolonged antibiotic therapy or with certain diseases (e.g., diabetes) and debilitating conditions (e.g., drug addiction).**
3. Streptococci would be responsive to antibiotic therapy and are not considered part of the normal flora.
4. The varicella zoster virus is not part of the normal flora.

CLASSIFICATION
Competency: **Foundations of Practice**
Taxonomy: **Knowledge/Comprehension**

144.
1. This response is evasive; the client is left without direction.
2. There are concerns with taking hormone replacement therapy (HRT), but this response would alarm Ms. Mengal.
3. Herbal supplements are not always the best option for treating the symptoms of surgical menopause.
4. **The use of hormones is controversial and needs to be discussed with a physician.**

CLASSIFICATION
Competency: **Foundations of Practice**
Taxonomy: **Application**

145.
1. No external surgical incision is made.
2. Most types of prostatic surgery result in some degree of retrograde ejaculation and it is not harmful.
3. **Bladder spasms are a distressing complication following TURP surgery.**
4. A cystocele is not a complication following TURP surgery.

CLASSIFICATION
Competency: **Foundations of Practice**
Taxonomy: **Application**

146.
1. An accurate specific gravity cannot be obtained when irrigating solutions are being instilled into the bladder.
2. Hourly outputs are indicated only if there is concern about renal failure or oliguria.
3. **The total amount of irrigation solution instilled into the bladder is eliminated with the urine and, therefore, must be subtracted from the total output to determine the volume of urine excreted.**
4. Twenty-four-hour urine tests would not be accurate if the client were receiving continuous irrigation.

CLASSIFICATION
Competency: **Foundations of Practice**
Taxonomy: **Application**

147.
1. Gauze dressing would not reinforce the suture line.
2. **Additional gauze at the base would ensure that drainage resulting from gravity would be absorbed.**

CLASSIFICATION
Competency: **Foundations of Practice**
Taxonomy: **Application**

3. Gravity during ambulation would cause the drainage to flow downward.
4. A pressure dressing is not necessary.

148.

1. Both physicians and nurses mutually accepted the practice.
2. Hospitals appreciate cost cutting, but evidence-informed practice was not a hospital initiative.
3. **This statement accurately reflects the origin of the concept.**
4. Although much information is shared over the Internet, this statement does not describe the origin of the concept.

CLASSIFICATION
Competency:
Professional Practice
Taxonomy:
Application

149.

1. **This action is the correct procedure. The direction of cleansing moves from the area of least contamination to the area of most contamination, preventing microorganisms from entering the urethra.**
2. The tip around the meatus is cleansed first.
3. The foreskin will need to be retracted, but the meatus is cleansed first.
4. Cleansing in upward strokes would move microorganisms toward the urethra.

CLASSIFICATION
Competency:
Foundations of Practice
Taxonomy:
Application

150.

1. He might not choose a safe helmet.
2. A preschool child may not be able to understand the safety implications.
3. Rewards may work but will not be effective if the child is riding a bike when the parent is not there to provide the reward.
4. **Children learn best from effective role models.**

CLASSIFICATION
Competency:
Foundations of Practice
Taxonomy:
Application

151.

1. The practical nurse is not permitted to change an ordered dose of medication unless there has been a previous medical directive.
2. **This is the most professional and legally acceptable choice. It enables the practical nurse to provide pain medication to the client in a timely fashion.**
3. This action is not professional.
4. These therapies are unlikely to provide the required level of pain relief.

CLASSIFICATION
Competency:
Collaborative Practice
Taxonomy:
Application

152.

1. Diphtheria, tetanus, pertussis (DtaP) is given at ages 2 months, 4 months, 6 months, and 18 months.
2. **Measles, mumps, rubella (MMR) is given at 12 months.**
3. Rota (Rotavirus) is most often administered at ages 2 months, 4 months, and 6 months of age.
4. Ava requires her MMR.

CLASSIFICATION
Competency:
Foundations of Practice
Taxonomy:
Knowledge/Comprehension

153.

1. **This response is factual.**
2. The fontanelle is not typically larger in children with Down's syndrome.
3. All infants have incomplete closure of the bones in their skulls at birth.
4. Children with Down's syndrome typically do not have premature closure of the fontanelle.

CLASSIFICATION
Competency:
Foundations of Practice
Taxonomy:
Application

154.
1. This inference is a stereotype.
2. Same as answer 1.
3. Same as answer 1.
4. **This inference recognizes that, above and beyond any cultural health practices, clients are individuals.**

CLASSIFICATION
Competency: **Professional Practice**
Taxonomy: **Application**

155.
1. Two days' time is too late. It will be assumed that the ampicillin was not administered.
2. This action is not necessary unless made so by an agency policy.
3. **Since there is no policy, the practical nurse must consult with a supervisor to determine the appropriate action.**
4. This action may be appropriate if determined so after consultation with the nursing supervisor.

CLASSIFICATION
Competency: **Professional Practice**
Taxonomy: **Application**

156.
1. **The practical nurse is responsible for providing the client with knowledge about all treatment options. As a first step, the practical nurse must assess and discuss the effectiveness of the herbal preparation.**
2. The practical nurse does not decide for clients what choices they should make about treatment.
3. This action can be done, but the client has already stated a preference for the herbal preparation. This response by the practical nurse indicates a bias for her own treatment preferences.
4. The practical nurse should support Ms. Holly's decision but only after the client is given all the information about the herbal preparation and the antihypertensive.

CLASSIFICATION
Competency: **Foundations of Practice**
Taxonomy: **Application**

157.
1. This finding is normal and is related to premenstrual syndrome.
2. These findings are normal in the third trimester of pregnancy. The yellowish fluid is colostrum.
3. **Although men do not have the same incidence of breast cancer as women, the finding of a lump in the breast area is of concern as it may be cancerous.**
4. These findings happen occasionally in newborn males as a result of hormones from the mother and will subside in several days.

CLASSIFICATION
Competency: **Foundations of Practice**
Taxonomy: **Critical Thinking**

158.
1. This consideration is important but not the priority.
2. Same as answer 1.
3. Same as answer 1.
4. **Clients with post-traumatic stress disorder may experience aggressive outbursts, use violence to solve problems, and display suicidal thoughts. The safety of the client and others is a priority.**

CLASSIFICATION
Competency: **Foundations of Practice**
Taxonomy: **Critical Thinking**

159.
1. Formal religion does not necessarily relate to spirituality. This question may be asked later in the interview.
2. This question should be asked but is not necessarily part of a spiritual assessment nor an initial question.

3. **Spirituality is unique to each adult. All people are considered to be spiritual whether or not they have a religious affiliation. This question would be appropriate as an initial question that could lead to gathering more specific information about the client's belief system.**

CLASSIFICATION
Competency:
Professional Practice
Taxonomy:
Critical Thinking

4. This question is important to ask but is not the best initial question when exploring spirituality with a client.

160.

1. This action would be Candace's decision. She would need to consent to this involvement prior to the practical nurse initiating contact with the police.
2. This recommendation may be appropriate at some point in her care but is not the first action.
3. **This action is the practical nurse's priority. The practical nurse needs more information to assess immediate safety and be able to determine the next action.**
4. This action would not be appropriate.

CLASSIFICATION
Competency:
Foundations of Practice
Taxonomy:
Critical Thinking

161.

1. This statement is not necessarily true and does not allow the client to voice her concerns.
2. **This response is open ended and allows the client to voice her concerns.**
3. This response assumes the woman's concerns are related to stages of labour and closes discussion.
4. This response makes an assumption that may not be correct.

CLASSIFICATION
Competency:
Professional Practice
Taxonomy:
Application

162.

1. This action will help the infant not to lose heat from the head but is not the most effective action to reduce heat loss and warm the baby.
2. This action will help warm the infant through body heat but is not the most effective method.
3. **This action is the most effective to prevent further heat loss and to warm the infant. Hypothermia is a danger for premature infants and places them at risk for other complications.**
4. This action is not the most effective for raising the body temperature of a premature infant and may cause further cooling due to loss of heat from evaporating water on the skin.

CLASSIFICATION
Competency:
Foundations of Practice
Taxonomy:
Critical Thinking

163.

1. This parent's situation is a stressor but does not necessarily predispose the parent to child abuse.
2. **A risk factor for abusing a child is having experienced previous abuse.**
3. Same as answer 1.
4. Same as answer 1.

CLASSIFICATION
Competency:
Foundations of Practice
Taxonomy:
Critical Thinking

164.

1. Such devices may likely be needed and are important to recommend to Mr. and Mrs. Cooke, but this is not the most important assessment.
2. This assessment is important to ensure that Mr. Cooke uses mild moisturizers that do not dry out sensitive skin.
3. The need for assistive devices should be determined once Mrs. Cooke's cognitive and musculoskeletal functions have been determined, but this is not the most important assessment.

4. Because Mrs. Cooke is in the early stages of Alzheimer's disease, she is likely able to manage many of her own hygiene needs. The practical nurse's primary responsibility is to determine if Mrs. Cooke has the cognitive ability and the coordination to bathe herself.

CLASSIFICATION
Competency:
Foundations of Practice
Taxonomy:
Critical Thinking

165.
1. The varicella vaccine does not provide protection against the mumps.
2. **The varicella vaccine provides protection against chicken pox.**
3. The varicella vaccine does not provide protection against whooping cough.
4. The varicella vaccine does not provide protection against rubella.

CLASSIFICATION
Competency:
Foundations of Practice
Taxonomy:
Application

166.
1. This action will promote regurgitation.
2. This action will probably have little effect on reflux.
3. This action will promote vomiting since it is too much formula for a week-old infant.
4. **Some mild reflux is common in newborn infants. Reflux results from an incompetent cardiac sphincter, which allows a reflux of gastric contents into the esophagus and eventual regurgitation. Although there is some research that finds positioning of the infant has no effect on regurgitation, the general practice is to place the infant in an upright position, which uses gravity to help keep the gastric contents in the stomach and also limits the pressure against the cardiac sphincter.**

CLASSIFICATION
Competency:
Foundations of Practice
Taxonomy:
Application

167.
1. During the 1970s, elevated estrogen and progesterone levels associated with pregnancy were viewed as protective against depression. This hypothesis is now known to be untrue.
2. Signs and symptoms of depression in pregnancy do not differ from depression at any other time of life.
3. Antenatal depression occurs most frequently in the last two trimesters.
4. **Women who have antenatal depression have an increased risk of postpartum depression.**

CLASSIFICATION
Competency:
Foundations of Practice
Taxonomy:
Knowledge/Comprehension

168.
1. This option is probably not realistic.
2. **A preceptor should assist with a learning plan, and the practical nurse should feel comfortable asking for learning resources and feedback on performance. The preceptor should assess the progress of the practical nurse and not intimidate her.**
3. This action does not aid in forming a supportive relationship, nor is it true.
4. Although the practical nurse is expected to engage in continuous learning, it would be unrealistic to assume that the practical nurse could learn everything about all the medications. The preceptor, however, would be able to suggest a learning plan.

CLASSIFICATION
Competency:
Professional Practice
Taxonomy:
Application

169.
1. This is a risk once the teeth have erupted.
2. **Honey should be avoided in the first 12 months because of the risk of infant botulism.**

CLASSIFICATION
Competency:
Foundations of Practice
Taxonomy:
Application

3. Sudden infant death syndrome is not a risk.
4. Toxic shock syndrome is not a risk.

170.

1. This calculation is incorrect; the dose is too low.
2. **Correct calculation:**

$$x \text{ mL} = \frac{1 \text{ mL}}{5 \not{\text{mg}}} \times \frac{2 \not{\text{mg}}}{1}$$

$$x \text{ mL} = \frac{2}{5} \text{ mL} = 0.4 \text{ mL}$$

3. This calculation is incorrect; the dose is too high.
4. Same as answer 3.

CLASSIFICATION
Competency:
Foundations of Practice
Taxonomy:
Application

171.

1. This is not the appropriate course of action.
2. Same as 1.
3. Same as 1.
4. **The practical nurse is aware that he does not have the emotional capacity to practice safely and competently and should withdraw from the provision of care after consulting with his supervisor.**

CLASSIFICATION
Competency:
Professional Practice
Taxonomy:
Application

172.

1. This recommendation will not solve the problem; besides, he cannot nap at work.
2. This recommendation does not solve the client's problem.
3. **These signs suggest sleep apnea, which needs to be investigated by a physician.**
4. The client has not stated that he has a problem with insomnia.

CLASSIFICATION
Competency:
Foundations of Practice
Taxonomy:
Application

173.

1. These foods are not rich sources of iron.
2. **Organ meats, green vegetables, and legumes are rich sources of iron.**
3. Pork is a rich source of iron, but these vegetables are not.
4. Meat and potatoes are rich sources of iron, but milk is not.

CLASSIFICATION
Competency:
Foundations of Practice
Taxonomy:
Application

174.

1. This response is not true. Acupuncture does help some clients with chronic pain.
2. Acupuncture is approved in some provinces.
3. **The practical nurse is functioning as a client advocate in assisting the client to act on his decision.**
4. This response ignores what the client has requested and assumes that he is not taking his pain medication correctly.

CLASSIFICATION
Competency:
Professional Practice
Taxonomy:
Application

175.

1. **This action is the most professional and safest for determining the correct client.**
2. The practical nurse does not know the clients. Mr. Masters may be confused or may not know his name.
3. It is not the responsibility of another client to provide client identification.
4. The individual practical nurse is responsible for ensuring that she has the correct client. Advice should be asked from other nurses if there is no other means of identification.

CLASSIFICATION
Competency:
Professional Practice
Taxonomy:
Application

176.

1. A child this age needs to know the seriousness of the illness and that recovery may not be possible.
2. Children of this age interpret death as separation and punishment. This response indicates the son will not care what happens to his sister.
3. This response only avoids the question.
4. **Children at early school age are not yet able to comprehend death's universality and inevitability, but they do fear it, often personifying death as a monster or dark angel. They need an opportunity to prepare for this situation.**

CLASSIFICATION
Competency: **Professional Practice**
Taxonomy: **Critical Thinking**

177.

1. It is unrealistic for the couple to refrain from sexual intercourse for the entire pregnancy.
2. Spermicides are of limited effectiveness with the herpes virus.
3. **There is evidence that the herpes virus is shed even when there are no symptoms. In case the client has not already contracted the virus from her husband, the couple should use a condom.**
4. Washing is not enough to prevent contraction of this virus; contact has already been made.

CLASSIFICATION
Competency: **Foundations of Practice**
Taxonomy: **Application**

178.

1. The immediate priority is to prevent harm to the client. Calling for assistance may or may not be indicated later.
2. **This action will provide stability as the practical nurse lowers the client to the floor.**
3. This action puts an unnecessary strain on the practical nurse and may cause injury to her.
4. This action may not be feasible and may be a strain for the practical nurse, causing injury to her.

CLASSIFICATION
Competency: **Professional Practice**
Taxonomy: **Application**

179.

1. This approach is threatening and nonprofessional.
2. **This approach is professional. The UCP may not be aware that she is not allowed to use the title "nurse."**
3. This action is not professional because it is not supportive of the role of the UCP and may confuse the client.
4. The situation involves only one UCP, and it is likely other caregivers are aware of "nurse" being a protected title.

CLASSIFICATION
Competency: **Collaborative Practice**
Taxonomy: **Application**

180.

1. **It is often more difficult to detect substance abuse in older persons since it may be masked by chronic disease.**
2. This statement is not true; misuse also involves alcohol and prescription medications.
3. Alcohol misuse is found in approximately 20% of the general population, not just older persons.
4. Older persons are generally reluctant to discuss the problem.

CLASSIFICATION
Competency: **Foundations of Practice**
Taxonomy: **Application**

181.
1. There is a strong familial link with keloid formation.
2. This statement offers false reassurance and dismisses Ms. Marie's concern.
3. **This statement supports Ms. Marie's concern and provides an option for her to discuss her worry about a scar with the physician.**
4. This outcome cannot be guaranteed.

CLASSIFICATION
Competency: **Foundations of Practice**
Taxonomy: **Application**

182.
1. These condoms should never be reused as they may retain traces of sperm or microorganisms and may sustain small tears.
2. **Only water-soluble lubricants should be used for body orifices.**
3. Male and female condoms should not be used together. It may promote tearing, and they do not work smoothly during intercourse.
4. It may be used for this purpose with the inner ring not placed inside.

CLASSIFICATION
Competency: **Foundations of Practice**
Taxonomy: **Application**

183.
1. **This response is best because it is truthful and provides reassurance about postoperative communication.**
2. This option is not possible.
3. There will be no voice production with a tracheotomy tube with an inflated cuff in place.
4. This response dismisses Ms. Grant's concerns.

CLASSIFICATION
Competency: **Foundations of Practice**
Taxonomy: **Application**

184.
1. This response is untrue. About 1 800 active cases are reported each year.
2. **This response is best. It answers Sally's concern and suggests a course of action toward determining if she has TB.**
3. This response is true but does not answer Sally's concern.
4. This response is not therapeutic, and the immune system cannot be assessed visually.

CLASSIFICATION
Competency: **Professional Practice**
Taxonomy: **Application**

185.
1. This approach is unhelpful and states the obvious.
2. **There may be other medications with fewer adverse effects that Ms. Pargeter could take. The situation must be evaluated and discussed with her physician.**
3. This approach is a threat to abandon care.
4. Ms. Pargeter has not mentioned stress, just that she was tired.

CLASSIFICATION
Competency: **Professional Practice**
Taxonomy: **Critical Thinking**

186.
1. Chart entries must never be removed or deleted.
2. **This action is the legally accepted correction.**
3. Same as answer 1.
4. This action is not necessary. Incident reports are generally required by agencies when a client's safety is at risk.

CLASSIFICATION
Competency: **Legal Practice**
Taxonomy: **Knowledge/Comprehension**

187.
1. **These signs are indicative of a cerebrovascular accident (stroke) and require emergency treatment. Immediate transportation to the nearest hospital is vital. If tissue plasminogen activator (tPA) is assessed to be the appropriate treatment, it must be administered within 3 to 4.5 hours of the stroke to prevent permanent cerebral damage.**

CLASSIFICATION
Competency: **Foundations of Practice**
Taxonomy: **Critical Thinking**

2. Mr. Leonard requires quick transport to services that only a hospital can provide.
3. This directive is not wise until it is established whether the stroke is hemolytic or thrombotic.
4. Same as answer 2.

188.

1. This action will need to be done but not until treatment has been initiated.
2. **This action is the correct emergency treatment. With anaphylactic responses, death can occur very quickly, even in minutes. The epinephrine should be given at the same time that 9-1-1 is called.**
3. This action is important, but the epinephrine is lifesaving.
4. Diphenhydramine hydrochloride is an antihistamine that is used to treat less critical allergies. It is not appropriate in this case.

CLASSIFICATION
Competency:
Foundations of Practice
Taxonomy:
Critical Thinking

189.

1. **Regular consumption of cranberry juice is believed to prevent bacteria from adhering to the lining of the urinary tract. Cranberry capsules or tablets are also helpful.**
2. These products may actually increase the incidence of UTIs.
3. This suggestion is the opposite of what is recommended. Increased fluids help to flush the bladder of bacteria.
4. This treatment is prescribed only in the case of chronic, serious UTIs (e.g., in clients with neurogenic bladders). The antiseptic must be ordered by a physician, not a nurse.

CLASSIFICATION
Competency:
Foundations of Practice
Taxonomy:
Application

190.

1. This option may not be possible if Mrs. Gingras is anorexic.
2. This option is possible; however, with anorexia, sometimes even favourite foods are not appealing or tolerated.
3. This option is possible but does not address the need for more protein.
4. **This strategy is the easiest and most consistent way to achieve a high-calorie, high-protein intake. Nutritional supplements come in a variety of flavours and serving them over ice may help improve acceptance.**

CLASSIFICATION
Competency:
Foundations of Practice
Taxonomy:
Critical Thinking

191.

1. It is not appropriate to prepare the body in view of the family. Only 15 minutes have passed; the family needs more time with their loved one.
2. This action is not respectful of the family's needs.
3. The family should be allowed to stay for as long as they require; however, it is not appropriate use of nursing financial resources to stay overtime for pay prior to consulting with the night staff.
4. **This action allows the family the necessary time with their loved one and uses nursing resources appropriately.**

CLASSIFICATION
Competency:
Professional Practice
Taxonomy:
Critical Thinking

192.

1. Alopecia does not result from steroid therapy.
2. An increase in appetite, not anorexia, results from steroid therapy.
3. Weight gain, not weight loss, results from steroid therapy.
4. **Euphoria and mood swings may result from steroid therapy.**

CLASSIFICATION
Competency:
Foundations of Practice
Taxonomy:
Application

---

193. **1. This action is the priority because the practical nurse must ensure he has the necessary equipment and supplies to treat clients, who may arrive at any time.**
2. While the practical nurse should have an idea of what types of clients have been treated on the previous shift, it is not a priority.
3. Unless there is a client requiring urgent care, head-to-toe assessments may not be necessary in this setting. If one is required, the practical nurse will need to take the time for a proper assessment.
4. This action is necessary; however, the medical directives are not likely to have changed since the nurse's previous shift.

CLASSIFICATION
Competency:
Professional Practice
Taxonomy:
Critical Thinking

---

194. **1. The affected areas of the intestines are in need of repair. Protein is required in the building and repairing of tissues.**
2. Increased protein will not significantly affect peristalsis.
3. Anemia may result from chronic bleeding; however, it usually is corrected with an increased iron intake and a normal intake of protein.
4. Protein is given to promote healing; once tissues are repaired, muscle tone may improve.

CLASSIFICATION
Competency:
Foundations of Practice
Taxonomy:
Application

---

195. **1. Denial is a pattern of defence often demonstrated in the self-protective stage of adaptation to illness. Thoughts and feelings are so painful and provoke such anxiety that the client rejects the existence of the paraplegia.**
2. From the information available, it cannot be assumed that the client is fantasizing; a fantasy is the transformation of undesirable experiences into imagined events to fulfill an unconscious wish or need.
3. Denial is a method of psychological adaptation.
4. Motivation involves the setting of realistic goals; this client is in denial.

CLASSIFICATION
Competency:
Foundations of Practice
Taxonomy:
Knowledge/Comprehension

---

196. 1. Nausea may occur but it is not a critical adverse effect.
2. Weight gain may occur but is not a critical adverse effect.
3. Thrombophlebitis (calf pain) has been associated with hormone therapy.
4. Breast tenderness is not a critical adverse effect.

CLASSIFICATION
Competency:
Foundations of Practice
Taxonomy:
Critical Thinking

---

197. 1. With a left-sided thrombus, right-sided weakness would be expected.
2. A decrease in tendon response would be the normal manifestation.
3. Urinary incontinence would be expected.
4. Anxiety and difficulty communicating are common physical findings since the primary speech centre is located in the left hemisphere.

CLASSIFICATION
Competency:
Foundations of Practice
Taxonomy:
Application

---

198. 1. This action may be warranted if a recent beating had occurred, but the neighbour has said this is a chronic situation occurring over many months. This action is not the most important unless the neighbour indicates to the practical nurse that the children have been severely injured.
2. This action could be taken by the practical nurse but is not the most important action.
3. This action is a helpful and therapeutic response but not the most important action.
4. By law, all nurses must report any actual or suspected cases of child abuse.

CLASSIFICATION
Competency:
Professional Practice
Taxonomy:
Critical Thinking

199. 1. Insertion into a vein would be intravenous therapy.

2. Hypodermoclysis catheters are inserted into the abdomen or upper thigh to allow for slow absorption through the tissue.

3. Same as answer 1.
4. Inserting a catheter into the pedal circulation may be harmful and is intravenous therapy.

CLASSIFICATION
Competency:
Foundations of Practice
Taxonomy:
Application

---

200. 1. There is no sex-related difference.

2. Nicotine is a powerful vasoconstrictor, which can lead to peripheral arterial disease.

3. This quantity of alcohol intake is a recommended allowance for women.
4. A high-fat diet may cause coronary rather than peripheral arterial problems.

CLASSIFICATION
Competency:
Foundations of Practice
Taxonomy:
Application

END OF ANSWERS AND RATIONALES TO PRACTICE EXAM 2

8 Practice Exam 3

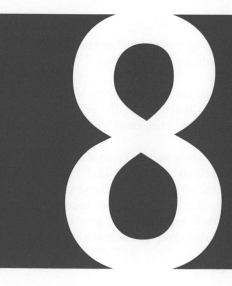

INSTRUCTIONS FOR PRACTICE EXAM 3

You will have 4 hours to complete the exam. The questions are presented as nursing cases or as independent questions. Read each question carefully, and then choose the answer that you think is the best of the four options presented. If you cannot decide on an answer to a question, proceed to the next question and return to this question later if you have time. Try to answer all the questions. Marks are not subtracted for wrong answers. If you are unsure of an answer, it will be to your advantage to guess.

Answers to Practice Exam 3 appear on page 174.

CASE-BASED QUESTIONS

CASE 1

Mr. Tolea, age 65, is in the terminal stage of liver failure resulting from hepatitis C. He has been unemployed for many years and lives below the poverty line in a low-income rooming house that has inadequate cooking and sanitation facilities. He is estranged from his former wife and two children.

QUESTIONS 1 to 4 refer to this case.

1. Mr. Tolea is seen by a practical nurse at a regional hepatitis C clinic. The practical nurse is aware that most new cases of hepatitis C are a result of which of the following?

1. Unprotected sexual activity
2. Blood transfusions
3. Coinfection with human immunodeficiency virus (HIV)
4. Intravenous drug use

2. The practical nurse is aware that Mr. Tolea has not been receiving the nutritional support he requires to manage his disease. How would the practical nurse best facilitate quality nutritional intake for him?

1. Encourage him to purchase liquid nutritional supplements
2. Suggest he add fresh fruit and vegetables to his diet
3. Consult with the clinic social worker to find a resource for a charitable meal service
4. Contact his family to persuade them to help provide him with nutritious food

3. Mr. Tolea's condition deteriorates, and he decides to be admitted to a palliative care unit. What is the most important aspect of care for the practical nurse to provide to Mr. Tolea?

1. Ensuring he has adequate sedation
2. Enabling him to make choices about his care
3. Managing symptoms related to pruritus
4. Preventing pressure injuries

4. The practical nurse is developing Mr. Tolea's nursing care plan. Which statement by the practical nurse would be most appropriate when establishing his goals of care?

1. "Don't worry we have a plan of care to help you through this difficult time in your life."
2. "Tell me what is important for you to achieve right now."
3. "We will contact your family to come see you."
4. "We will make sure we give you pain medication regularly to keep you comfortable."

END OF CASE 1

CASE 2

A practical nurse works in a pediatric obesity clinic. Rickhelm, age 11 years, is a new client in the clinic.

QUESTIONS 5 to 11 refer to this case.

5. What causes obesity?

1. Eating high-calorie foods
2. Lack of physical exercise
3. Caloric intake that exceeds caloric requirements
4. Sedentary lifestyle

6. Which of the following factors would be the most predictive etiology for Rickhelm's obesity?

1. A birth weight of 5.5 kg
2. Obese parents
3. A culture that considers fat children to be healthy children
4. A parenting style that provides food as a reward for good behaviour

7. Rickhelm has screening tests relating to his obesity. Which of the following results would be of most concern to the practical nurse?

1. Total cholesterol: 4.4 mmol/L
2. Fasting blood sugar: 7.8 mmol/L

3. Blood pressure: 105/63 mm Hg
4. Spirometry: 85% of predicted values

8. The practical nurse weighs Rickhelm. His mother asks what his weight is in pounds. The formula for converting kilograms to pounds is weight in kilograms multiplied by 2.2. Rickhelm weighs 57.5 kg. What is Rickhelm's weight in pounds?

1. 116
2. 114.5
3. 126.5
4. 115

9. The practical nurse begins a therapeutic plan for managing Rickhelm's obesity and goal of losing weight. What approach would likely have the most positive results?

1. Behaviour modification
2. A calorie-reduced diet
3. Appetite-suppressant drugs
4. Gastric bypass surgery

10. Rickhelm asks the practical nurse if he can still go to fast-food restaurants after school with his friends. What should the practical nurse recommend?

1. "Yes, I'll give you a list of low-calorie options from fast-food restaurants."
2. "Yes, you can go, but limit what you eat to just one hamburger and a small fries."
3. "It is probably not wise for you to go because you will be tempted to eat fatty foods."
4. "Fast-food restaurants serve high-fat, high-calorie foods, so you should never eat there."

11. Knowing that obese children are often teased by other children and may suffer low self-esteem, the practical nurse performs a psychosocial assessment of Rickhelm. Which question asked of Rickhelm would best approach this topic?

1. "Who are your friends?"
2. "Do you find that you are teased because you are overweight?"
3. "Do you feel bad about yourself because you are overweight?"
4. "Tell me how you feel about being overweight."

END OF CASE 2

CASE 3

Mr. Jason, age 79 years, is admitted to the medical unit with pneumonia. He has a tracheostomy from a neck tumour removal 3 years ago. He is to receive IV antibiotics for pneumonia. The treatment has been explained to him in detail by the physician, but he remains very anxious.

QUESTIONS 12 to 16 refer to this case.

12. Which of the following approaches by the practical nurse would help to reduce Mr. Jason's anxiety?

1. Talk with him to discover his specific concerns
2. Explain, in simple terms, what the physician already told him
3. Demonstrate how the IV equipment operates
4. Include Mr. Jason in developing a plan for additional home care after discharge

13. What position should the practical nurse place the client in for tracheostomy care.

1. Lateral
2. Trendelenburg
3. Sim's
4. Semi-Fowlers

14. Which of the following nursing actions would the practical nurse take when performing tracheal suctioning on Mr. Jason?

1. Preoxygenate before suctioning
2. Apply negative pressure as the catheter is being inserted
3. Ensure the catheter reaches well beyond the base of the tube
4. Instill acetylcysteine (Mucomyst) into the tracheotomy prior to suctioning to loosen secretions

15. What is the maximum length of time that the practical nurse should suction the tracheostomy tube?

1. 10 seconds
2. 30 seconds
3. 1 minute
4. 20 seconds

16. Mr. Jason communicates to the practical nurse that his tracheostomy ties are too tight and are choking him. Which of the following initial actions by the practical nurse would be most appropriate?

1. Assess Mr. Jason's neck for signs of constriction
2. Observe the tracheostomy dressing for drainage
3. Explain to Mr. Jason that the tight tracheostomy ties are necessary
4. Remove the tracheostomy ties to relieve the pressure.

END OF CASE 3

CASE 4

An Indigenous practical nurse begins employment at a community health clinic in the northern reserve where she grew up.

QUESTIONS 17 to 20 refer to this case.

17. The practical nurse understands that the objective of Indigenous health care is to bring balance to the body, mind, emotions, and spirit. Which of the following terms is used to describe this type of health care?

1. Holistic health care
2. Primary health care
3. Spiritual health care
4. Socioenvironmental health care

18. Shortly after the practical nurse begins work on the reserve, an outbreak of respiratory syncytial virus (RSV) occurs. Why is there a high incidence of RSV in northern Indigenous communities?

1. There is a lack of adequate housing, and the resulting overcrowding contributes to the disease's spread.
2. Indigenous infants are particularly susceptible to the virus.
3. The cold weather in the north favours the spread of the virus.
4. Members of the population have a depressed immune system related to poor diet.

19. The practical nurse is concerned that several members of the community have a poor diet, consuming many foods that have little nutritional value. Which of the following is the underlying reason for the poor diet?

1. Indigenous people do not like the taste of fruits and vegetables.
2. Genetic makeup causes Indigenous people to crave foods with a high sugar content.
3. In northern Canada, sugar-filled foods and soft drinks are less expensive than foods that have a higher nutritional value.
4. There has been inadequate education regarding the dangers of poor nutrition.

20. On the reserve, many of the people are related. The practical nurse's 14-year-old niece comes to the community clinic for advice on birth control because she is sexually active. The other nurse who works in the clinic will not be on duty for another week. The practical nurse is concerned about confidentiality issues in treating a relative. What should she do?

1. Advise her niece to return to the clinic when the other nurse is on duty
2. Tell her niece that because she is a relative, she is not allowed to provide care to her
3. Attempt to arrange a physician consultation in a nearby community via a telehealth link
4. Provide the necessary health teaching to her niece while ensuring confidentiality and professional boundaries

END OF CASE 4

CASE 5

Ms. Bennett, a resident of a group home for young adults, has a history of bipolar 1 disorder. One day, she tells the practical nurse she has a date with a counsellor who works at the group home. Ms. Bennett says she has bought the counsellor a gold ring and they will go to an expensive restaurant because she is "very wealthy" and appreciates the help the counsellor has given her.

QUESTIONS 21 to 22 refer to this case.

21. Following the conversation with Ms. Bennett, what would be the most appropriate initial response by the practical nurse?

1. Set boundaries for Ms. Bennett by telling her that it is not appropriate to engage in social activities with her counsellor
2. Advise Ms. Bennett that the counsellor is not allowed to accept any type of gift from a client
3. Report the counsellor to his immediate supervisor and regulatory body
4. Document the conversation and clarify her perceptions with the counsellor directly

22. Which of the following statements would reflect the practical nurse's immediate concerns relating to the conversation with Ms. Bennett?

1. An inappropriate relationship has developed between Ms. Bennett and the counsellor.
2. Ms. Bennett is experiencing a manic episode of her mental health disorder.
3. The counsellor will be placed in an awkward, unprofessional position by Ms. Bennett.
4. The practical nurse will have no immediate concerns since she will understand that there is no truth in Ms. Bennett's claim.

END OF CASE 5

CASE 6

Mr. Braun, age 47 years, is brought to the hospital by ambulance after his wife found him unconscious. Following a computed tomography (CT) scan, he is diagnosed as having experienced a ruptured aneurysm with a prognosis of no hope of recovery. He has been admitted to a medical unit.

QUESTIONS 23 to 27 refer to this case.

23. Mr. Braun's practical nurse has never experienced the death of a client. What is his priority action to facilitate his competence to care for Mr. Braun and his family?

1. Reflect on his own beliefs and feelings about death
2. Research recent publications about death and dying
3. Talk with his co-workers about caring for a dying client
4. Ask for assistance with care for Mr. Braun

24. There is nothing written in Mr. Braun's health record concerning resuscitation. The practical nurse does not know what to do if Mr. Braun should "code." What should be the first step in determining action by the nursing staff in this situation?

1. Have the physician write a do-not-resuscitate order (DNR)
2. Ensure that all staff members are prepared to resuscitate Mr. Braun
3. Speak with the family regarding Mr. Braun's previously stated wishes or advance directive concerning end-of-life care
4. Research directives from the Canadian Council for Practical Nurse Regulators' *Code of Ethics for Licensed Practical Nurses in Canada* regarding end-of-life decision making

25. The physician has spoken with Mrs. Braun regarding the fact that her husband will most likely die within 48 hours. The practical nurse overhears Mrs. Braun telling her young-adult children in the family waiting room, "The doctors and nurses are doing everything they can. I know he is going to be okay, so don't worry." When the practical nurse speaks with Mrs. Braun, what would be an appropriate question to ask?

1. "Why did you tell your family that your husband is going to get better?"
2. "Tell me about your discussion with the physician."
3. "Would you like me to explain to you what the physician told you about your husband?"
4. "Have you told your children that their father is going to die?"

26. Mr. Braun dies shortly after being on the medical unit and is pronounced dead. What does the practical nurse need to document in the health record after his death?

1. Whether an autopsy will be conducted
2. Time of death and who pronounced the death
3. All specific hygiene care provided to the body
4. What time the family left the bedside

27. The practical nurse is having difficulty managing the grief he feels upon the death of Mr. Braun, and he has lingering feelings of inadequacy with regard to his support of the family. What should be the practical nurse's initial action to work through his grief?

1. Register for a course in palliative care
2. Discuss his feelings with colleagues
3. Recognize the feelings of inadequacy as normal grieving
4. Ask the unit manager how he could have done a better job of supporting the Braun family

END OF CASE 6

CASE 7

Ms. Hudson brings her 2-week-old infant, Jeremy, to the well-baby clinic. She requests help with breastfeeding from the practical nurse.

QUESTIONS 28 to 34 refer to this case.

28. Ms. Hudson does not think she is providing enough milk for Jeremy because she has small breasts. The practical nurse tells her that there are very few reasons why a woman cannot successfully breastfeed. Which of the following maternal conditions is a contraindication to breastfeeding?

1. Substance use
2. Inverted nipples
3. Mastitis
4. A diagnosis of cancer

29. Ms. Hudson is worried about Jeremy because she says her girlfriend's baby, who is bottle-fed, is putting on much more weight than Jeremy. What explanation should the practical nurse provide to Ms. Hudson?

1. Babies who are fed formula are generally overfed, and that is why they gain more weight.
2. Although breast milk is better for the baby's immune system, it lacks enough fat for adequate growth during the first 6 months.
3. Breastfed infants tend to be leaner and have less body fat, but this is not an indication of inadequate nutritional status.
4. Infant formulas have more calories per millilitre, so infants who are bottle-fed gain more weight.

30. What suggestion should the practical nurse provide to Ms. Hudson to increase her milk supply?

1. "Give more frequent feedings."
2. "Drink at least 15 glasses of water per day."
3. "Massage your breasts prior to feeding."
4. "Use oxytocin nasal spray to induce milk production."

31. How will Ms. Hudson best evaluate whether Jeremy is receiving adequate breast milk and fluids?

1. He will have six to eight wet diapers per day.
2. He will have good skin turgor.
3. She will weigh him before and after she breastfeeds him to determine how much he drinks at each feeding.
4. Jeremy will have at least one stool per day.

32. Ms. Hudson reports that sometimes Jeremy wakes up crying and cannot focus on feeding because he is so fussy. What should the practical nurse recommend in this situation?

1. "Change his diaper before feeding."
2. "Apply a cool cloth to his face."
3. "Increase the lighting to focus his attention on you."
4. "Hold him skin-to-skin and have him suck on your finger."

33. Ms. Hudson wonders if there is any point in continuing with breastfeeding because she wants to return to work in a few months. What is the most appropriate action for the practical nurse to suggest?

1. "After 2 months, you should gradually decrease breastfeeding so that your milk supply will have dried up when you return to work."
2. "Discuss with your partner the possibility of not returning to work."
3. "Feed Jeremy formula during the day and breastfeed at night so that this feeding pattern will be established when you return to work."
4. "I'll arrange a meeting with the lactation consultant for strategies to enable you to continue breastfeeding when you return to work."

34. Which of the following organizations has as its primary function the provision of support and education to breastfeeding women?

1. La Leche League International
2. Lamaze International
3. Public Health Agency of Canada
4. Victorian Order of Nurses (VON)

END OF CASE 7

CASE 8

Ms. Loates, age 67 years, has a subtotal gastrectomy for cancer of the stomach. After surgery, she returns to the acute medical unit with an IV and a nasogastric tube set to low intermittent suction (a Gomco pump).

QUESTIONS 35 TO 37 refer to this case.

35. Two hours after the subtotal gastrectomy, the practical nurse observes a small amount of bright red drainage from Ms. Loates's nasogastric tube. What should the practical nurse do?

1. Notify the physician immediately
2. Clamp the nasogastric tube for 1 hour
3. Recognize that this is an expected finding
4. Irrigate the nasogastric tube with iced saline

36. The practical nurse notes that there has been no nasogastric drainage for 30 minutes and determines that irrigation is required. There is an order to irrigate the nasogastric tube prn. How should the practical nurse irrigate the nasogastric tube?

1. Instill 30 mL of normal saline and withdraw slowly
2. Instill 20 mL of air and clamp off the suction for 1 hour
3. Instill 50 mL of saline and increase the pressure of the suction
4. Instill 15 mL of distilled water and disconnect the suction for 30 minutes

37. After a subtotal gastrectomy, pulmonary complications may occur. During the first 24 hours postoperatively, how would the practical nurse help to prevent pulmonary complications in Ms. Loates?

1. Frequent oral suctioning
2. Maintaining a consistent oxygen flow rate
3. Ambulating Ms. Loates to increase respiratory exchange
4. Promoting frequent turning, moving, and deep breathing

END OF CASE 8

CASE 9

Juanita is a 17-year-old woman who was diagnosed with a rare type of cancer at age 4 years. Although there have been several remissions, she has lived most of her life with pain and repeated hospitalizations. She experienced a terminal relapse and while in hospital decides she wishes no further treatment.

QUESTIONS 38 to 42 refer to this case.

38. The practical nurse needs to ensure Juanita is making an informed decision regarding refusal of treatment. What should the practical nurse say to best confirm Juanita is making an informed decision?

1. "Are you aware of what will happen if you refuse treatment?"

2. "Explain your understanding of what will happen if treatment is stopped."
3. "This is a very hard decision for you to make, isn't it?"
4. "I will make arrangements for you to speak with a client advocate so you are aware of the information you need to know before you make this decision."

39. Juanita's parents disagree with her decision. The practical nurse, who has a daughter close to Juanita's age, disagrees as well. According to the Canadian Council for Practical Nurse Regulators' *Code of Ethics for Licensed Practical Nurses in Canada* what is the practical nurse's primary role in this situation?

1. To be an advocate for Juanita after she has made an informed decision
2. To provide counselling to Juanita's parents to help them persuade Juanita to change her decision
3. To refrain from being Juanita's primary nurse because she has an ethical disagreement with her
4. To call a meeting of the health care team, including Juanita and her parents, to discuss her decision

40. Juanita's family is large and includes, in addition to her mother and father, five siblings. All of them visit and call requesting information about Juanita. At times, the family becomes frustrated with the nurses and complains that they are receiving confusing information about Juanita. How should the practical nurse best manage this situation?

1. Tell the family that only the parents will receive information about Juanita
2. Request that Juanita and her family choose a designated person to communicate with health care staff
3. Have Juanita be the person to provide all her family with relevant information
4. Ask the family to choose one primary nurse to speak with for all information about Juanita

41. Juanita is transferred to the palliative care service at her request. On the palliative unit, her family angrily tells the practical nurse that Juanita is receiving inadequate care. What would be the most helpful response from the practical nurse?

1. "I know how you feel. It is difficult when a loved one is in pain."
2. "I am sorry. We are understaffed and haven't been able to provide the best care."
3. "I will discuss your concern with the other nurses, and we will change her plan of care."
4. "Tell me what it is that is bothering you about your daughter's care."

42. Juanita has chosen a DNR status, which is documented on the health record. One night while the family is with Juanita, she stops breathing. Her mother screams at the practical nurse, "She's stopped breathing! Do something or I'll sue!" What should the practical nurse do?

1. Shake Juanita, as per CPR sequence, to stimulate her to breathe
2. Call a code
3. Take Juanita's pulse
4. Comfort her mother by reminding her this was Juanita's stated wishes and informed decision

END OF CASE 9

CASE 10

Mr. Partilucci, age 58 years, has type 2 diabetes. Several weeks ago, a pebble lodged in his shoe while he and his wife were hiking. He developed a large gangrenous area on his left foot and has been admitted to hospital.

QUESTIONS 43 to 45 refer to this case.

43. Mrs. Partilucci says that she cannot understand how this happened so rapidly. She asks the practical nurse what will happen to her husband's foot. Which of the following responses would provide her with the most accurate information?

1. "The blackened areas of the foot indicate that the tissue in these areas has died. The physician will probably remove those areas to keep the rest of the foot healthy."
2. "Your husband will likely have an amputation below the knee to ensure the disease does not progress any further."
3. "The doctor will have to explain what he will do for your husband. I cannot say what he will decide."
4. "It looks pretty serious. You probably should have sought medical attention before now."

44. Mrs. Partilucci would like to know more about diabetes and wants to be involved in her husband's care. How would the practical nurse best facilitate her learning at this time?

1. Provide her with handouts and the address of the local diabetes association
2. Arrange a meeting with Mrs. Partilucci and the diabetes nurse educator
3. Encourage Mrs. Partilucci to assist with all aspects of his in-hospital diabetes management
4. Tell Mrs. Partilucci that her husband will be able to manage his disease by himself after discharge, so she need not worry

45. Mr. Partilucci's son asks if he will get diabetes like his father. Which of the following responses by the practical nurse would best answer his question?

1. "You will not develop diabetes. There is no increase in your risk because your father has it."
2. "Yes, but probably not until you are over 40 years of age. The severity varies from person to person."
3. "Diabetes tends to have a familial link. I will give you some information about some of the risk factors and preventive strategies."
4. "Diabetes runs in families. Your mother does not have it, so your chance of developing diabetes is reduced by 50%."

END OF CASE 10

CASE 11

Mr. O'Morrissey works for a hydroelectric company and spends most of his time outdoors. He makes an appointment to see the practical nurse at the company health unit because he is concerned about a mole on his neck that has recently changed shape and colour. The practical nurse examines the lesion and finds it has an irregular border and looks very dark. She refers him to the company physician.

QUESTIONS 46 to 48 refer to this case.

46. The physician tells Mr. O'Morrissey he believes the mole may be malignant melanoma. Mr. O'Morrissey asks the practical nurse what this means. Which of the following responses by the practical nurse would be most accurate?

1. "It is a cancerous tumour that starts in the cells that produce pigment."
2. "It is a rare type of superficial skin cancer."
3. "It is caused by radiation from the sun."
4. "It is a tumour that grows from a freckle."

47. Mr. O'Morrissey is referred to a cancer specialist, who will perform a surgical excision of the melanoma. Prior to surgery, Mr. O'Morrissey returns to the company health clinic to speak with the practical nurse. He asks her whether she thinks the surgery will cure him of the cancer. Which of the following responses by the practical nurse would be most accurate?

1. "Malignant melanoma can generally be cured by surgery with little chance of relapse."
2. "Surgical removal will take care of only that one lesion; others are likely to develop."
3. "It is possible to cure malignant melanoma with surgery; however, this type of cancer is known to spread rapidly."
4. "Chemotherapy or radiation will follow the surgery."

48. Mr. O'Morrissey's surgery is successful, and he receives follow-up care at the company health clinic. The practical nurse teaches him about prevention of further melanomas. Which of the following would be most important for the practical nurse to teach Mr. O'Morrissey?

1. To stay out of direct sunlight
2. To wear protective headgear when outside
3. To routinely monitor skin and moles for any changes
4. To wear sunscreen with a sun protection factor (SPF) of at least 20

END OF CASE 11

CASE 12

Mr. Nigel, age 26, has a history of moderate to severe asthma since childhood. He presents at the community health clinic with chest tightness, dyspnea, and anxiety and states that he feels as though he is suffocating.

QUESTIONS 49 to 55 refer to this case.

49. What is the definition of asthma?

1. A genetic disorder that produces airway obstruction because of changes in glandular secretions
2. A condition characterized by destructive changes that result in a loss of lung elasticity
3. Chronic inflammation of the mucous membranes of the bronchi, causing excessive secretion of mucus
4. A chronic lung condition characterized by variable airflow obstruction as a result of airway hyper-responsiveness and airway inflammation

50. The practical nurse performs a chest assessment on Mr. Nigel. Which of the following manifestations would be of most concern to the practical nurse?

1. Wheezing on expiration
2. Wheezing on inspiration and expiration
3. Use of accessory muscles to breathe
4. Diminished or absent breath sounds

51. The practical nurse takes Mr. Nigel's vital signs and evaluates Mr. Nigel to be in a state of status asthmaticus. What should be the practical nurse's initial action?

1. Administer the ordered bronchodilator
2. Ask the client more questions to identify causative factors
3. Notify the physician of an emergency situation
4. Provide a bolus of IV fluid, as per protocol

52. Mr. Nigel is transferred to hospital and blood gas readings are taken. Evaluate the following arterial blood gases: partial pressure of oxygen (PaO_2) 72 mm Hg; partial pressure of carbon dioxide ($PaCO_2$) 50 mm Hg; pH 7.28.

1. Hypoxia, hypercapnia, and acidosis
2. Hypoxia, hypocapnia, and alkalosis
3. Hyperoxia, hypercapnia, and acidosis
4. Normal oxygen, hypocapnia, and alkalosis

53. Mr. Nigel is admitted to a medical unit at the hospital, where he receives health teaching prior to discharge. Which of the following strategies best demonstrates client-centred learning?

1. Immediately provide all necessary information on asthma to the client.
2. Use the teach-back technique when demonstrating the use of the inhaler.
3. Provide health teaching on how to use his medications at the nurse's station.
4. Use closed-ended questions to ensure the client understands the content.

54. According to best practice guidelines for the treatment of asthma, which of the following interventions is the most important component of Mr. Nigel's asthma management?

1. Eliminating or avoiding triggers
2. Education and the use of an action plan
3. Appropriate pharmacotherapy
4. Regular follow-up with a respirologist

55. The practical nurse demonstrates to Mr. Nigel the appropriate administration of his inhaled bronchodilator and inhaled steroid. Which of the following procedures is correct concerning the use of metered dose inhalers?

1. Shake the inhaler vigorously twice; then give two quick puffs of the inhaler
2. Put lips around the inhaler, and breathe out while depressing the canister
3. Use a spacer, such as an AeroChamber, if coordination cannot be achieved
4. Inhale as deeply as possible, and then depress the canister

END OF CASE 12

CASE 13

Ms. Wilmox, a 46-year-old mother of two adolescent children, has been admitted to an inpatient psychiatric unit. She is accompanied by her sister, who states that Ms. Wilmox has been using crack cocaine, alcohol, and possibly marijuana. The sister reports that Ms. Wilmox has a history of intermittent substance use but that she has been "clean" for almost 4 years. The practical nurse performs an admission assessment.

QUESTIONS 56 to 59 refer to this case.

56. What would be the practical nurse's primary concern with regard to Ms. Wilmox?

1. History of self-harm
2. Previous use of crack cocaine
3. Current substance use
4. Lack of support systems

57. During the assessment, Ms. Wilmox looks at the practical nurse intently and blinks her eyes in a rhythmic pattern. Ms. Wilmox states that she is answering his questions mentally and is projecting her responses directly into his mind. What would be the most appropriate action by the practical nurse?

1. Remind Ms. Wilmox that this is impossible and that she should answer his questions verbally
2. Advise Ms. Wilmox that she is suffering from the effects of drug use, and it would be better for her if she would answer questions appropriately
3. Excuse himself from the assessment and seek clarification from Ms. Wilmox's sister
4. Advise Ms. Wilmox that he is only able to understand spoken replies

58. The sister appears to know a significant amount of information relating to Ms. Wilmox's drug-use history. Which of the following actions by the practical nurse would ensure he is able to obtain the sister's information?

1. Ensure Ms. Wilmox is present when the sister is questioned
2. Ask Ms. Wilmox's permission to seek information from her sister
3. Speak to the sister separately without advising Ms. Wilmox, to avoid upsetting her
4. Insist that Ms. Wilmox sign a "confidentiality disclosure" document before he speaks to the sister

59. Later that evening, Ms. Wilmox becomes verbally abusive toward the sister and the practical nurse. Which of the following interventions is the most appropriate?

1. Place Ms. Wilmox in four-point restraints for the safety of herself and others
2. Advise Ms. Wilmox that abusive behaviour is not appropriate and will not be tolerated
3. Ignore the behaviour since it is most likely attention seeking
4. Give Ms. Wilmox the maximum ordered antianxiety medication

END OF CASE 13

CASE 14

A practical nurse works at a large manufacturing company and conducts weekly educational sessions with employees regarding a wide variety of health and wellness topics.

QUESTIONS 60 to 64 refer to this case.

60. The practical nurse discusses smoking cessation with a group of employees who are heavily dependent on nicotine. What should the practical nurse recommend as the most effective method to quit smoking?

1. Nicotine-replacement therapy
2. Hypnosis combined with aversion therapy
3. Group support programs and behavioural interventions
4. Any method that individuals feel will be effective for them

61. Mr. Louis, an employee, asks the practical nurse why he should get the seasonal influenza vaccine this year when he already got one last year. How should the practical nurse respond?

1. "The vaccine effect lasts for only 8 to 12 months."
2. "Because, as with your childhood immunizations, with the flu vaccine, you need a booster."
3. "The influenza viruses change into new strains every year, and there is a different vaccine for each specific strain."
4. "Each year, the process for refining the vaccine improves so that you will have better immunity with this year's vaccine."

62. The practical nurse talks about the importance of sleep. Mr. Steele, who works 12-hour shifts, complains that he has chronic insomnia. What strategies should the practical nurse recommend to help Mr. Steele improve his sleep?

1. A bedtime ritual combined with relaxation techniques
2. Moderate exercise 1 hour before bedtime
3. A mild over-the-counter sedative
4. A spicy meal 2 hours before bedtime

63. The practical nurse conducts WHMIS training for all employees. What is WHMIS?

1. Safety education to prevent accidents with manufacturing equipment
2. Training in infection control
3. Workplace Health Ministry Instructions for Safety
4. A system to control hazardous substances in the workplace

64. Many of the men and women at the company complain about the stress in their lives. The practical nurse discusses how stress affects the health and wellness of individuals. Which of the following statements is true regarding stress?

1. Men are more likely than women to experience stress.
2. Stress-management techniques should be tailored to the individual's stressors.
3. Stress is always harmful and causes physical and emotional illness.
4. Stress is primarily an urban myth and is not as prevalent as portrayed by the media.

END OF CASE 14

CASE 15

Ms. Magnusson, age 69 years, has been admitted to a medical unit with atrial fibrillation.

QUESTIONS 65 to 66 refer to this case.

65. Ms. Magnusson is to have an electrocardiogram (ECG). As the practical nurse explains the procedure, Ms. Magnusson asks if this test is really necessary because she does not want electricity going through her. Which of the following responses by the practical nurse would be most appropriate?

1. "The doctor has ordered this test, so you need to have it."
2. "The ECG provides necessary information about your heart's electrical patterns. It does not send electricity through you."
3. "Don't worry; only a small amount of electricity actually comes from the machine. The test is necessary so that there will be a baseline record of your heart's function."
4. "A lot of people ask about the electrical charge, but you will be fine and probably won't feel a thing."

66. Ms. Magnusson asks the practical nurse if her atrial fibrillation is a rare condition that can be prevented from recurring. Which of the following answers would be the practical nurse's best response?

1. "This is the most common heart rhythm disturbance in Canada. Reducing your alcohol and caffeine intake may help to prevent attacks."
2. "It is not rare. There are no lifestyle changes that can help to prevent it happening again."
3. "Many people have only one episode in their life. It is not really known why it happens."
4. "This is a rare condition caused by scarring in the heart, so it is uncertain whether it will recur."

END OF CASE 15

CASE 16

The Nursing Practice Committee at Mount Summit Hospital reviews medication policies and practice at its facility.

QUESTIONS 67 to 69 refer to this case.

67. At Mount Summit, nurses must complete an agency medication incident report when they discover a medication error. What is the intended and most important reason for medication incident reports?

1. Tracking errors and trends to improve client safety
2. Identifying nurses who require remediation in medication administration
3. Documentation of facts in case of future legal action
4. A record of client reaction and adverse effects of error

68. The committee would like to draft a policy concerning clients taking their own medication they have brought from home. What is the most important guiding principle when deciding if clients should administer their own medication?

1. Whether the physician has ordered the medication
2. Whether the medication interacts with any of the other ordered medications
3. Whether the drugs are considered to be high risk for error
4. Whether the client has the knowledge, skill, and judgement to self-administer

69. The committee discovers that many medication errors are caused by nurse fatigue. Which of the following has research shown to be the most effective strategy in decreasing nurse fatigue?

1. Limiting shift length to 8 hours
2. Prohibiting overtime shifts
3. Promoting equal day and night shifts
4. Providing choice of shift type and length

END OF CASE 16

CASE 17

Mrs. Douglas, age 83, lives in a long-term care facility. She has a history of dementia, hypertension, and right knee osteoarthritis. The unregulated care provider (UCP) tells the practical nurse that Mrs. Douglas complained of right knee stiffness when the UCP was providing personal care. The UCP also reports that Mrs. Douglas has dry skin on her lower legs and seems increasingly agitated and restless. Her vital signs are T 37. 3, HR 84, RR 18, and B/P 130/84.

QUESTIONS 70 to 74 refer to this case.

70. Which of the following findings should the practical nurse assess first?

1. B/P 130/84
2. Dry skin on her lower legs
3. Stiffness of right knee
4. Increasing agitation and restlessness

71. The practical nurse plans to obtain a urine sample to assess for a urinary tract infection (UTI). What is the most common pathogen leading to a UTI?

1. *Escherichia coli (E. coli)*
2. *Helicobacter pylori (H. pylori)*
3. *Candida albicans*
4. *Streptococcus pneumoniae*

72. The practical nurse performs a dipstick urine analysis test for initial assessment. What finding on the test strip would indicate that Mrs. Douglas may have a UTI?

1. Platelets
2. Leukocytes
3. Ketones
4. Potassium

73. What characteristics are common in the urine when a UTI is present?

1. Clear and odourless
2. Amber and sweet odour
3. Orange and odourless
4. Cloudy with a foul odour

74. Mrs. Douglas' urine sample comes back showing she has a urinary tract infection, and she is started on antibiotics. Which of the following nursing interventions would be recommended?

1. Apply an ice pack to the lower abdomen
2. Frequently offer her a glass of water or cranberry juice.
3. Leave her favorite drink, a cup of coffee, at her bedside table for her sip on
4. Stop the antibiotic therapy once her symptoms resolve

END OF CASE 17

CASE 18

Charlie, age 9 months, is admitted to the pediatric unit with diarrhea and dehydration related to gastroenteritis. He has been breastfed but has lost a great deal of fluid due to numerous watery stools. The practical nurse assesses Charlie.

QUESTIONS 75 to 78 refer to this case.

75. Which of the following organisms is the most common causative organism for infant gastroenteritis?

1. *Escherichia coli* (*E. coli*)
2. Shigella
3. Rotavirus
4. Salmonella

76. The practical nurse assesses Charlie for dehydration. Which of the following manifestations would be of most concern to the practical nurse?

1. Poor skin turgor
2. A sunken fontanelle
3. Dry mucous membranes
4. A rapid, thready pulse

77. Charlie needs intravenous rehydration. The physician orders a bolus of 0.9% sodium chloride, then IV+ p.o. to equal 20 mL/kg per hour. Charlie weighs 9 kg. He drinks 120 mL of oral electrolyte solution and will be fed again in 3 hours. At what hourly rate should the IV be infused for the next 3 hours?

1. 60 mL
2. 120 mL
3. 140 mL
4. 220 mL

78. Charlie responds well to IV treatment, and his vital signs stabilize. He is discharged. What nutrition would be recommended for Charlie to maintain hydration?

1. Breast milk and oral rehydration solutions
2. Soy formula and glucose water
3. BRAT diet and breast milk
4. Half-strength lactose-free formula and apple juice

END OF CASE 18

CASE 19

Mr. Clarkson, age 40 years, has been brought to an emergency psychiatric facility by the police after he assaulted his neighbour. He has had numerous episodes of violent behaviour in the past. He is diagnosed as having an antisocial personality disorder. He is placed in the close observation unit.

QUESTIONS 79 to 82 refer to this case.

79. The practical nurse performs an admission assessment on Mr. Clarkson. Mr. Clarkson says he is concerned about confidentiality and does not want anyone listening to what he tells her. Where is the best setting for the practical nurse to conduct the interview?

1. In a private interview room, situated close to the rest of the clients but with the door closed
2. In an open area, where there are others to provide safety
3. In a room close to the nursing station, with the practical nurse seated between Mr. Clarkson and the door
4. In a room with a police officer beside her

80. Which concept about antisocial personality disorders should the practical nurse consider when planning care for Mr. Clarkson?

1. He may suffer from a great deal of anxiety.
2. He probably cannot postpone gratification.
3. He will rapidly learn by experience and punishment.
4. He will have a great sense of responsibility toward others.

81. Which of the following is characteristic of people who have an antisocial personality disorder?

1. They have a history of chronic depression.
2. They do not easily become frustrated.
3. They are motivated to change their behaviour.
4. They have a lifelong pattern of maladaptive behaviour.

82. Mr. Clarkson asks the practical nurse for her phone number so that he can call her for a date. How should the practical nurse respond?

1. "We are not permitted to date clients."
2. "No, you are the client, and I am the nurse."
3. "Thank you, but our relationship is professional."
4. "It is against my personal and professional ethics to date clients."

END OF CASE 19

CASE 20

A practical nurse is a preceptor for a recent practical nursing graduate Ms. Baldassarian. He teaches the new graduate practical nurse about the care of a peripherally inserted central catheter (PICC).

QUESTIONS 83 to 85 refer to this case.

83. Prior to changing a PICC line dressing, which of the following preparatory steps is important in preventing infection?

1. Donning an N-95 mask
2. Preparing a clean area with appropriate supplies

3. Using antimicrobial swabs to cleanse the exit site and catheter
4. Wearing nonsterile gloves

84. The new graduate documents a dressing change in the client's health record. Which of the following examples is the most accurate documentation?

1. 10/29/21 1000 PICC dressing changed right upper arm. Skin intact, no signs of infection. Site cleansed with chlorhexidine gluconate swabs. New securement device and dressing applied. S. Baldassarian, RPN.
2. 10/29/21 1000 PICC line site healthy, taught client care of dressing. S. Baldassarian, RPN.
3. 10/29/21 1000 PICC line dressing changed right upper arm. New dressing applied after site cleansed with chlorhexidine as per Dr. Ogden's orders, pt. tolerated procedure well. S. Baldassarian, RPN.
4. 10/29/21 1000 Old transparent semipermeable dressing changed, catheter in place. S. Baldassarian, RPN.

85. As a learner, which of the following guidelines does the new graduate understand?

1. She must clarify her knowledge and limitations with her preceptor.
2. Her preceptor is co-responsible for the care she provides to clients.
3. Her preceptor has the responsibility to identify the need for supervision in client care situations.
4. She is solely accountable for all errors even if she is directed by the preceptor to provide care beyond her level of competency.

END OF CASE 20

CASE 21

Ms. Baverstock, age 94 years, is a resident in a long-term care facility. She is in the midstage of Alzheimer's disease and has dysphagia. Her nurse is the preceptor for a second-year practical nursing student who is interested in the care of older persons.

QUESTIONS 86 to 89 refer to this case.

86. The nurse teaches the practical nursing student about dysphagia. Which of the following statements would be accurate information?

1. "Always give liquids with a straw so that the client can place them more accurately in the mouth."
2. "Dysphagic clients are best fed by gastrostomy tube."
3. "Spices and seasonings should be kept to a minimum as they may stimulate the gag reflex."
4. "Dysphagic assessment and teaching are usually performed by a trained speech therapist."

87. Ms. Baverstock has a pressure injury on her ankle. During the dressing change, the practical nursing student asks the nurse why she is using a hydrogel dressing. Which of the following explanations would provide the correct information?

1. It allows the nurses to see the wound without having to change the dressing.
2. It maintains a moist environment to promote wound healing.
3. It provides a surface that will resist the irritation of bed linens.
4. It is used to remove moisture from the wound

88. Ms. Baverstock's husband died many years ago. She tells the student that when her husband comes to take her home, she would like her to visit them for dinner. Which of the following approaches by the student would be most therapeutic?

1. Gently explain to Ms. Baverstock that her husband died, and she now lives in a residence
2. Tell Ms. Baverstock that she is very kind, but it would be unethical for her to arrange a visit outside the facility
3. Ask Ms. Baverstock what her favourite foods are for dinner
4. Sit quietly with Ms. Baverstock and hold her hand

89. Ms. Baverstock often wanders at night, disturbing other clients. Which of the following nursing actions would be the safest approach to care for Ms. Baverstock when she wanders?

1. Request that a relative come in to sit with her at night
2. Repeat her nighttime sedation when she starts to walk around
3. Apply restraints to ensure that she remains in bed
4. Encourage her to stay near the nursing station rather than wander elsewhere

END OF CASE 21

CASE 22

A practical nurse works at a summer camp for children who have chronic illnesses.

QUESTIONS 90 to 94 refer to this case.

90. Several of the children begin experiencing fever and runny noses. What action should the practical nurse initially implement?

1. Notify the parents of the affected children
2. Arrange for the affected children to be treated with antipyretics and fluids

3. Isolate the affected children in a separate cabin
4. Examine the rest of the children in the camp for similar symptoms

91. A counsellor brings Hunter, age 9, to the first aid room because a wasp has stung him. What is the priority consideration by the practical nurse in this situation?

1. Determine if Hunter has had any previous anaphylactic or allergic response to insect bites
2. Give Hunter an antihistamine, as per medical directive
3. Provide comfort and reassurance to Hunter
4. Attempt to remove the stinger

92. The practical nurse realizes at 0830 hours that he has administered the 0800 furosemide (Lasix) to Madison instead of Meghan, for whom the furosemide not lasix was ordered. What is the priority action by the practical nurse?

1. Notify the prescribing physician
2. Document the error on the health forms of Madison and Meghan
3. Assess and monitor Madison for any adverse reactions to the furosemide not lasix
4. Administer the correct dose of furosemide to Meghan

93. The family of Fatima gives the practical nurse gift certificates from a local coffee shop for looking after their child. What is the most appropriate response by the practical nurse to Fatima's family?

1. "I am not allowed to accept gifts."
2. "You are very kind, and I will take good care of Fatima."
3. "Why are you giving me a gift?"
4. "I will share this gift with the rest of the health care staff."

94. After working at the camp for 2 weeks, a practical nurse discovers that he was exposed to chicken pox just prior to leaving home for the camp. He has never had chicken pox. What is the most appropriate action by the practical nurse?

1. Withdraw from providing care to the children at the camp
2. Contact his personal physician for advice
3. Ensure appropriate infection control practices, such as an N-95 mask
4. Obtain immunization for chicken pox from the camp physician

END OF CASE 22

CASE 23

Ms. Anderson, a postmenopausal woman, discovers a lump in her breast while bathing. She delays going to the doctor for several weeks until her husband insists that she have the lump examined. A fine-needle aspiration confirms that the lump is malignant.

QUESTIONS 95 to 97 refer to this case.

95. The physician suggests that Ms. Anderson have breast conservation surgery (a lumpectomy), followed by radiation therapy. Ms. Anderson asks the practical nurse if she should have a modified radical mastectomy instead of the lumpectomy in case there has been spread of the cancer to her lymph nodes. Which of the following responses by the practical nurse would provide the most accurate information?

1. "Both surgical approaches remove lymph nodes."
2. "Research indicates that both surgeries have similar results."
3. "I think you require more information from your physician to clarify these options."
4. "The decision is really up to you; I'm not sure what I would do."

96. Ms. Anderson states that she cannot think of anyone else in her family who has had breast cancer. She tells the practical nurse that she has been on hormone replacement therapy (HRT) and asks if this puts her at a higher risk for developing breast cancer. Which of the following responses by the practical nurse would be most accurate?

1. "Studies indicate that long-term use may put a woman at greater risk."
2. "Most women who develop breast cancer have no identifiable risk factors."
3. "Estrogen is naturally occurring in your body, so I don't think it would be a cause."
4. "It is probably genetic, and you could not have prevented it."

97. Ms. Anderson's husband asks if there are any observations he should be alert for while his wife receives treatment for her cancer. What would be the most appropriate response by the practical nurse?

1. "Make sure she comes in for her scheduled treatment, and everything should be fine."
2. "Your wife will know if she is experiencing serious problems and will seek medical attention."
3. "There are a number of facts you should know about the surgery and chemotherapy. I will give you a complete list before she is discharged."
4. "It is great that Ms. Anderson has someone who is concerned for her."

END OF CASE 23

CASE 24

Mr. Thompson, age 60 years, makes an appointment with his family physician because his dentist told him to have the sore on the undersurface of his tongue examined by a doctor. Mr. Thompson has not had regular dental care for many years.

QUESTIONS 98 to 100 refer to this case.

98. The physician diagnoses oral cancer, and Mr. Thompson has a hemiglossectomy. Which of the following assessments would be a priority when Mr. Thompson returns to the unit from the postanesthetic care unit?

1. Pulse oximetry
2. Level of pain
3. Airway clearance
4. Level of consciousness

99. Postoperatively, which of the following positions would be most suitable for Mr. Thompson?

1. Supine with his head immobilized
2. A semi-Fowler position
3. Sims position
4. A left lateral position

100. Mr. Thompson asks the practical nurse what he can do in the future to reduce the risk of the cancer recurring. Which of the following points would the practical nurse cover in health teaching?

1. Preventive dental care
2. Eating a diet according to *Canada's Food Guide*
3. Drinking plenty of fluid to keep well hydrated
4. Exercising at least three times a week

END OF CASE 24

INDEPENDENT QUESTIONS

QUESTIONS 101 to 200 do not refer to a particular case.

101. Some competitive athletes have been known to abuse central nervous system stimulants such as the amphetamine methylphenidate hydrochloride (Ritalin). Which of the following effects do these drugs have on an athlete's performance?

1. Enhance muscle strength and performance
2. Improve fine and gross motor coordination
3. Increase the ability to manage the stress of competition
4. Increase alertness and provide relief from fatigue

102. An infant has torticollis. Which of the following therapeutic interventions would be recommended by the practical nurse to treat this condition?

1. Gentle stretching exercises in the neck
2. Range-of-motion exercises for the legs
3. Positioning of the infant in the supine position when asleep
4. Extra padding in the diapers to hold the hips in adduction

103. Carys, age 8 years, is brought to the pediatrician's office displaying manifestations of allergic rhinitis. What initial question should the practical nurse performing the health assessment ask of the parents?

1. "Do you have pets at home?"
2. "Does anyone in the household smoke cigarettes?"
3. "Is there a family history of allergies?"
4. "Can you tell me the history and pattern of her symptoms?"

104. The parents of a 10-year-old child have just been informed that their son's disease is terminal. They will need to learn some skills associated with his palliative care needs. What is the initial consideration for the practical nurse when she plans teaching with his parents?

1. Individualizing the teaching plan
2. Assessing their readiness to learn
3. Planning evaluation criteria
4. Determining their baseline knowledge

105. Which of the following clients would be at greatest risk for developing delirium when admitted to an acute care facility?

1. A 21-year-old male with renal colic and a history of drug abuse
2. An 87-year-old male with congestive heart failure
3. A 42-year-old male with appendicitis and depression
4. A 53-year-old female with ovarian cancer

106. Why do corticosteroids increase a client's risk for infections?

1. Corticosteroids increase the production of leukocytes.
2. Corticosteroids interfere with antibody production in the lymphatic tissues.
3. Corticosteroids promote the growth and spread of enteric viruses.
4. Corticosteroids suppress the inflammatory response of the body.

107. Ms. Pitre, age 35 years, tells the practical nurse she is very worried because her doctor has found a condyloma during her annual gynecological exam. She is waiting for biopsy results to see if it is cancerous. Which of the following statements by the practical nurse would be the most therapeutic?

1. "Sexually transmitted condylomas are a risk factor for developing cervical cancer."
2. "It is very upsetting to have to wait for a biopsy report."
3. "You probably don't have cancer because a condyloma is usually benign."
4. "Even if it's cervical cancer, you don't have to worry much because the cure rate is high."

108. When auscultating Ms. Gash's lungs, the practical nurse hears a dry, grating sound on inspiration. Ms. Gash is asked to cough, but the sound persists and is loudest over the lower, lateral, anterior surface. Which of the following conditions would most likely explain what the practical nurse is hearing?

1. A wheeze due to a narrowed bronchus
2. A pericardial friction rub
3. A pleural friction rub
4. An atelectatic lobe

109. The practical nurse plans to take the blood pressure of Emma, a preschool-age child prior to surgery. Which approach by the practical nurse indicates an understanding of growth and development?

1. Provide Emma with verbal instructions explaining blood pressure.
2. Provide Emma with pictures showing her how blood pressure is taken.
3. Allow Emma to help the practical nurse take the blood pressure of a teddy bear.
4. Encourage Emma to ask questions about the procedure.

110. Which of the following recordings is the most accurate and objective example of client documentation?

1. "Mr. Tang has a history of alcohol misuse."
2. "Ms. Gileppo has a large sacral pressure injury."
3. "Ms. Lok's urine specific gravity is 1.030."
4. "Mr. Halsey showed a high level of anxiety."

111. A practical nurse must prioritize client care when beginning a night shift at 1945 hours. Which of the following clients should be seen first?

1. A client who was scheduled for turning every 2 hours, on the even hours
2. A client who is receiving a continuous gastrostomy tube feeding by infusion pump
3. A client who had a hypoglycemic episode at 1900 hours
4. A client who was medicated for pain at 1930 hours

112. A practical nurse works at a community clinic where most of the clients are from countries other than Canada. In caring for these multiethnic clients, what is the most important cultural principle that the practical nurse should follow?

1. The client is the primary source of data.
2. Family members should always be included in care.
3. Health beliefs and practices of clients may be different from those of the practical nurse.
4. Culturally sensitive care may be provided only if the practical nurse has knowledge of the culture.

113. Which of the following points about alcohol consumption would be included in health teaching for a client with newly diagnosed type 2 diabetes mellitus?

1. No alcohol should be consumed while taking diabetic medications.
2. Alcohol increases the ability of the pancreas to produce insulin.
3. Both diabetics and nondiabetics should observe the same precautions about moderation of alcohol consumption.
4. Alcohol may be consumed, but the client must monitor the effects on his blood sugar and incorporate the calories into his meal plan.

114. Ms. Davis has a urinary tract infection. Which of the following teaching points would the practical nurse review with her?

1. "Take a daily shower, not a tub bath."
2. "Increase your intake of apple juice."
3. "Void every hour during the day."
4. "Do not have intercourse until urine cultures are negative."

115. Prostate cancer is the most common cancer in Canadian men, excluding skin cancer Which of the following statements about prostate cancer is true?

1. It is reliably diagnosed by the prostate-specific antigen (PSA).
2. Surgical removal is the treatment of choice.
3. Cancer must be confirmed by a prostate biopsy.
4. Treatment causes impotence and incontinence.

116. Mr. Laszlo, age 21 years, is brought to the health clinic because he has been hearing voices. The practical nurse is concerned that this is a sign of schizophrenia. When considering Mr. Laszlo's manifestations, which of the following factors should the practical nurse take into consideration?

1. Substance misuse can mimic some of the symptoms of schizophrenia.
2. He should be assessed by a psychiatrist immediately.
3. The nurse needs to implement safety precautions because the client may be violent.
4. He is too young to display any type of first-episode psychosis.

117. Ms. Dougherty, age 76 years, has aphasia. The practical nurse did not obtain a written consent before inserting an indwelling urinary catheter. Which of the following statements accurately reflects this situation?

1. The catheter was necessary, so written consent was not required.
2. This treatment requires a specific written consent form.
3. This situation is an example of treatment without consent, which is contrary to Canadian laws.
4. Consent may be obtained by nonverbal communication.

118. Mr. Peter has obstructive sleep apnea. He has been evaluated in a sleep clinic and has been told he must use a continuous positive airway pressure (CPAP) machine at night. Mr. Peter asks the practical nurse what this machine will do for him. Which of the following statements would be the practical nurse's best response?

1. "It is a machine that will stop you from snoring and waking up in the night."
2. "The machine uses air pressure to keep your airways open so that you will be able to breathe normally and get a better night's sleep."
3. "The machine increases air flow to the lungs so that your oxygen saturation does not drop, and you sleep better."
4. "The machine delivers oxygen to you all night, taking the strain off your lungs and heart."

119. Audrey, age 7 years, has pediculosis. What treatment would the practical nurse recommend to Audrey's parents?

1. A specifically formulated pediculicide shampoo
2. An antifungal cream
3. An over-the-counter antibiotic cream (Polysporin)
4. A salicylic acid preparation

120. Mr. Prahdeep, an 83-year-old male living in a long-term care facility with moderate Alzheimer's disease, is experiencing sundowning. What is the best approach by the practical nurse when caring for this client?

1. Provide him with an evening snack of cookies and coffee or tea
2. Ensure he receives a large evening meal
3. Give him a bath each evening
4. Close the curtains in the evening and turn on the lights.

121. Jaymee, age 11 years, has exercise-induced asthma. Which of the following recommendations relating to exercise would the practical nurse suggest to Jaymee?

1. She should participate in sports such as swimming rather than soccer.
2. She should self-administer her beta-2 agonist shortly before exercise.
3. She can participate in sports, but not during cold weather.
4. If her peak flow readings are within normal ranges, she may exercise as tolerated.

122. Ms. Gianopoulos is ordered complete bedrest because she is experiencing a pregnancy complication. She begins to cry and states, "I have two small children at home. Who is going to look after them?" How should the practical nurse respond?

1. "Let's talk about how you can get the help you need."
2. "You are worried about how you will be able to manage?"
3. "You'll be able to fix meals, and the children can go to day care."
4. "Your husband will be able to look after the children."

123. Ms. Jaffer comes to the emergency department experiencing rapid heartbeat, shakiness, shortness of breath, and dizziness. She is diagnosed with panic disorder. Which of the following therapeutic interventions would be most effective during the initial treatment of Ms. Jaffer?

1. Biofeedback
2. Identification of anxiety triggers
3. Medication with lorazepam (Ativan)
4. Initiation of selective serotonin reuptake inhibitors

124. Mr. Loek has been diagnosed with a borderline personality disorder. What therapeutic approach by the practical nurse is appropriate during counselling with Mr. Loek?

1. Provide solutions for his behavioural problems
2. Modify therapeutic approaches depending on his mood

3. Discuss his ambivalent feelings toward staff members
4. Reinforce acceptable behaviour

125. The practical nurse is preparing to administer isophane insulin suspension (NPH) and regular insulin to Mr. Blanche. How should the practical nurse administer these two insulin preparations?

1. "Administer the two insulins in the same syringe only if the ratio is 1:1."
2. "Mix the two insulins in the prescribed doses in the same syringe."
3. "Administer the two insulins in the different syringes and at different times."
4. "Administer each insulin in a separate syringe, using different sites for injection."

126. Clients on sodium-reduced diets need to be aware that sodium occurs naturally in foods and is added during processing. Which of the following foods would be highest in sodium?

1. Canned vegetable soup
2. Natural cheese
3. Fresh fish
4. Whole-wheat pasta

127. Which of the following behaviours is an example of passive–aggressive behaviour?

1. Pounding a wall
2. Chronic lateness
3. Sarcasm
4. Piercing stares

128. Mrs. Willona is day 1 postpartum following the delivery of a healthy 4 100-g infant. What instructions should the practical nurse provide to her about Kegel exercises?

1. "When you are urinating or having a bowel movement, hold your breath and bear down."
2. "Delay urinating for as long as you can to strengthen the sphincter muscles."
3. "Tighten the muscles in your anus before you have a bowel movement."
4. "To target the muscles, pretend you are stopping the flow of urine in midstream."

129. A practical nurse is performing a sterile wound irrigation wearing goggles, a gown, and gloves. After removing and disposing of the soiled dressings, what is the next action the practical nurse must perform?

1. Discard the gloves
2. Open the dressing tray
3. Perform hand hygiene
4. Close the room door or bed curtains

130. Ms. Vernon is hospitalized with active pulmonary tuberculosis. Which of the following diagnostic results would be the most important in determining whether respiratory isolation and airborne precautions can be discontinued?

1. The two-step Mantoux tuberculin skin test is negative.
2. Ms. Vernon's chest radiograph shows improved consolidation.
3. A sputum sample is clear of acid-fast bacteria.
4. Ms. Vernon's temperature has returned to normal for 24 hours.

131. Ms. Diniz, age 85 years, is a client in a long-term care facility. The practical nurse suspects Ms. Diniz has developed fecal impaction. Which of the following statements by Ms. Diniz might indicate fecal impaction?

1. "I have a lot of gas pains."
2. "I don't have much of an appetite."
3. "I feel like I have to go and just can't."
4. "I haven't had a bowel movement for 2 days."

132. Toxoplasmosis in a pregnant woman can cause fetal anomalies. To prevent toxoplasmosis, which of the following measures should the practical nurse advise pregnant clients to avoid?

1. Contact with cat feces
2. People who have viral illnesses
3. Ingestion of freshwater fish
4. Exposure to children who have not been immunized

133. A practical nurse encounters a motor vehicle accident on the way home from work. Mr. Cahuas is found under the wreckage of his car. He is conscious and breathing satisfactorily. He is lying on his back complaining of pain in his back and an inability to move his legs. What should be the first action by the practical nurse?

1. Leave Mr. Cahuas lying on his back with instructions not to move, and then seek help
2. Gently raise Mr. Cahuas to a sitting position to see if the pain either diminishes or increases in intensity
3. Roll Mr. Cahuas onto his abdomen, place a pad under his head, and cover him with any material available
4. Gently lift Mr. Cahuas onto a flat piece of lumber and call 9-1-1

134. Ms. Chu is diagnosed with expressive aphasia. Which of the following difficulties related to the aphasia should the practical nurse include in the nursing care plan?

1. Speaking or writing
2. Following specific instructions
3. Understanding speech
4. Recognizing words for familiar objects

135. A community practical nurse speaks with a father who is concerned that there is a yellow-crusted discharge around the glans penis of his recently circumcised newborn. How should the practical nurse advise the father?

1. "This is a sign of an infection, and he will require antibiotics."
2. "If he is voiding normally, this is part of the healing process and just needs daily cleansing with water."
3. "This is a sign that there needs to be better cleansing of the area, so soak the penis in half-strength hydrogen peroxide."
4. "Problems such as these are one of the reasons health care providers do not recommend circumcision."

136. Mr. Edwards has a midthigh amputation following a severe snowboarding accident. One week after the amputation, how would the practical nurse best control edema in the residual limb?

1. Administer the prescribed diuretic
2. Restrict Mr. Edwards's oral fluid intake
3. Keep his residual limb elevated on a pillow
4. Rewrap the elastic bandage as necessary

137. North Beaver Creek Hospital is on alert to receive victims of an explosion in a manufacturing plant. The health care team reviews the triage procedure. Which of the following injuries would be the highest priority to receive care?

1. Closed fractures of major bones
2. Partial-thickness burns of 10% of the body
3. Epistaxis
4. Severe lacerations involving open fractures of major bones

138. Ms. Moss is a practical nurse who works on a busy surgical unit. This is her fourth 12-hour night shift in a row. Although she has already had her break at 0400 hours, she feels ill and is so tired that she is having difficulty staying awake. All her clients are stable, and do not require any care until 0500 hours. What would be the practical nurse's most appropriate action?

1. Contact her immediate nursing supervisor
2. Put her head down on the desk at the nurse's station
3. Attempt to stay awake
4. Have a co-worker who is presently on break care for her clients while she sleeps

139. Jackson, age 4 days, is brought to the health clinic by his mother. The practical nurse assesses that the baby has a purulent discharge from the eyes. What is the most likely cause for the discharge?

1. A *Chlamydia trachomatis* infection
2. Congenital syphilis
3. An allergic reaction to allergens in the home
4. A reaction to the ophthalmic antibiotic ointment instilled after birth

140. A practical nurse works in a busy outpatient department where a team of nurses is responsible for all clients. The practical nurse finds that with this system, there is very little continuity of care, some interventions are missed or unnecessarily repeated, and clients are anxious because they do not have one specific nurse to speak with. What is the most appropriate action by the practical nurse?

1. Advocate for a system that provides better consistency of care
2. Ask to be assigned to a limited and specific number of clients at each shift
3. Complain to the nursing manager that this system of care is not optimum
4. Understand that the present system of care is necessary to efficiently manage the client numbers

141. Mrs. Scales asks the practical nurse what she should do to cure the upper respiratory infection (cold) she has. What would be the practical nurse's best advice?

1. Go to the doctor to get a prescription for an antibiotic
2. Ask the doctor for a prescription for an antiviral medication
3. Drink warm fluids and try alternative therapies such as echinacea and zinc lozenges.
4. Do nothing since there is no cure for the common cold

142. A practical nurse discusses menstruation with a young teenage girl. Which of the following practices would be included in the counselling regarding menstruation?

1. "Do not bathe during menstruation."
2. "Change tampons every 2 to 4 hours."
3. "Use only sanitary napkins because tampons cause toxic shock syndrome."
4. "Douche regularly with a commercial product or vinegar and water."

143. Mrs. Kyros is being treated for infertility due to endometriosis. Which of the following manifestations is characteristic of endometriosis?

1. Amenorrhea
2. Anovulation
3. Dysmenorrhea
4. Pelvic inflammation

144. A practical nurse observes another nurse fondling the breasts of an unresponsive female client. What should be the practical nurse's initial action?

1. Intervene by requesting that her colleague leave the client's room
2. Immediately report what she has observed to the unit manager
3. Report her colleague to the provincial regulatory body
4. Make a written report of what she has observed

145. Which of the following pathological conditions is a common complication of osteoporosis?

1. Spiral fractures of the radius
2. Compression fractures of the spine
3. Displaced fractures of the tibia
4. Avulsed fracture of the phalanges

146. Nurses working in a nephrology unit use automatic equipment for vital sign monitoring. At the beginning of a shift, the practical nurse obtains a blood pressure reading of 195/120 mm Hg for Mr. Fernandes. His readings have previously been in the range of 132/94 to 140/96 mm Hg. He displays no other symptoms of hypertension. What should be the practical nurse's initial action?

1. Notify the physician
2. Administer the ordered prn antihypertensive medication
3. Change the cuff to his other arm
4. Retake the blood pressure again using the automated equipment, then compare using a manual sphygmomanometer and cuff

147. Mr. Alberto has Parkinson's disease. The practical nurse overhears his wife say to him, "If you take your medicines, you will be able to walk better, and you will be cured." What should the practical nurse say to Mr. Alberto's wife?

1. "I am glad to hear you encouraging your husband to take his medications."
2. "Has there been a problem with your husband taking his medications?"
3. "Why are you saying this to your husband when you know that, although the medications will help him, there is no cure for Parkinson's?"
4. "What is your understanding about how Parkinson's disease is affecting your husband?"

148. Which type of cancer causes the highest death rate in the Canadian population?

1. Lung
2. Breast
3. Prostate
4. Colorectal

149. The practical nurse repositions a client in bed and observes a blistered area on the client's heel. What is the classification of this pressure injury?

1. Stage 1
2. Stage 2
3. Stage 3
4. Stage 4

150. Linda, age 15 years, is diagnosed with moderate idiopathic scoliosis. What is the treatment of choice for moderate idiopathic scoliosis?

1. An external spinal orthosis such as the Boston Brace
2. Surgical correction of the curve
3. Therapeutic exercises
4. External electrical stimulation of the spinal muscles

151. Ms. Benergan has had unprotected sex and obtains emergency contraception from a pharmacy in the form of a high-dose estrogen–progestin combination (Plan B). How does this emergency contraception prevent pregnancy?

1. If taken before ovulation, it prevents or delays ovulation.
2. If taken after ovulation, it stimulates menstruation.
3. If taken after ovulation, it causes the fertilized ovum to stop developing.
4. If taken after fertilization, it causes the ovum to abort.

152. Mr. Chask has severe pain. Which medication would be the most appropriate treatment for the pain?

1. Acetaminophen (Tylenol)
2. Lorazepam (Ativan)
3. Aacetylsalicylic acid (ASA)
4. Morphine sulphate (Morphine)

153. Mr. Leslie works as an unregulated care provider in a chronic care facility. He has been trained to suction

the tracheotomy of a stable long-term client and has performed this routine care for many years. Another client with a tracheotomy develops pneumonia. Mr. Leslie tells the practical nurse that to save her time, he can suction the client with pneumonia. Which of the following answers would be the practical nurse's best response?

1. Explain to Mr. Leslie that if she is very busy, he may perform the procedure but that she is ultimately responsible
2. Tell Mr. Leslie that he may not suction this client because suctioning a client with pneumonia is different from suctioning a client who has a permanent, well-established tracheotomy and is not considered routine care
3. Thank Mr. Leslie for understanding that she has a very heavy workload and let him perform the procedure
4. Tell Mr. Leslie that she will do all the suctioning in the future and that he should not be performing suctioning at all

154. A public education campaign that occurred during the 1990s following research findings about sudden unexpected infant death syndrome (SUIDS) is credited with reducing the mortality from SUIDS by 50%. What action did the public education campaign recommend to parents?

1. Position infants in the supine position for sleep
2. Breastfeed the infant until 6 months to confer maternal antibodies
3. Place infants in the prone position to prevent aspiration
4. Use baby monitors for high-risk infants

155. A hospitalized client, Mr. Morgan, refuses his prescribed medication because it upsets his stomach. Which of the following actions by the practical nurse would be most appropriate?

1. Ask Mr. Morgan's wife to convince him to take the medication
2. Put the medication in his juice as this will disguise the taste
3. Tell Mr. Morgan that if he does not take the medication, he will not get better
4. Consult with the physician or pharmacist about Mr. Morgan's refusal of the medication

156. Which of the following manifestations would be most indicative of an early sign of cervical cancer?

1. Abdominal heaviness and discomfort
2. Foul-smelling vaginal discharge
3. Pressure on the bladder
4. Bloody spotting after intercourse

157. Ms. Coton has breast cancer. She asks the practical nurse what the term estrogen receptor–positive (*ER-positive*) refers to. Which of the following responses by the practical nurse provides correct information?

1. "It indicates whether axillary lymph nodes are involved."
2. "It states the need for supplemental estrogen."
3. "It refers to a potential response to hormone therapy."
4. "It refers to the degree of metastasis that has occurred."

158. Mr. Lemone takes nitroglycerine in the form of Nitrolingual translingual spray. How would the effectiveness of the nitroglycerine best be evaluated?

1. By the relief of anginal pain
2. By improved cardiac output
3. By a decrease in blood pressure
4. By the dilation of superficial blood vessels

159. The parents of a child who has had open-heart surgery are informed that their child is in the postanaesthetic care unit and is stable. They are crying and extremely worried. How can the practical nurse best help decrease the parents' anxiety?

1. Reassure them that their child is doing well
2. Allow them to continue to express their feelings
3. Bring them to the postanaesthetic care unit for several minutes
4. Encourage them to return in 1 hour when the child is transferred to the intensive care unit

160. Ms. Li has an arteriovenous fistula (AVF) in her left forearm for her hemodialysis treatments. What is an important nursing consideration when caring for Ms. Li?

1. IV insertion may be performed in either arm
2. Routine blood tests are best taken in the left arm
3. Take the blood pressure only in the right arm
4. The AVF should never be palpated

161. Which of the following behaviours produces the highest risk for the transmission of HIV?

1. Vaginal intercourse
2. Man-to-man oral sex
3. Sexual intercourse with a bisexual individual
4. Anal intercourse

162. A practical nurse has been nominated to participate on a task force for environmentally responsible health care at the hospital. How would the task force members best promote environmental awareness in their institution?

1. Institute agency policies that incorporate "green" strategies
2. Develop brief workshops to educate the employees about environmental issues
3. Colour code green all supplies that are environmentally safe
4. Purchase recycling containers to be placed throughout the agency.

163. In the middle of an operation, a surgeon yells at a practical nurse, "This is the wrong instrument, you stupid nurse." What should the practical nurse do initially?

1. Recognize this as abuse and report the surgeon to his supervisor
2. Say to the surgeon, "This is abuse, and you will not speak to me this way."
3. File a complaint with the hospital authorities
4. After the operation is over, speak privately with the surgeon about the behaviour

164. Scott, age 16 years, participates in many athletic activities at his school. Which food would be the quickest source of energy for him during his sporting events?

1. Glass of 2% milk
2. Slice of bread
3. Chocolate bar
4. Glass of fruit juice

165. A client with a hiatal hernia complains about having difficulty sleeping at night. What should the practical nurse recommend?

1. Sleeping on two or three pillows to raise his upper body
2. Reducing carbohydrates in his diet
3. Drinking a glass of milk before retiring
4. Taking an antacid such as sodium bicarbonate

166. A client is receiving intermittent feedings via a nasogastric tube. How would the practical nurse best evaluate whether a prior feeding has been absorbed?

1. Evaluate the intake in relation to the output
2. Aspirate for residual volume
3. Instill air into the nasogastric tube while auscultating the stomach
4. Compare the client's body weight with baseline data

167. Mr. Braccio has been admitted to hospital for alcoholic cirrhosis of the liver and portal hypertension. The practical nurse should be alert for which of the following potential complications?

1. Liver abscesses
2. Intestinal obstruction
3. Perforation of the duodenum
4. Hemorrhage from esophageal varices

168. A 5-month-old, pale, unresponsive infant is brought to the emergency department by his parents. Which of the following factors is the strongest indicator for a suspicion of child abuse?

1. The story of how the child became unresponsive is not credible.
2. The infant is thin and shows signs of failure to thrive.
3. The parents have a previous history of neglect toward their other children.
4. The infant has had previous fractures confirmed by X-ray.

169. Which of the following skin lesions would be of most concern to a practical nurse working in a dermatological clinic?

1. A scaly erythematous patch on the elbow of Mr. LeClerc, age 24 years
2. A sudden appearance of an oval balding patch with smooth, soft skin underneath on Venetia, age 10 years
3. Flat, brown macules on the hands of Ms. Parsons, age 83 years
4. A mixed pigmentation lesion with irregular borders on the back of Mr. Priestly, age 42 years

170. Following a transurethral resection of the prostate, Mr. Burn's indwelling catheter becomes obstructed. Which of the following solutions would be most appropriate for irrigating the catheter?

1. Sterile water
2. Hypertonic saline
3. Sterile normal saline
4. Tap water

171. Mr. Beauclerc is in hospital after experiencing two transient ischemic attacks. The physician discussed with him the dangers of smoking, and Mr. Beauclerc stated that he quit 2 weeks ago, after the first attack. The practical nurse discovers a pack of cigarettes in Mr. Beauclerc's bathrobe pocket. What would be the most appropriate action of the practical nurse in addressing this situation?

1. Let Mr. Beauclerc know the cigarettes were found
2. Admonish Mr. Beauclerc for having cigarettes

3. Notify the physician
4. Discard the cigarettes without making a comment

172. What is the Canadian Nurses Association?

1. The provincial and territorial organization responsible for registering all nurses in Canada
2. A federation of provincial and territorial associations whose mission is to advance the quality of nursing
3. The national association whose mission is to provide collective bargaining and labour relations collaboration
4. An association that has been delegated by federal statutes to provide self-governance within the profession of nursing

173. Ms. Serena is discharged home with her infant, who has a severe genetic disorder. When the practical nurse arrives to visit, Ms. Serena is crying and appears tired. Which of the following comments by the practical nurse would be most therapeutic?

1. "Is everything all right? You look tired."
2. "Tell me a little about your daily routine."
3. "Are you having trouble looking after the baby?"
4. "You appear upset. Tell me what is going on."

174. Mrs. O'Deli, age 89, lives with her son and is unable to drive. The son does not allow her to go out to socialize. Therefore, she has no contact with any friends or family. She is told by her son she is lucky to live with him and if she complains he will put her in a long-term care facility. What form of abuse is this considered?

1. Physical abuse
2. Neglect
3. Financial abuse
4. Emotional abuse

175. A mother brings her 3-day old infant to the breastfeeding clinic. The practical nurse notice that the infant looks slightly jaundiced. What is the appropriate action by the practical nurse?

1. Advise the mother to discontinue breastfeeding
2. Have the mother position the infant's cot beside a sunny window
3. Advise the mother to supplement breastfeeding with glucose and water for increased fluids
4. Arrange for the infant to have a serum bilirubin test

176. Mr. and Mrs. Fenton have been married for 48 years. Recently, Mr. Fenton had a cerebrovascular accident that has left him with partial right-sided paralysis. At the rehabilitation unit, Mrs. Fenton insists on doing everything for her husband. Mr. Fenton appears quite sad. Which of the following emotions is Mr. Fenton probably feeling?

1. He is losing hope for the future.
2. He is feeling the loss of his independence.
3. He is feeling guilty about being a burden to his wife.
4. He is feeling loss of his masculine role.

177. Mrs. Hoagy, age 63, has been diagnosed with herpes zoster (shingles). Mrs. Hoagy asks the practical nurse if she is a risk of spreading the infection. What is the best response by the practical nurse?

1. "You need to avoid contact with someone who has never had measles."
2. "You need to avoid contact with someone who has never had chicken pox."
3. "You need to avoid contact with someone who has never had the Epstein-Barr virus."
4. "You need to avoid contact with someone who has never had rubella."

178. The practical nurse is monitoring an adult client's intake and output to calculate fluid balance. What is the normal urine output expected?

1. 1 L/day
2. 1.5 L/day
3. 3 L/day
4. 4 L/day

179. Mrs. Carter sustained a Colles fracture of her wrist when she fell on an icy sidewalk. She asks the practical nurse why she has to have her elbow in the cast, as it is her wrist that is broken. Which of the following responses by the practical nurse would be the most accurate?

1. "The cast will help to keep the wrist bones aligned."
2. "The cast will stop you from rotating your hand."
3. "It is easier to maintain this longer cast than one just on the wrist."
4. "You will soon get used to it, and it will provide support."

180. Mr. Cameron is experiencing hives and respiratory difficulty after a bee sting. Which of the following medications is most important to be given to Mr. Cameron initially?

1. Glucocorticoids
2. Epinephrine (Adrenalin)
3. Bronchodilators
4. Narcotic analgesics

181. John Byth is admitted to an orthopedic unit with a fractured left radius. Following a pain scale, the nurse learns his discomfort is 4/10. The practical nurse reviews his MAR to see that he is due for more medication in one half hour. The practical nurse encourages him to elevate the limb and do some deep breathing exercises to help relieve some of the discomfort while waiting for his next dose of pain medication. Which principle is the practical nurse demonstrating towards her client?

1. Justice
2. Nonmaleficence
3. Autonomy
4. Beneficence

182. Mr. Petrie, age 55 years, is about to be discharged home following recovery from a myocardial infarction. Mr. Petrie's partner is concerned about resuming sexual relations. Which of the following would be correct information for the practical nurse to give Mr. Petrie and his partner?

1. "When you feel comfortable climbing two flights of stairs, sexual activity may be resumed."
2. "This is a personal matter for both of you to discuss. You know how physical your relations are, so you can best judge when to resume sexual activity."
3. "It is usually recommended to wait about 4 to 6 months before resuming sexual relations."
4. "Sexual relations may be resumed when you can jog around a block without experiencing any significant chest pain."

183. Mr. Phillion, age 21, is on a swim team that competes internationally. He develops sinusitis, for which he receives treatment at the sports facility health clinic. He is scheduled to be in a high-profile race in 2 days. What health teaching should the practical nurse provide to Mr. Phillion?

1. "Have warm showers twice a day, and call if you develop a fever."
2. "Take over-the-counter analgesics to relieve the pain and stay out of the pool."
3. "Blow your nose often to keep your nasal passages open."
4. "Keep your head above the water when swimming."

184. In a group of older persons, a practical nurse discusses nutrition. Which of the following statements represents correct information about older persons and nutrition?

1. Older persons with diseases such as diabetes and depression have a decreased risk of malnutrition.
2. Older persons may experience age-related gastrointestinal changes that impact nutrition.
3. Many older persons are on a fixed income so they have enough money to eat well.
4. Because of the decreased metabolic needs of older persons, most are able to achieve sufficient nutrition in their diet.

185. Ms. Cooke developed pleuritis on her right side following an automobile accident. She experiences pain when she coughs or breathes deeply. Which suggestion by the practical nurse would help Ms. Cooke to alleviate her pain?

1. "Turn frequently onto the unaffected side and use a pillow as a splint when you cough."
2. "Sit up with two pillows behind you and use the palms of your hands as a splint."
3. "Turn frequently onto the affected side and use a pillow as a splint."
4. "Try not to breathe too deeply, and drink extra fluids to thin the secretions."

186. By what age should a newborn infant regain his or her birth weight?

1. 5 to 7 days
2. 7 to 10 days
3. 10 to 12 days
4. 14 to 21 days

187. After 4 days on an inpatient psychiatric unit, a client on suicide precautions tells the practical nurse, "Hey, look! I was feeling pretty depressed for a while, but I'm certainly not going to kill myself." What would be the practical nurse's best response?

1. "Were you really thinking of killing yourself?"
2. "You do seem to be feeling better."
3. "Why don't we sit down and talk some more about this?"
4. "That's good, but the staff will continue to observe you very carefully, just in case."

188. A practical nurse working in an emergency department in a small rural hospital received information that a 20-vehicle collision occurred nearby. Numerous casualties are being reported, and aid is requested to triage the victims at the scene. What other health care professional, other than nurses and physicians, would be beneficial to travel to the area to assist with triage?

1. The social worker
2. The rehabilitation therapist
3. The respiratory therapist
4. The paramedic

189. A client is experiencing a manic episode of her bipolar disorder. What would be the best approach for the practical nurse to assist her with her personal appearance?

1. Encourage her to dress appropriately in her own clothing
2. Allow her to apply makeup in whatever manner she chooses
3. Keep cosmetics away from her because she will apply them too freely
4. Suggest that she wear hospital clothing

190. A practical nurse is concerned about privatization of health care in her province, which has several private clinics where wealthy residents may pay for immediate diagnostic radiography, magnetic resonance imaging, and positron emission tomography scans. What is the most professional and effective action for the practical nurse to initiate?

1. Speak with the owners of the private clinics
2. Organize a protest march outside of a clinic
3. Initiate a letter-writing campaign to the appropriate member of provincial or federal government
4. Discuss her concerns with her health care colleagues

191. A focus for health programming in a community is maternal–child health. It is recognized that there is a need to decrease the number of unplanned teen pregnancies. What is the best approach to decrease the number of pregnancies in this community?

1. Education about abstinence as a birth-control choice
2. Teaching men about the use of condoms to prevent unwanted pregnancies
3. Providing information about abortions
4. Increasing the availability of contraceptives

192. Mr. Jackes tells the practical nurse at the medical clinic that he was "throwing up horribly all night long and couldn't keep anything down." What would be the practical nurse's best initial question?

1. "How many times, and how much did you vomit?"
2. "What did you have to eat last night?"
3. "Did you take your temperature?"
4. "Does anyone else in your family have the same symptoms?"

193. Mr. Burgess is diagnosed with gonorrhea. Which of the following statements is correct concerning this sexually transmitted infection (STI)?

1. Gonorrhea is not a common STI.
2. Cases of gonorrhea must be reported to health authorities.
3. Antibiotic treatment takes several weeks to ensure a cure.
4. Permanent damage to the testes is common.

194. Baby Liam is born at 28 weeks' gestation. What is the most common complication of prematurity?

1. Hemorrhage
2. Brain damage
3. Aspiration of mucus
4. Respiratory distress

195. Ms. LeBlanc is at 32 weeks' gestation in her first pregnancy. What would be a symptom of developing preeclampsia?

1. Hypotension
2. Proteinuria
3. Weight loss
4. Excessive thirst

196. Mr. Brankston is HIV positive. He asks the practical nurse what antiretroviral therapy will do. Which of the following explanations by the practical nurse would correctly state the purpose of the therapy?

1. "The antiretrovirals remove the virus from your body."
2. "The antiretrovirals reduce the amount of HIV in your body and increase CD4 cells, which improve your immunity."
3. "The antiretrovirals kill the virus just as an antibiotic does with bacteria."
4. "The antiretrovirals prevent duplication of the virus by altering the DNA–RNA transcription phase."

197. Mr. Levy has a venous thromboembolism and is to begin a heparin infusion. The infusion rate will be adjusted based on the results of his activated partial thromboplastin (aPTT) time. The practical nurse assigned to care for Mr. Levy is not competent in heparin infusion adjustments. What should the practical nurse do?

1. Initiate the heparin infusion as ordered
2. Consult the RN supervisor
3. Refuse to provide all care to the client
4. Ask the physician for instruction on heparin infusion adjustment

198. The nurse manager of a busy medical–surgical unit is concerned about meeting staffing needs over the Christmas holiday period. Many nurses have requested the same time off, and the hospital does not hire agency staff. Which of the following actions would be most successful in solving this problem?

1. Call a meeting of the nursing staff and ask members to provide possible solutions
2. Implement a holiday schedule that the manager feels is fair to all staff

3. Provide senior nurses with the first opportunity to schedule their holidays
4. Hold a lottery for nurses to win their preferred vacation days

199. Ms. Pratha, age 77 years, has been recently diagnosed with hypertension. She asks the practical nurse what type of exercise program she should begin. What would be the practical nurse's best response?

1. "Now that you have high blood pressure, it would be unwise for you to exercise."
2. "Begin by walking around your block, and then increase the distance as you can tolerate it."
3. "Working out in a gym for 45 minutes three times a week under the supervision of a personal trainer would be best."
4. "You should do all of your exercise in the evening, when your blood pressure is at its lowest."

200. A practical nurse receives the client care assignment for the day shift at the hospital. Which client should the practical nurse assess first?

1. A client hoping to go home once she climbs the stairs with physiotherapy.
2. A client who prefers to have assistance with personal care completed before 0800.
3. A client whose Foley catheter was emptied of 1800 mL of cloudy urine overnight.
4. A client with chronic obstructive pulmonary disease (COPD) who was short of breath when getting up to the bathroom during the night.

END OF PRACTICE EXAM 3

9 Answers and Rationales for Practice Exam 3

CASE–BASED QUESTIONS ANSWERS AND RATIONALES

CASE 1

1.

1. Unprotected sex is a transmission route for hepatitis C but is not the most common one.
2. Transfusions of contaminated blood were the cause of some cases of hepatitis C prior to the late 1990s, but this is not presently the most common source.
3. There is frequently coinfection with hepatitis C and human immunodeficiency virus (HIV), but one disease does not result in the other.
4. **Hepatitis C is transmitted via blood and body fluids. More than half of hepatitis C clients are intravenous drug users.**

CLASSIFICATION
Competency:
Foundations of Practice
Taxonomy:
Knowledge and Comprehension

2.

1. While nutritional supplements are what he needs, it is unlikely Mr. Tolea would have the financial ability to buy them.
2. His diet does require fruit and vegetables, but it is unlikely he would be able to afford them or store them in his rooming house.
3. **Mr. Tolea requires nutritional support beyond what he can purchase himself. The strategy that has the best chance of success is to find public or private resources to provide his meals. The social worker is the health care provider with the knowledge to access appropriate resources.**
4. While it may be an option for the nurse to have the social worker try to contact his family, Mr. Tolea is estranged from them, and they may not want to support him.

CLASSIFICATION
Competency:
Collaborative Practice
Taxonomy:
Critical Thinking

3.

1. Sedation is not pain management. Mr. Tolea may prefer to be awake and alert, not sedated.
2. **The purpose of palliative care is to help the client achieve a dignified, comfortable death on his own terms. The client may make decisions about sedation, analgesia, skin care, nutrition, spiritual support, and so on.**
3. Care for itchy skin that may be a result of liver failure is included in client choice.
4. Pressure injury is a risk in the palliative care client, but care for these is included in provision of client choice.

CLASSIFICATION
Competency:
Foundations of Practice
Taxonomy:
Critical Thinking

4.

1. This statement dismisses the client's feelings. The statement does not allow the client to express his concerns.
2. **Probing what is important to the client is helpful to establish the appropriate goals of care.**
3. While family is an important part of the client's circle of care, this may not be what he wants since he has been estranged from them. This statement is not allowing Mr. Tolea to express his wishes or desires.
4. This statement does not allow Mr. Tolea to express his feelings regarding pain control and how he would like to receive it.

CLASSIFICATION
Competency:
Professional Practice
Taxonomy:
Application

CASE 2

5.

1. This factor may cause obesity but only if it is not offset by calorie expenditure.
2. This factor may cause obesity but only if calories are not restricted.

3. When the caloric intake consistently exceeds the expenditure of calories, the excess calories will be stored in the body in the form of fat.

4. Same as answer 2.

CLASSIFICATION
Competency:
Foundations of Practice
Taxonomy:
Knowledge and Comprehension

---

6. 1. There is no correlation between birth weight and future obesity.

2. The incidence of obese children born to obese parents is significantly higher than that of obese children born to parents of normal weight.

3. This factor is predictive but is not as significant as obesity in parents.
4. Same as answer 3.

CLASSIFICATION
Competency:
Health and Wellness Foundations of Practice
Taxonomy:
Critical Thinking

---

7. 1. This cholesterol value is normal for an 11-year-old.

2. This value is higher than expected and may be indicative of type 2 diabetes. Childhood obesity is related to an increase in type 2 diabetes.

3. This blood pressure is normal for an 11-year-old.
4. Breathing problems do occur in overweight children, but these spirometry values are normal.

CLASSIFICATION
Competency:
Foundations of Practice
Taxonomy:
Application

---

8. 1. This calculation is incorrect.
2. Same as answer 1.

3. This calculation is correct: $57.5 \times 2.2 = 126.5$

4. Same as answer 1.

CLASSIFICATION
Competency:
Foundations of Practice
Taxonomy:
Application

---

9. **1. Successful behaviour-modification programs assist children to identify inappropriate eating habits and to incorporate suitable physical activity, which may lead to lifelong management of the obesity.**

2. Diet is one part of therapy, but it should not be severely reduced because the child will not be able to maintain the restrictions.
3. These drugs are not recommended for children.
4. This surgery is not recommended for children.

CLASSIFICATION
Competency:
Foundations of Practice
Taxonomy:
Critical Thinking

---

10. **1. Denying Rickhelm social interaction with his friends is a poor approach. If he is denied foods he finds enjoyable, he is not likely to stick to a diet. Many fast-food restaurants supply pamphlets with the nutritional information of their menus.**

2. A hamburger and fries are high in fat and calories.
3. Same as answer 1.
4. Same as answer 1.

CLASSIFICATION
Competency:
Professional Practice
Taxonomy:
Application

---

11. 1. This question is close ended. It may also be seen by Rickhelm as intrusive.
2. This question is close ended and will elicit a yes or no answer.
3. This question is close ended and implies that Rickhelm should feel bad about himself.

4. This question is open ended and allows Rickhelm to discuss any problems that are occurring as a result of his weight.

CLASSIFICATION
Competency:
Professional Practice
Taxonomy:
Critical Thinking

CASE 3

12. **1. Various aspects of hospitalization and diagnosis could cause the client anxiety. The practical nurse should determine what disturbs the client most.**
2. Anxiety is a barrier to learning. The client would not be receptive.
3. This approach may serve to increase his anxiety.
4. It is possible that additional home care will be required after discharge; however, the practical nurse should initially determine what Mr. Jason's specific anxieties are.

CLASSIFICATION
Competency: **Collaborative Practice**
Taxonomy: **Application**

---

13. 1. This position will not allow lung expansion, making breathing difficult.
2. Same as answer 1.
3. Same as answer 1.
4. This position promotes lung expansion during tracheostomy care.

CLASSIFICATION
Competency: **Foundations of Practice**
Taxonomy: **Knowledge and Comprehension**

---

14. **1. Administration of oxygen for a few minutes prior to suctioning reduces the risk of hypoxia, the major complication associated with suctioning.**
2. Negative pressure is applied as the catheter is withdrawn.
3. The tip of the catheter should reach the base of the tube but not far beyond.
4. When ordered, this drug is usually given by inhalation, not instillation; 3 to 5 mL of normal saline can be instilled into the tracheotomy tube to loosen secretions.

CLASSIFICATION
Competency: **Foundations of Practice**
Taxonomy: **Application**

---

15. **1. Suctioning time should be limited to 10 seconds to prevent hypoxemia.**
2. Suctioning for more than 10 seconds may lead to hypoxemia.
3. Same as answer 2.
4. Same as answer 2.

CLASSIFICATION
Competency: **Foundations of Practice**
Taxonomy: **Application**

---

16. **1. If the tracheostomy ties are too tight, impaired cerebral circulation may result.**
2. Discharge would not cause the client to complain of tightness.
3. This statement is untrue; impaired cerebral circulation may result from too tight tracheostomy ties.
4. Removing the tracheostomy ties could cause accidental displacement of the tube.

CLASSIFICATION
Competency: **Foundations of Practice**
Taxonomy: **Critical Thinking**

CASE 4

17. **1. Holistic health care encompasses the health of the whole person—body, mind, emotions, and spirit.**
2. Primary health care is a philosophy and model for improving health that focuses on promoting health and preventing illness.
3. Spiritual health care primarily concerns the health of the spiritual aspect of the individual but does not include the physical components.
4. In socioenvironmental health care, health is closely tied to the social structure of a population.

CLASSIFICATION
Competency: **Professional Practice**
Taxonomy: **Knowledge/Comprehension**

18.
1. **Like many infectious diseases, respiratory syncytial virus (RSV) is more readily transmitted in overcrowded conditions.**

CLASSIFICATION
Competency:
Foundations of Practice
Taxonomy:
Critical Thinking

2. Premature infants and new babies of any ethnicity are particularly at risk for the virus, but this is not the reason for the increase in incidence in Indigenous communities.
3. Warm or changeable weather favours transmission.
4. A depressed immune system is possibly a factor but does not explain the high incidence in these communities.

19.
1. This statement is not true, although the taste of high-sugar foods appeals to many.
2. This statement is not true. High-sugar foods are sweet to taste and appealing, but there is no genetic makeup that causes a craving.
3. **Because of the high cost of transportation of food to the north, nutritional foods such as milk and fresh produce are often scarce. Sugar-filled products tend to be less expensive than those of higher nutritional value.**
4. While there does need to be increased and continual nutrition education, this is not the primary reason for the poor diet. The cause is socioeconomic.

CLASSIFICATION
Competency:
Foundations of Practice
Taxonomy:
Application

20.
1. This option is not realistic, nor is it provision of optimum care. The niece may need timely information regarding birth control and may not be able to wait for several days.
2. This statement is not necessarily true. Care should be transferred to a nonrelated caregiver if possible; however, if one is not available, care may be delivered to a relative.
3. This option is a possibility but may not provide timely care, and a physician consultation is not necessary.
4. **A practical nurse may have to care for a family member or friend as part of her professional employment; however, this should occur only when no other caregiver is available. The practical nurse should reflect on whether she can maintain the boundary between professional and personal roles, clarify the boundaries to the client, and maintain confidentiality.**

CLASSIFICATION
Competency:
Legal Practice
Taxonomy:
Critical Thinking

CASE 5

21.
1. The practical nurse is not yet aware if the conversation between Ms. Bennett and the counsellor is true.
2. It is true that it is not ethical for the counsellor to accept gifts, but the practical nurse first needs to consult the counsellor to establish any truth to Ms. Bennett's story.
3. It is necessary to talk to the counsellor first to establish any truth to Ms. Bennett's story.
4. **Given the potential for Ms. Bennett to misunderstand or misinterpret the nature of the relationship, it is the practical nurse's obligation to clarify the circumstances around the conversation.**

CLASSIFICATION
Competency:
Ethical Practice
Taxonomy:
Application

22.
1. More information is required before this assumption can be made.
2. **Grandiosity is associated with a manic episode of bipolar disorder. This often includes elaborate plans with individuals in positions of power, excessive spending of money, and misperceptions relating to the nature of relationship boundaries.**

CLASSIFICATION
Competency:
Foundations of Practice
Taxonomy:
Application

3. Same as answer 1.
4. Although the practical nurse will understand that Ms. Bennett's claims are likely unfounded, she will realize that they are a sign of grandiosity, characteristic of the manic phase, which is a concern.

CASE 6

23.

1. **Prior to being able to assist a grieving family, the practical nurse must be aware of his own feelings about death.**
2. This action may be applicable but only after the practical nurse reflects on his own feelings.
3. Same as answer 2.
4. Same as answer 2.

CLASSIFICATION
Competency:
Ethical Practice
Taxonomy:
Critical Thinking

24.

1. Most agencies do require a do-not-resuscitate order (DNR), but the important first step is to determine the wishes of the client.
2. This step may be taken if there are no directives, but the practical nurse should determine Mr. Braun's (or his family's) wishes so that he does not experience unwanted intervention.
3. **The practical nurse should determine the family and client wishes as soon as possible and communicate these to the health care team. Nurses ethically abide by the expressed wishes of the client or the client's substitute decision maker.**
4. While directives regarding end-of-life decision making are included in the Canadian Council for Practical Nurse Regulators' *Code of Ethics for Licensed Practical Nurses in Canada*, the practical nurse should first consult the family.

CLASSIFICATION
Competency:
Ethical Practice
Taxonomy:
Critical Thinking

25.

1. This question is not therapeutic and may cause Mrs. Braun to feel defensive.
2. **This question does not accuse Mrs. Braun of denial or misunderstanding the physician's prognosis and should elicit information about what Mrs. Braun understands about her husband's situation.**
3. With this question, Mrs. Braun is able to answer yes or no, which may end the discussion and not provide the practical nurse with the opportunity to explore Mrs. Braun's grief.
4. Mrs. Braun may deny her discussion with the children or may answer only yes or no; this question may make her feel defensive.

CLASSIFICATION
Competency:
Collaborative Practice
Taxonomy:
Application

26.

1. This documentation is a physician responsibility and does not need to be made by the nurse.
2. **This documentation is a legal requirement.**
3. Specific hygiene care—for example, washing the body, closing the eyes—does not need to be itemized. Documentation would need to include that care of the body was performed and by whom as well as which tubes were left in place and any personal articles left on the body.
4. Family participation should be documented, but it is not necessary to note the time of their departure.

CLASSIFICATION
Competency:
Legal Practice
Taxonomy:
Knowledge/Comprehension

27.

1. This action may be helpful to help the practical nurse to work through conflicts about caring for dying clients, but it should not be his first action.

2. Talking with respected colleagues may help the practical nurse reflect on his feelings, find support from his peers, and put his feelings of inadequacy in perspective.

3. Feelings of inadequacy are not part of normal grieving for a health care provider. The practical nurse should be able to reflect on what actions he might have performed differently, but this should not be accompanied by guilt.
4. It may help to discuss his performance with the unit manager after he has had time for self-reflection and dialogue with colleagues.

CLASSIFICATION
Competency:
Professional Practice
Taxonomy:
Critical Thinking

CASE 7

28. **1. Breastfeeding is contraindicated when the mother has a chemical use problem, most specifically involving alcohol, marijuana, or cocaine, as these substances are transmitted in breast milk.**

2. Women with inverted nipples are able to breastfeed.
3. Mastitis is not a contraindication unless the discomfort is intolerable to the mother.
4. Cancer is a contraindication only if the mother is receiving chemotherapy.

CLASSIFICATION
Competency:
Foundations of Practice
Taxonomy:
Knowledge/Comprehension

---

29. 1. This statement is not necessarily true. Not all bottle-fed infants are overfed.
2. Breast milk does not lack enough fat for growth.

3. This statement is true of breastfed infants.

4. Infant formulas are generally of equal caloric content to breast milk.

CLASSIFICATION
Competency:
Foundations of Practice
Taxonomy:
Application

---

30. **1. Milk supply depends on demand. The more feedings that are required, the more milk the mother will produce. The nursing mother should be feeding her infant 8 to 12 times per day initially.**

2. Increased fluids have not been shown to increase milk production. Fifteen glasses is too much fluid.
3. This action may stimulate the letdown reflex or help with engorgement but does not increase milk supply.
4. This action may be of help in stimulating the letdown reflex.

CLASSIFICATION
Competency:
Foundations of Practice
Taxonomy:
Application

---

31. **1. Jeremy should have six to eight wet diapers per day if he is receiving sufficient breast milk.**

2. This statement is correct, but this measure is not objective.
3. This method of determining intake is outdated and has been evaluated to cause undue anxiety in mothers who are concerned about their ability to breastfeed. As well, it evaluates the intake only at one feeding.
4. Breastfed infants at this age should have a minimum of three stools per day. However, the number of stools is not a reliable indicator of nutrition and hydration.

CLASSIFICATION
Competency:
Foundations of Practice
Taxonomy:
Application

---

32. 1. This action may cause him to become more distressed.
2. This action may help to wake a sleepy baby, but it will distress a fussy baby.
3. Environmental stimuli need to be decreased, not increased.

4. Holding him skin-to-skin and allowing him to suck will help Jeremy to calm down so that he is better able to latch on to the breast.

CLASSIFICATION
Competency:
Foundations of Practice
Taxonomy:
Application

---

33. 1. This option is not the best since there is not necessarily any need to discontinue breastfeeding.
2. This option may have been viable if Ms. Hudson were conflicted about returning to work, but she has said that she wants to return to work. It would be better to explore her feelings about her job and the necessity of returning to work.
3. This option is a possibility but is unnecessary since Jeremy is still just 2 weeks of age. She should continue breastfeeding exclusively for the time being.

4. Continuing with breastfeeding after returning to work is a viable option. A lactation consultant will work with Ms. Hudson to provide individualized strategies for her and Jeremy.

CLASSIFICATION
Competency:
Collaborative Practice
Taxonomy:
Application

---

34. **1. The La Leche League is the internationally recognized organization that provides education about breastfeeding and support to professionals and mothers.**

2. This organization provides education and support for natural childbirth.
3. This government agency mandates to protect the health and safety of Canadians; it is not specifically focused on breastfeeding.
4. This not-for-profit agency provides health care services to Canadians in the community. Breastfeeding support may be provided but is not the primary focus of the agency.

CLASSIFICATION
Competency:
Collaborative Practice
Taxonomy:
Knowledge/Comprehension

CASE 8

35. 1. Bloody drainage is expected this soon after surgery, and the physician does not need to be notified.
2. Nasogastric suction must be working, and the tube must remain patent to prevent stress on the suture line.

3. Nasogastric drainage is expected to be bright red at first and gradually darkens within the first 24 hours after surgery.

4. The nasogastric tube would be irrigated with iced saline only if a physician specifically orders it.

CLASSIFICATION
Competency:
Foundations of Practice
Taxonomy:
Application

---

36. **1. Physiological normal saline is used in gastric irrigation to prevent electrolyte imbalance. Because of the fresh gastric sutures, irrigation should be slow and gentle.**

2. The purpose of irrigation is to maintain the patency of the tube for gastric decompression; with a disconnection from the suction, a buildup of secretions and air can occur, or the tube can become blocked by viscous drainage.
3. Increasing the pressure may cause damage to the suture line.
4. Same as answer 2.

CLASSIFICATION
Competency:
Foundations of Practice
Taxonomy:
Application

---

37. 1. This action is not necessary unless Ms. Loates is unable to expectorate secretions.
2. Oxygen administration is generally not required unless the client has an underlying cardiac or respiratory disease.
3. Although ambulation will help to decrease the risk of pulmonary complications and a pooling of pulmonary secretions, individuals with abdominal incisions often revert to shallow breathing during physical effort. Ambulation during the first 24 hours may be limited.

4. To promote drainage of different lung regions, clients should turn every 2 hours. Deep breathing inflates the alveoli and promotes fluid drainage.

CLASSIFICATION
Competency:
Foundations of Practice
Taxonomy:
Application

CASE 9

38. 1. This question is close ended and would not yield the information the practical nurse requires.

2. This question is open ended and will inform the practical nurse of Juanita's understanding of what will occur when she stops treatment.

CLASSIFICATION
Competency:
Legal Practice
Taxonomy:
Critical Thinking

3. This question sympathizes with Juanita but does not provide the practical nurse with the information she needs to confirm informed consent.
4. This action may occur but is not necessary at this point. The practical nurse first needs to collect assessment data on Juanita's understanding of refusing treatment.

---

39. **1. According to the Canadian Council for Practical Nurse Regulators' *Code of Ethics for Licensed Practical Nurses in Canada*, the practical nurse's first responsibility is to advocate for the client's wishes once an informed decision has been made.**

CLASSIFICATION
Competency:
Ethical Practice
Taxonomy:
Critical Thinking

2. It may be appropriate to refer Juanita's parents for counselling but not for the purpose of having Juanita change her mind.
3. This action may occur if the practical nurse is not able to resolve her ethical dilemma, but it is not the practical nurse's primary role in this situation.
4. This action may be a therapeutic approach to resolve the parents' issues but is not the primary role of the practical nurse.

---

40. 1. The parents may not want to be, nor may Juanita want them to be, the designated people to receive information. This action makes the decision the practical nurse's choice, not the family's.

2. This action achieves client and family choice and provides a clear communication route for the health care staff.

CLASSIFICATION
Competency:
Collaborative Practice
Taxonomy:
Critical Thinking

3. Juanita may not be able, particularly in her weakened state, to communicate with her family.
4. This action does not solve the problem since the primary nurse still must communicate with all family members.

---

41. 1. The practical nurse does not know how the family feels.
2. It is not professional to blame poor care on staffing. The practical nurse does not know what is inadequate about the care.
3. The practical nurse cannot change the plan of care until she has discussed with the family exactly what is wrong with the care.

4. This question asks the family to identify what they feel is inadequate about Juanita's care. By asking this question, the practical nurse may be able to determine if there are facets of care that need to be improved or if the family's lashing out is a symptom of their grief.

CLASSIFICATION
Competency:
Collaborative Practice
Taxonomy:
Application

---

42. 1. This action is contrary to Juanita's documented wishes.
2. Same as answer 1.

3. Same as answer 1.
4. **The practical nurse may not interfere with Juanita's documented wish for no resuscitation. The mother is manifesting anger in her grief and needs comforting. There is no legal basis for a lawsuit.**

CLASSIFICATION
Competency:
Ethical Practice
Taxonomy:
Critical Thinking

CASE 10

43.
1. **This information is practical and honest.**
2. There is no indication that the amputation would have to be below the knee.
3. This response avoids answering the question.
4. This response can be construed as blaming the wife for not bringing her husband in sooner.

CLASSIFICATION
Competency:
Foundations of Practice
Taxonomy:
Application

44.
1. This action may be helpful but will not provide Mrs. Partilucci with the best learning experience at this time.
2. **The diabetes nurse educator is the best source of education for Mrs. Partilucci. This is a practical step to help her learning.**
3. This action will only help her understand what is happening during this acute episode.
4. This action dismisses Mrs. Partilucci's question and ignores her need to help her husband.

CLASSIFICATION
Competency:
Collaborative Practice
Taxonomy:
Application

45.
1. There is a familial link.
2. This information may not be completely correct. The timing of onset of diabetes cannot be predicted, although, in most cases, it does start to manifest after 40 years. Often the severity depends on lifestyle choices and therapeutic management.
3. **This response is factual but not threatening and provides some information about how the son can help prevent developing type 2 diabetes.**
4. This information is not correct.

CLASSIFICATION
Competency:
Foundations of Practice
Taxonomy:
Application

CASE 11

46.
1. **It arises from melanocytes but may metastasize to any organ.**
2. It is not rare and causes a large majority of skin cancer deaths. It is not superficial and becomes invasive if untreated.
3. Radiation is a risk factor, not a cause.
4. This information is incorrect.

CLASSIFICATION
Competency:
Foundations of Practice
Taxonomy:
Knowledge/Comprehension

47.
1. It isn't known if his cancer can be cured by surgery until the extent of the tumour is known.
2. While the surgery will remove the cancerous lesion, there is no indication that other melanomas will develop.
3. **The cure rate for cutaneous melanoma by excision is nearly 100% if the malignant cells are restricted to the epidermis and only if the entire lesion is removed prior to metastasis. At this time, it is not possible to know if there has been metastasis.**

CLASSIFICATION
Competency:
Foundations of Practice
Taxonomy:
Application

4. This step would be unnecessary if surgery removed all the cancerous cells. This response does not answer Mr. O'Morrissey's question.

48.
1. This advice is not reasonable since he works outdoors.
2. This advice is good but does not include covering for his arms and hands.
3. **This advice is most important since, with early detection and treatment, melanoma can be cured.**
4. Sunscreen is necessary but is not as important as skin monitoring; also, the SPF should probably be 30 for increased protection.

CLASSIFICATION
Competency:
Foundations of Practice
Taxonomy:
Critical Thinking

CASE 12

49.
1. This description defines cystic fibrosis.
2. This description defines emphysema.
3. This description defines chronic bronchitis.
4. **This description defines asthma.**

CLASSIFICATION
Competency:
Foundations of Practice
Taxonomy:
Knowledge/Comprehension

50.
1. Wheezing is a classic manifestation of asthma as air passes over narrowed airways. However, wheezing is an unreliable sign to gauge the severity of an attack. Minor attacks may cause audible wheezing.
2. As the attack progresses, there may be inspiratory and expiratory wheezing, but this is not the most severe symptom.
3. People experiencing an asthma attack will sit forward and use accessory muscles to attempt to get more air into their lungs. It is not an indicator of the severity of the attack.
4. **Severely diminished or absent breath sounds, often referred to as a "silent chest," are an ominous sign indicating severe obstruction and impending respiratory failure.**

CLASSIFICATION
Competency:
Foundations of Practice
Taxonomy:
Critical Thinking

51.
1. A bronchodilator would be ordered by the physician and should be administered as quickly as possible. Oxygen may be administered prior to the order for a bronchodilator.
2. The clients breathing requires immediate assistance first. It is important to identify triggers once client acute episode is stabilized. It is not the most crucial action.
3. **Status asthmaticus is a life-threatening situation and could quickly lead to respiratory failure. A physician is needed immediately to direct care. Mechanical ventilation may be necessary.**
4. An IV fluid bolus is not necessary for status asthmaticus.

CLASSIFICATION
Competency:
Collaborative Practice
Taxonomy:
Critical Thinking

52.
1. **Normal values are PaO_2 80 to 100 mm Hg; $PaCO_2$ 35 to 45 mm Hg; and pH 7.35 to 7.45. These gases indicate a low oxygen (hypoxia), a high CO_2 (hypercapnia), and a low pH (acidosis).**
2. Same as answer 1.
3. Same as answer 1.
4. Same as answer 1.

CLASSIFICATION
Competency:
Foundations of Practice
Taxonomy:
Critical Thinking

---

53. 1. Content is only part of the new learning and can be overwhelming if presenting all the information on asthma at once.

2. Client-centred learning involves actively educating persons with asthma on correct inhaler device through client demonstration and feedback until the skill is mastered.

CLASSIFICATION
Competency:
Collaborative Practice
Taxonomy:
Knowledge and Comprehension

3. Teaching should be done in a safe, quiet environment free of distraction. The nurse's station may be too noisy for client learning to take place.
4. Closed-ended questions make it difficult for the client to express his concerns or misunderstandings.

---

54. 1. This intervention is a component of asthma management but not the most important one.

2. The Registered Nurses' Association of Ontario developed best practice guidelines for the management of asthma. The key component identified was appropriate education and self-management training that includes an asthma action plan.

CLASSIFICATION
Competency:
Foundations of Practice
Taxonomy:
Critical Thinking

3. This intervention is a component of the appropriate treatment of asthma but requires education for the client to manage the medication regime.
4. This intervention is an important component for monitoring the client's management of and the severity of the asthma and would be part of an action plan.

---

55. 1. The metered dose inhaler should be shaken five to six times, and the client should use one puff at a time.
2. Mr. Nigel should inhale as he is depressing the canister.

3. AeroChambers break up and slow down the medication particles, enhancing the amount of medication received by the client. Their use is often advantageous for children, older persons, and clients who have difficulty coordinating the use of the metered dose inhaler.

CLASSIFICATION
Competency:
Foundations of Practice
Taxonomy:
Application

4. The canister should be depressed as the client is inhaling.

CASE 13

56. 1. This information is important but not the practical nurse's primary concern during admission.
2. Current substance use is of greater importance.

3. The most immediate risk to Ms. Wilmox's life is what substances she may currently have in her system. All other options are valid; however, the client's medical status must be stable in order to proceed with a mental health evaluation.

CLASSIFICATION
Competency:
Foundations of Practice
Taxonomy:
Critical Thinking

4. Ms. Wilmox has a sister and two children, so she is not without support.

---

57. 1. This action is confrontational and may prevent further cooperation.
2. This action would not be appropriate.
3. The client is always the main source of information.

4. **Presenting boundaries in a nonconfrontational, nonchallenging manner reduces the possibility that the client will feel threatened. As a result, the potential for building a therapeutic relationship with the client increases significantly.**

CLASSIFICATION
Competency:
Collaborative Practice
Taxonomy:
Application

---

58. 1. This action is not necessary.

2. **A client always retains the right to disclosure of information; therefore, the practical nurse must seek permission to speak to family members or significant others. Verbal permission is adequate, and in obtaining it, the practical nurse builds trust and enhances the therapeutic relationship with the client. The practical nurse must always document a verbal consent on the client's chart.**

CLASSIFICATION
Competency:
Ethical Practice
Taxonomy:
Application

3. This action breaks confidentiality and could prevent further cooperation from Ms. Wilmox.
4. This action is not necessary.

---

59. 1. Four-point restraints are not indicated and have not been ordered. They may prove counterproductive.

2. **The practical nurse's primary response should be to verbally clarify with the client that abuse of any kind is not appropriate and will not be tolerated. This gives the client the opportunity to alter her behaviour to what is more appropriate. Immediately following the practical nurse's verbal boundary-setting, the practical nurse may investigate any potential reasons for the client's change in presentation.**

CLASSIFICATION
Competency:
Legal Practice
Taxonomy:
Application

3. This behaviour will escalate if ignored.
4. This intervention is not indicated in this situation.

CASE 14

60. 1. This method is highly recommended, particularly for heavy smokers who have not been successful with prior attempts to quit. However, one approach is not necessarily the best for all smokers.
2. This method is effective for some, but not all, smokers.
3. Same as answer 2.

4. **Many factors are recognized to be important in the cessation of smoking. One method is not necessarily the best for all. By choosing an option they feel will be successful, individuals will be more motivated to continue with that method.**

CLASSIFICATION
Competency:
Foundations of Practice
Taxonomy:
Application

---

61. 1. This statement is not true.
2. This statement is not true; it is one-shot immunity.

3. **There are two groups of seasonal influenza viruses, which have an ability to change over time. With each influenza season, epidemiologists predict which will be the prevalent strain and develop a vaccine particular to that strain.**

CLASSIFICATION
Competency:
Foundations of Practice
Taxonomy:
Knowledge/Comprehension

4. While the vaccines are increasingly purified, this is not the reason for the need for annual immunizing.

62.
1. **Rituals and relaxation encourage sleep.**
2. Exercising too close to bedtime releases epinephrine, which is a stimulant.
3. Over-the-counter sleep remedies are not recommended, especially for chronic insomnia.
4. Spicy meals may cause indigestion, which could interfere with sleep.

CLASSIFICATION
Competency:
Foundations of Practice
Taxonomy:
Application

63.
1. This description does not define WHMIS.
2. WHMIS does not train for infection control.
3. This description does not define WHMIS.
4. **Chemicals are a source of environmental risk. The Workplace Hazardous Materials Information System (WHMIS) sets the standard for control of hazardous substances in the workplace, including health care agencies.**

CLASSIFICATION
Competency:
Foundations of Practice
Taxonomy:
Knowledge/Comprehension

64.
1. Women are more likely than men to experience stress.
2. **Each individual experiences stress differently, and there are differing stressors for each individual. Therefore, strategies must be adapted to the individual and her particular stressors.**
3. Stress is always present and is necessary for life. It is how an individual copes with stress that causes health problems.
4. Stress is a reality for all people.

CLASSIFICATION
Competency:
Foundations of Practice
Taxonomy:
Knowledge/Comprehension

CASE 15

65.
1. This response does nothing to relieve Ms. Magnusson's anxiety.
2. **This response addresses the client's concern about the electricity and provides a reason for the test.**
3. This response dismisses Ms. Magnusson's concerns and does not give accurate information.
4. This response is dismissive.

CLASSIFICATION
Competency:
Collaborative Practice
Taxonomy:
Application

66.
1. **This response is accurate and provides information to Ms. Magnusson about how she may prevent future episodes.**
2. This response is inaccurate.
3. This response offers incorrect information.
4. Same as answer 3.

CLASSIFICATION
Competency:
Foundations of Practice
Taxonomy:
Application

CASE 16

67.
1. **Agency incident or risk reports are for the purpose of tracking errors and identifying system failures or deficiencies, with the purpose of decreasing medication errors.**
2. This situation may occur but would more likely be identified at a unit manager or employee level.

CLASSIFICATION
Competency:
Professional Practice
Taxonomy:
Critical Thinking

3. The medication error may be subpoenaed, but this is not the primary reason for their completion.
4. Although client information is included in the medication error report, specific health information related to any adverse effects should be documented in the client's health record.

68.
1. The physician must have ordered the medication unless it is an over-the-counter preparation, but this is not the guiding principle.
2. This consideration is important for any medication administration but is not the guiding principle for self-administration.
3. Same as answer 2.
4. **The nurse must evaluate if the individual clients have the competency to administer their own medications. If not, self-administration cannot be considered.**

CLASSIFICATION
Competency:
Professional Practice
Taxonomy:
Critical Thinking

69.
1. Many nurses work and prefer 12-hour shifts. With 8-hour shifts, they work more days, which for some may be just as tiring.
2. Working too many overtime shifts can lead to nurse fatigue. But there may be times and situations in which overtime is an effective use of personnel, and if not overused, it does not contribute to nurse fatigue.
3. This strategy has not been shown to prevent fatigue. Many nurses find that the change from days to nights contributes to fatigue.
4. **Research has shown that individual nurses, when given an option of shift length and type, choose shifts that fit into their lifestyle and their circadian rhythm, thus decreasing fatigue.**

CLASSIFICATION
Competency:
Professional Practice
Taxonomy:
Critical Thinking

CASE 17

70.
1. Mrs. Douglas' blood pressure is stable.
2. Although her skin will require assessment, this is not a priority concern.
3. Although her knee will require assessment, this is not a priority.
4. **A change in behaviour such as agitation and restlessness is important to assess as it may be indicative of an acute illness such as an infection or electrolyte imbalance.**

CLASSIFICATION
Competency:
Foundations of Practice
Taxonomy:
Critical Thinking

71.
1. ***E. coli* is the most common pathogen leading to a UTI.**
2. *H. pylori* is a bacterium that is usually found in the stomach.
3. *Candida albicans* is a fungus that causes candidiasis, vaginitis, and thrush.
4. *Streptococcus pneumoniae* is a bacterium that causes pneumococcal pneumonia.

CLASSIFICATION
Competency:
Foundations of Practice
Taxonomy:
Knowledge and Comprehension

72.
1. Not indicative of potential UTI and not found on the test strip
2. **Indicative of a potential UTI**
3. Not indicative of potential UTI
4. Same as answer 1

CLASSIFICATION
Competency:
Foundations of Practice
Taxonomy:
Application

---

73. 1. Not a characteristic of a UTI in the urine sample
2. Same as answer 1
3. Same as answer 1

4. Urine characteristic of a UTI

CLASSIFICATION
Competency:
Foundations of Practice
Taxonomy:
Knowledge and Comprehension

---

74. 1. This will not treat the urinary infection.

2. Encouraging her to regularly drink water or other fluids will help flush the bacteria from her urinary tract. The nurse needs to help her drink; otherwise, the client will not know to drink due to her dementia.

3. Coffee is a bladder irritant and she may not know or remember to drink it, due to her dementia.
4. Clients must finish all their antibiotic treatments to prevent recurrence of the infection.

CLASSIFICATION
Competency:
Foundations of Practice
Taxonomy:
Application

CASE 18

75. 1. *E. coli* causes diarrhea but is not as common as rotavirus.
2. Shigella causes diarrhea but is not as common as rotavirus.

3. Rotavirus is a common cause of gastroenteritis in children and infants, particularly those in daycare settings.

4. Salmonella causes diarrhea but is not as common as rotavirus.

CLASSIFICATION
Competency:
Foundations of Practice
Taxonomy:
Critical Thinking

---

76. 1. This manifestation suggests moderate dehydration.
2. Same as answer 1.
3. Same as answer 1.

4. A rapid, thready pulse is a sign of severe dehydration and requires immediate treatment to prevent cardiovascular collapse.

CLASSIFICATION
Competency:
Foundations of Practice
Taxonomy:
Critical Thinking

---

77. 1. This calculation is incorrect.
2. Same as answer 1.

3. This calculation is correct: Total fluid intake: 20 mL × 9 kg = 180 mL/hr

Oral fluids averaged over 1 hour = 120 mL ÷ 3 hours = 40 mL
IV rate = 180 mL – 40 mL = 140 mL/hr

4. Same as answer 1.

CLASSIFICATION
Competency:
Professional Practice
Taxonomy:
Application

---

78. **1. Oral rehydration solutions (e.g., Pedialyte, Rehydralyte, and Infalyte) are the treatment of choice for most cases of dehydration caused by diarrhea. They are safe, reduce diarrheal volume loss, provide nutrients and fluids, and shorten the duration of the disease. Infants who are breastfeeding should continue to do so, alternating feeds with the oral rehydration solution.**

2. Soy formula is not necessary or recommended if he is breastfeeding. Glucose water will not treat the potential electrolyte imbalance.

CLASSIFICATION
Competency:
Foundations of Practice
Taxonomy:
Application

3. The BRAT (*b*ananas, *r*ice, *a*pplesauce, and *t*oast) diet is no longer used for infants because it has poor nutritional value. Charlie requires more fluids than the BRAT diet and breast milk provide.
4. A lactose-free formula is not indicated since Charlie is not lactose intolerant. Breast milk will provide the necessary fluids, and its nutrients will be better digested. Apple juice may be given if tolerated, but oral rehydration solutions are more effective.

CASE 19

79.
1. A private room with a closed door may not be safe for the practical nurse, and she will not want to conduct a confidential interview close to other clients.
2. Safety is the most important issue, but the assessment should provide safety and the assurance of confidentiality. This setting is not appropriate.
3. **When interviewing a psychiatric client with a history of violence, the first concern for the practical nurse should be her own safety. If she conducts the interview in a room that provides some privacy, yet she is positioned close to a door, she will be safe, and the assessment will not be overheard by others.**
4. This precaution is not necessary unless Mr. Clarkson is being violent at the time. The presence of a police officer may escalate his behaviour or intimidate him. The police officer at this point is not part of the health care team; thus, his presence would breach confidentiality.

CLASSIFICATION
Competency:
Collaborative Practice
Taxonomy:
Critical Thinking

80.
1. Generally, the opposite is true.
2. **Individuals with this personality disorder tend to be self-centred and impulsive and often require immediate gratification. They lack judgement and self-control and do not profit from their mistakes.**
3. These people tend not to learn from their mistakes, experiences, or punishment.
4. These people are self-centred and do not have a sense of responsibility to others.

CLASSIFICATION
Competency:
Foundations of Practice
Taxonomy:
Application

81.
1. People with this disorder do not generally have a history of depression.
2. They tend to be easily frustrated.
3. They lack insight into their behaviour as well as empathy for others, which is essential in order to motivate them to change.
4. **Individuals with an antisocial personality disorder have a history of self-motivated and maladaptive behaviour.**

CLASSIFICATION
Competency:
Foundations of Practice
Taxonomy:
Knowledge/Comprehension

82.
1. This response shifts responsibility from the issue at hand to the institution.
2. This response does not address the statement; the client is aware of their roles.
3. **This response politely confirms the relationship as professional rather than social.**
4. Dating a client may be against her ethics, but it is the professional reason that takes precedence.

CLASSIFICATION
Competency:
Ethical Practice
Taxonomy:
Critical Thinking

CASE 20

83. 1. This type of mask is not necessary. A sterile mask is required.
2. The practical nurse needs to prepare a sterile field for the dressing change.
3. **Skin preparation is necessary using a back-and-forth motion to prevent introducing microbes into the system. This is the most important step in preventing infection.**
4. Sterile gloves are necessary.

CLASSIFICATION
Competency: **Foundations of Practice**
Taxonomy: **Critical Thinking**

---

84. 1. **This entry provides the most complete information about the actions taken.**
2. This information is incomplete.
3. No assessment of the PICC line site documented. The doctor's name is not necessary.
4. This entry provides no assessment data regarding the PICC line site or information about the dressing change.

CLASSIFICATION
Competency: **Legal Practice**
Taxonomy: **Critical Thinking**

---

85. 1. **The learner is responsible for recognizing her knowledge, skills, abilities, and limits of responsibilities. The nurse preceptor must be aware of the student's abilities and knowledge base in order for the two of them to mutually develop a learning plan and provide safe care to clients.**
2. Learners are responsible and accountable for their own practice. The nurse preceptor is not co-responsible if he has fulfilled his responsibilities as a preceptor and not put the learner in a position where she is functioning beyond her abilities.
3. The learner must identify the need for and act to obtain appropriate supervision.
4. The learner and the preceptor share the responsibility for errors if she is directed to provide care that the preceptor knows is beyond her level of competency.

CLASSIFICATION
Competency: **Professional Practice**
Taxonomy: **Knowledge/Comprehension**

CASE 21

86. 1. Straws should never be used because they increase the risk of aspiration.
2. This information is not necessarily accurate. Insertion of a gastrostomy tube is recommended if a full assessment by the speech therapist has shown a risk for aspiration or inadequate swallowing.
3. There is no reason for bland food if the client prefers spicy foods.
4. **This information is correct. Speech therapists perform a complete assessment of the client's eating and swallowing skills and develop a plan of care for the dysphagia.**

CLASSIFICATION
Competency: **Collaborative Practice**
Taxonomy: **Application**

---

87. 1. Hydrogel is covered with a cotton gauze to help secure it in place and prevent dehydration of the hydrogel.
2. **The moist environment promotes more rapid healing.**
3. This type of dressing does provide some protection, but it is not the main reason for choosing it.
4. Hydrogel is not suitable for wounds with a large amount of drainage because it is designed to add moisture rather then remove moisture.

CLASSIFICATION
Competency: **Foundations of Practice**
Taxonomy: **Critical Thinking**

---

88. 1. Trying to reorient the client to the present will only distress her.
2. This response is too complex for this type of client to understand.
3. This response provides distraction and allows the client to express herself.
4. This response may be appropriate if Ms. Baverstock cannot be distracted.

CLASSIFICATION
Competency:
Collaborative of Practice
Taxonomy:
Application

---

89. 1. This action is impractical and may not be possible.
2. This action is not an independent nursing action.
3. Same as answer 2.
4. This action will ensure that she is safe and provide her with some company and interest.

CLASSIFICATION
Competency:
Professional Practice
Taxonomy:
Application

CASE 22

90. 1. This action must be done but is not the initial action.
2. This action will be done of there is a medical directive for the antipyretics. It is not the first action.
3. These children most likely have a communicable disease. It is particularly important when working with chronically ill children that the symptomatic children be isolated to prevent transmission of the microorganisms.
4. Same as answer 1.

CLASSIFICATION
Competency:
Professional Practice
Taxonomy:
Critical Thinking

---

91. **1. If the child has had a previous anaphylactic response to an insect bite, the practical nurse must be prepared to treat the expected similar response, which could be life threatening.**
2. This action may be done if necessary.
3. This action will be done but is not the priority.
4. Wasps do not generally leave stingers; however, the area should be inspected to see if there is one. If visible, the practical nurse may attempt to remove it. This is an important action but an assessment for anaphylaxis is more critical.

CLASSIFICATION
Competency:
Foundations of Practice
Taxonomy:
Critical Thinking

---

92. 1. This action will need to be done but is not the priority.
2. Same as answer 1.
3. The practical nurse has an initial and primary responsibility to ensure that the medication error has not caused any adverse effects in Madison.
4. Same as answer 1.

CLASSIFICATION
Competency:
Professional Practice
Taxonomy:
Critical Thinking

---

93. 1. Nurses may be allowed to accept a gift, depending on the circumstances and purpose of the gift. People of some cultures would be offended by the nurse refusing the gift.
2. This response implies that the practical nurse will take better care of Fatima because she has received a gift.
3. The family may be offended by this question.
4. This answer does not offend the family, does not imply Fatima will get special treatment, and does not create bad feelings among the rest of the health care team.

CLASSIFICATION
Competency:
Ethical Practice
Taxonomy:
Application

94.
1. **This action is the most important initial action to protect the children from being infected by the practical nurse. Chicken pox in chronically ill, immunosuppressed children can be very serious.**
2. This action should be done but is not the priority.
3. If the practical nurse must be in contact with anyone, he should use proper infection control practices, but it is more important that he isolate himself from the children.
4. Since the contact was 2 weeks prior, it is too late for immunization to be effective if he has contracted the disease.

CLASSIFICATION
Competency: **Professional Practice**
Taxonomy: **Critical Thinking**

CASE 23

95.
1. This response is correct but does not address Ms. Anderson's lack of information.
2. Same as answer 1.
3. **This response recognizes that Ms. Anderson still requires information before she can make an informed decision.**
4. This response may be true but avoids the issue. Ms. Anderson has not asked what the practical nurse would do.

CLASSIFICATION
Competency: **Legal Practice**
Taxonomy: **Critical Thinking**

96.
1. **This information is correct.**
2. This information is correct but does not answer the question.
3. Production of estrogen ceases after menopause.
4. Only 5 to 10% of breast cancer cases are thought to be due to genetic causes.

CLASSIFICATION
Competency: **Foundations of Practice**
Taxonomy: **Application**

97.
1. This response offers false reassurance.
2. This response is too vague and has not answered Mr. Anderson's question.
3. **This response is practical and reliable.**
4. This response does not answer Mr. Anderson's question.

CLASSIFICATION
Competency: **Collaborative Practice**
Taxonomy: **Application**

CASE 24

98.
1. This assessment is necessary but is not the most important.
2. Same as answer 1.
3. **Ensuring that the client has a patent airway and is able to breathe adequately is the most important assessment.**
4. Same as answer 1.

CLASSIFICATION
Competency: **Foundations of Practice**
Taxonomy: **Critical Thinking**

99.
1. This position would encourage aspiration and make it difficult for mucus to drain.
2. **This position allows fluid to drain and permits suctioning.**
3. Same as answer 1.
4. Same as answer 1.

CLASSIFICATION
Competency: **Changes in Health**
Taxonomy: **Application**

100.

1. **The client must be encouraged to practise good oral hygiene and have regular dental exams.**
2. This information is not specific to this condition.
3. Same as answer 2.
4. Same as answer 2.

CLASSIFICATION
Competency:
Collaborative Practice
Taxonomy:
Application

INDEPENDENT QUESTIONS ANSWERS AND RATIONALES

101.

1. This description describes the effect of anabolic steroids.
2. Amphetamines may actually decrease coordination.
3. Over time, use of amphetamines would cause the athlete to have a decreased ability to manage stress.
4. **This effect of central nervous stimulants like amphetamines results in their substance use by athletes. Obscuring of fatigue can lead to the exceeding of physical limits and a resulting collapse.**

CLASSIFICATION
Competency:
Foundations of Practice
Taxonomy:
Knowledge/Comprehension

102.

1. **Torticollis is limited neck motion, in which the neck is flexed and turned to the affected side. Treatment consists of gentle stretching exercises for the neck.**
2. This intervention does not treat torticollis.
3. This intervention does not treat torticollis and is contraindicated due to the risk of sudden infant death syndrome.
4. This intervention is a treatment for dislocation of the hips.

CLASSIFICATION
Competency:
Foundations of Practice
Taxonomy:
Application

103.

1. This question is part of the environmental assessment but is not the first question.
2. Same as answer 1.
3. Same as answer 1.
4. **This question will yield baseline information on the pattern and extent of the allergies. This information can then lead to a possible identification of triggers and a plan for management of the allergies.**

CLASSIFICATION
Competency:
Professional Practice
Taxonomy:
Critical Thinking

104.

1. This action must be done but is not the initial step.
2. **This consideration is the priority for the practical nurse. People who are not ready to learn will not be able to learn, regardless of the individualization, the teaching plan, their baseline knowledge, and so on. These parents have just received a terminal diagnosis for their child and, thus, are not likely to be able to learn skills.**
3. Same as answer 1
4. Same as answer 1.

CLASSIFICATION
Competency:
Professional Practice
Taxonomy:
Critical Thinking

105.

1. Drug use does not necessarily lead to delirium.
2. **Delirium, temporary but acute mental confusion, is common in older persons admitted to hospital.**

CLASSIFICATION
Competency:
Foundations of Practice
Taxonomy:
Critical Thinking

3. Depression is not an indicator for the development of delirium.
4. Ovarian cancer is not a risk for delirium.

106.

1. Immunosuppressant action causes bone marrow depression, which decreases the number of leukocytes.
2. They do not interfere with antibody production.
3. Glucocorticoids interfere with the body's response to microorganisms but do not directly promote the spread of enteroviruses.
4. **These agents are classified as anti-inflammatory or immunosuppressive. They interfere with the release of enzymes responsible for the inflammatory response.**

CLASSIFICATION
Competency: **Foundations of Practice**
Taxonomy: **Knowledge/Comprehension**

107.

1. This statement is true, but because of the reference to sexually transmitted condylomas, the statement may be perceived as assigning blame and may inhibit the expression of feelings.
2. **This statement recognizes Ms. Pitre's feeling of anxiety as valid.**
3. This statement offers false reassurance. Although a condyloma is a benign wart, the papilloma virus that causes it can bring about neoplastic changes in the cervical tissue, which, if not interrupted, lead to cervical carcinoma.
4. This statement is true, but any cancer diagnosis is worrisome for people. The practical nurse's statement does not recognize Ms. Pitre's concerns or give her a chance to discuss her feelings.

CLASSIFICATION
Competency: **Professional Practice**
Taxonomy: **Application**

108.

1. A wheeze is a high-pitched sound, usually louder on expiration.
2. This sound would be heard over the precordium and would be synchronized with the heartbeat.
3. **A pleural friction rub would make this sound when the parietal pleura rubs against the visceral pleura.**
4. Atelectasis has greatly reduced air entry and does not produce a rubbing sound.

CLASSIFICATION
Competency: **Foundations of Practice**
Taxonomy: **Application**

109.

1. Discussion and questioning are not an appropriate teaching strategy for toddlers. This is recommended for adolescents and adults.
2. Pictures may be helpful but may also increase the toddler's anxiety.
3. **Play is an appropriate teaching demonstration method for a toddler.**
4. Same as answer 1.

CLASSIFICATION
Competency: **Foundations of Practice**
Taxonomy: **Critical Thinking**

110.

1. There is no specific or factual information about the history of substance use.
2. This documentation does not describe the pressure injury or provide any factual information about it.
3. **This documentation is specific and objective.**
4. Feelings cannot be uniformly measured.

CLASSIFICATION
Competency: **Legal Practice**
Taxonomy: **Critical Thinking**

111.

1. The client will not require turning for another 15 minutes.
2. This client should be checked hourly but can wait until 2000 hours.

3. **This client has the greatest acuity. The practical nurse must ensure that the hypoglycemia has been properly treated and the blood sugar is now within normal ranges.**
4. The client will not have the full effect of pain medication as yet, and this is not the most acute situation.

CLASSIFICATION
Competency:
Professional Practice
Taxonomy:
Critical Thinking

112.

1. **Each client should be treated as an individual regardless of any aspect of diversity.**
2. Family should be included if this is desired by the client.
3. Differences in health beliefs and practices are common but are not the most important cultural principle.
4. The practical nurse may not be able to have knowledge of every culture. Appropriate care may still be provided by requesting information and assistance from the client.

CLASSIFICATION
Competency:
Professional Practice
Taxonomy:
Critical Thinking

113.

1. Alcohol may be consumed in moderation.
2. Alcohol does not have this effect on the pancreas.
3. Although people with type 2 diabetes may be allowed alcohol in similar amounts to people without the disease, there are other factors of which the client must be aware.
4. **The client will need to monitor the effects of alcohol on his blood sugar so that he may adjust his intake accordingly. Alcohol contains calories, which must be calculated into his daily caloric intake.**

CLASSIFICATION
Competency:
Foundations of Practice
Taxonomy:
Application

114.

1. **Showers are preferable to tub baths since bacteria in the water may enter the urethra.**
2. An increase in cranberry juices, not apple, prevents bacteria from adhering to the wall of the bladder.
3. Voiding every hour is probably not possible or necessary. Voiding every 2 hours is recommended.
4. Intercourse is not forbidden, but it is recommended that the client void immediately afterward.

CLASSIFICATION
Competency:
Foundations of Practice
Taxonomy:
Application

115.

1. The prostate-specific antigen (PSA) is a screening test but does not necessarily confirm the presence of cancer.
2. There are several treatments recommended depending on the type and progress of the cancer: surgery, watchful waiting, external radiation, hormone therapy, insertion of radioactive pellets (brachytherapy), and others.
3. **A biopsy determines if there is cancer and provides information for staging of the cancer.**
4. Depending on the treatment, impotence and incontinence may be avoided.

CLASSIFICATION
Competency:
Foundations of Practice
Taxonomy:
Critical Thinking

116.

1. **Often, substance misuse can trigger auditory and visual hallucinations, depending on the substance use pattern.**
2. The client must be assessed, but there is not an immediate need.

CLASSIFICATION
Competency:
Foundations of Practice
Taxonomy:
Application

3. There is no indication that he will become violent.
4. He is in the most likely age range for schizophrenia to appear.

117.

1. Unless the care is provided in an emergency situation, consent for treatment is required; however, written consent is not necessary.
2. A signed consent is not required.
3. Same as answer 2.
4. **A practical nurse must ask for and be granted consent before undertaking any procedure. If the procedure has been explained to the client, the client may indicate consent verbally or nonverbally by nodding the head yes or positioning the body for the procedure to be carried out.**

CLASSIFICATION
Competency:
Legal Practice
Taxonomy:
Application

118.

1. The pressure will help with snoring, but this is not the machine's main purpose.
2. **The positive pressure prevents airway collapse so that the client does not have oxygen desaturation.**
3. The machine does help with oxygen saturation, but this is not its main purpose.
4. The machine is used to keep the airway patent, not to reduce the workload of the heart.

CLASSIFICATION
Competency:
Foundations of Practice
Taxonomy:
Critical Thinking

119.

1. **Pediculosis is infestation by lice. Infestation by *Pediculus humanus capitis*, or head lice, is a common condition among school-aged children. The condition is treated with specifically formulated over-the-counter shampoos that kill the lice and nits.**
2. Pediculosis does not involve a fungus. It involves an arthropod (parasitic animal).
3. This treatment is used for mild abrasions and superficial infections.
4. This treatment may be used for psoriasis, not pediculosis.

CLASSIFICATION
Competency:
Foundations of Practice
Taxonomy:
Application

120.

1. Requires well balanced snacks. Caffeine is a stimulant that will affect his sleep pattern
2. A large meal in the evening will increase his agitation and keep him up all night.
3. This should be done routinely during the day when less agitated.
4. **Light will reduce agitation and fear that occurs around darkness and shadows.**

CLASSIFICATION
Competency:
Foundations of Practice
Taxonomy:
Application

121.

1. The goal of asthma management is that control should allow for participation in all activities.
2. **This action has been shown to be effective in preventing exercise-induced asthma in children.**
3. Some children have attacks during cold weather, but if the asthma is adequately controlled, such attacks can be managed in most cases.
4. Peak flow rates may be within normal ranges in a child, but an attack can still occur during exercise.

CLASSIFICATION
Competency:
Foundations of Practice
Taxonomy:
Application

122.

1. **The therapeutic regimen of bedrest includes peace of mind, which can best be achieved if the children are adequately cared for. Exploring possible options may provide practical solutions to the childcare problem.**
2. This response explores the client's feelings but does not address the therapeutic regimen.

CLASSIFICATION
Competency:
Professional Practice
Taxonomy:
Application

3. Complete bedrest has been prescribed, so the client should not fix meals.
4. This response offers a solution that may not be possible or acceptable rather than exploring the situation with the client.

123.

1. This intervention does help clients to manage panic disorders but requires counselling, which is not initially appropriate in an emergency department.
2. The client's anxiety triggers will be explored during counselling but identifying them is not an initial intervention.
3. **Lorazepam (Ativan) is used as an initial treatment because it provides a rapid reduction in symptoms.**
4. Selective serotonin reuptake inhibitors are often prescribed for clients with panic disorders; however, they would not be the initial treatment and are not as likely to be prescribed in an emergency department.

CLASSIFICATION
Competency:
Foundations of Practice
Taxonomy:
Critical Thinking

124.

1. Clients with a borderline personality disorder take little responsibility for themselves or their actions. They should be encouraged to solve their own problems.
2. With this disorder, it is important to maintain a consistent approach in all interactions and ensure that other staff members do so as well.
3. Clients with borderline personality disorder may idolize some staff members and devalue others. The practical nurse should not take sides in his disputes with other staff members.
4. **Consistent reinforcement of acceptable behaviour will enable Mr. Loek to better function in society.**

CLASSIFICATION
Competency:
Foundations of Practice
Taxonomy:
Application

125.

1. The ratio does not affect compatibility.
2. **These types of insulin are compatible and are administered in the same syringe.**
3. The two insulins may be given together at the same time.
4. This action is not required; unnecessary injections increase the risk of infection as well as cause additional discomfort.

CLASSIFICATION
Competency:
Foundations of Practice
Taxonomy:
Application

126.

1. **Canned vegetable soup is high in sodium, containing approximately 1 060 mg of sodium per 250 mL.**
2. Natural cheese does contain sodium but not as much as canned tomato juice.
3. Fresh fish is not high in sodium.
4. Whole-wheat pasta, if cooked in unsalted water, is low in sodium.

CLASSIFICATION
Competency:
Foundations of Practice
Taxonomy:
Knowledge/Comprehension

127.

1. This example portrays aggressive behaviour.
2. **The essential feature of passive–aggressive behaviour is resistance to meeting the demands of others in terms of social and occupational functioning. Chronic lateness is an excellent example of this.**
3. This example portrays anger or aggression but is not passive.
4. Same as answer 3.

CLASSIFICATION
Competency:
Foundations of Practice
Taxonomy:
Knowledge/Comprehension

128.

1. This instruction is for the Valsalva manoeuvre.
2. It is not wise to delay voiding with a full bladder because this weakens the sphincter muscles.
3. Kegel exercises involve the urinary sphincter, not the anal sphincter.
4. **This method is correct for targeting the correct muscles used in Kegel exercises, which strengthen the urinary sphincter.**

CLASSIFICATION
Competency:
Foundations of Practice
Taxonomy:
Application

129.

1. **The gloves have become contaminated by the soiled dressing and must be immediately removed to prevent transmission of microorganisms.**
2. The dressing tray should not be opened while the nurse is wearing soiled gloves.
3. Hand hygiene will be performed but not until after the removal of the soiled gloves.
4. The door or curtain should have been closed prior to applying the gown, gloves, and goggles.

CLASSIFICATION
Competency:
Professional Practice
Taxonomy:
Application

130.

1. This test determines exposure to the tubercle bacillus. Once an individual has been infected, the test will always be positive.
2. This test does not provide information about communicability.
3. **The absence of bacteria in the sputum indicates that the disease can no longer be spread by the airborne route.**
4. Absence of fever is not evidence that the disease cannot be transmitted.

CLASSIFICATION
Competency:
Foundations of Practice
Taxonomy:
Knowledge/Comprehension

131.

1. Flatulence may occur as a result of immobility, not just obstruction.
2. Anorexia may occur with an impaction, but it may also be caused by other conditions.
3. **Because of the presence of feces in the colon, a client with a fecal impaction has the urge to defecate but is unable to.**
4. The frequency of bowel movements varies for individuals; it may be normal for this individual not to have one for several days.

CLASSIFICATION
Competency:
Foundations of Practice
Taxonomy:
Application

132.

1. ***Toxoplasma gondii*, a protozoan, can be transmitted by exposure to infected cat feces or by ingestion of undercooked, contaminated meat.**
2. Toxoplasmosis is not related to viral illnesses.
3. *Toxoplasma gondii* is a parasite of warm-blooded animals; fish are not considered the source of contamination.
4. Toxoplasmosis is not related to diseases included in childhood immunizations.

CLASSIFICATION
Competency:
Foundations of Practice
Taxonomy:
Knowledge/Comprehension

133.

1. **To avoid additional spinal cord damage, the victim must be moved with great care. Moving a person whose spinal cord has been injured could cause irreversible paralysis. The practical nurse requires assistance from emergency health care workers who have the appropriate equipment.**
2. A back injury is suspected; therefore, the person should not be moved.
3. A back injury precludes changing the person's position.
4. A flat board would be indicated; however, one rescuer alone could not safely move the victim.

CLASSIFICATION
Competency:
Foundations of Practice
Taxonomy:
Critical Thinking

134.

1. **Damage to Broca's area, located in the posterior frontal region of the dominant hemisphere, causes problems in the motor aspect of speech.**
2. This difficulty is associated with receptive aphasia, not expressive aphasia; receptive aphasia is associated with disease of Wernicke's area of the brain.
3. Understanding speech is associated with receptive aphasia.
4. Same as answer 2.

CLASSIFICATION
Competency:
Foundations of Practice
Taxonomy:
Knowledge/Comprehension

135.

1. This manifestation is not a sign of infection.
2. **This manifestation is part of the normal healing process. The penis does not require any further care, other than gentle cleansing with water.**
3. This manifestation is not a sign of a need for better cleansing. Hydrogen peroxide is not necessary and would irritate the skin.
4. This statement is implied criticism of the father for having the child circumcised and is not a therapeutic response.

CLASSIFICATION
Competency:
Foundations of Practice
Taxonomy:
Application

136.

1. This action would have a systemic effect on fluid balance; edema of the residual limb is a localized response to inflammation.
2. Same as answer 1.
3. Prolonged immobilization of the residual extremity in one position can lead to a flexion contracture of the hip.
4. **Elastic bandages compress the residual limb, preventing edema and promoting residual limb shrinkage and moulding; the bandage must be rewrapped when it loosens.**

CLASSIFICATION
Competency:
Foundations of Practice
Taxonomy:
Application

137.

1. Individuals with these injuries could wait for treatment per the health care team triage routine.
2. Same as answer 1.
3. Same as answer 1.
4. **Individuals with these injuries require urgent care as they may experience severe blood loss and risk of infection.**

CLASSIFICATION
Competency:
Professional Practice
Taxonomy:
Critical Thinking

138.

1. **This action is the professional choice. If she is ill or too tired to function, she must consult with the supervisor, who will decide what solution is appropriate.**
2. This action would be considered professional misconduct.
3. The practical nurse may not be able to stay awake. She is jeopardizing the safety of her clients, particularly if she is ill.
4. This action is not reasonable. The co-worker is in need of a break and should not be asked or told to look after the practical nurse's clients. If the co-worker offers to cover for the practical nurse and the co-worker is feeling refreshed, it may be allowable.

CLASSIFICATION
Competency:
Professional Practice
Taxonomy:
Critical Thinking

139.

1. **This type of conjunctivitis occurs about 3 to 4 days after birth. If it is not treated, chronic follicular conjunctivitis with conjunctival scarring will likely result.**
2. Congenital syphilis does not manifest as eye discharge.

CLASSIFICATION
Competency:
Foundations of Practice
Taxonomy:
Knowledge/Comprehension

3. Allergies are uncommon in newborns due to the transmission of maternal antibodies.
4. This chemical conjunctivitis occurs within the first 48 hours, and the discharge is not purulent.

140.

1. **The role of the practical nurse includes advocating for quality environments to promote safe, holistic client care.**
2. This problem is with the system and will not be solved by the nurse's having a limited client assignment.
3. It is more professional and effective to advocate than to complain. The manager may not be receptive to complaints.
4. The status quo does not allow for the provision of quality care. There may be alternatives that would address quality care and client numbers.

CLASSIFICATION
Competency:
Professional Practice
Taxonomy:
Critical Thinking

141.

1. Colds are caused by viruses; therefore, antibiotics have no effect.
2. Antiviral medications are neither recommended nor effective for colds.
3. **Warm or hot fluids help keep mucus fluid and clear the nose. Anecdotal and some research evidence suggest that echinacea and zinc lozenges work for some people.**
4. Although there is no cure, Mrs. Scales can be encouraged to rest, increase her fluids, and treat specific symptoms.

CLASSIFICATION
Competency:
Foundations of Practice
Taxonomy:
Knowledge/Comprehension

142.

1. This statement repeats a myth. Regular bathing is even more important during menstruation.
2. **Changing tampons every 2 to 4 hours helps prevent toxic shock syndrome.**
3. Tampons may be worn, provided they are changed frequently.
4. Douches are not recommended because they alter the natural flora of the vagina and may introduce microorganisms.

CLASSIFICATION
Competency:
Collaborative Practice
Taxonomy:
Application

143.

1. Endometriosis does not cause amenorrhea.
2. Endometriosis does not cause anovulation.
3. **Endometriosis is the presence of aberrant endometrial tissue outside the uterus. The tissue responds to ovarian stimulation, bleeds during menstruation, and causes severe pain.**
4. Pelvic inflammation usually results from infection.

CLASSIFICATION
Competency:
Foundations of Practice
Taxonomy:
Knowledge/Comprehension

144.

1. **The practical nurse's initial action is to stop the abuse.**
2. This action will have to be done but is not the priority.
3. Reporting the abuse to the regulatory body is a nurse's legal responsibility, but it is not the initial action.
4. A written report will have to be made, but stopping the abuse is the most important action initially.

CLASSIFICATION
Competency:
Legal Practice
Taxonomy:
Critical Thinking

145.

1. This type of fracture is caused by twisting of the limb. It is seen in cases of child abuse.
2. **Bone fragility causes the spinal vertebrae to weaken, leading to multiple compression fractures that cause pain and reduce height.**

CLASSIFICATION
Competency:
Foundations of Practice
Taxonomy:
Application

3. This type of fracture is caused by direct force to the bone.
4. This type of fracture pulls bone and other tissues from the usual attachments and does not commonly occur with osteoporosis.

146.

1. This action is not the initial action. The physician would likely request that the nurse retake the client's blood pressure using a manual system.
2. The client's blood pressure should be retaken manually to confirm the findings prior to medication administration.
3. This action is an option but is unlikely to change the reading.
4. **It is best practice for the practical nurse to retake the reading and compare results. Automatic monitoring systems malfunction on occasion. Aberrant recordings should be checked manually.**

CLASSIFICATION
Competency:
Professional Practice
Taxonomy:
Critical Thinking

147.

1. This statement would indicate to the wife that she was correct in what she was telling her husband.
2. This question voices an assumption and may make Mrs. Alberto feel defensive.
3. This question is aggressive and sounds punitive.
4. **There may be many reasons for Mrs. Alberto's telling her husband incorrect information. By using an open-ended question asking for information, the practical nurse should be able to identify and correct misinformation.**

CLASSIFICATION
Competency:
Professional Practice
Taxonomy:
Application

148.

1. **According to the Canadian Cancer Society, lung cancer is the leading cause of cancer deaths in Canada.**
2. Breast cancer accounts for a high incidence of cancer in women, but in the overall population, it does not cause as many deaths as lung and colon cancers.
3. Prostate cancer accounts for a high incidence of cancer in men, but in the overall population, it does not cause as many deaths as lung and colon cancers.
4. Colorectal cancer, which may be effectively treated if caught in the early stages, is the second-largest cause of cancer death in men and third leading cause of death in women.

CLASSIFICATION
Competency:
Foundations of Practice
Taxonomy:
Knowledge/Comprehension

149.

1. Incorrect answer. Stage 1 pressure injuries have intact skin.
2. **Correct answer. Stage 2 pressure injuries may present as an intact serum-filled blister. These injuries commonly result from shear in the skin of the heel.**
3. Incorrect answer. Stage 3 pressure injuries have full thickness loss of skin with exposed adipose tissue.
4. Incorrect answer. Stage 4 pressure injuries have full thickness skin and tissue loss with potential exposed fascia, bone, ligament, tendon, cartilage, or muscle present.

CLASSIFICATION
Competency:
Foundations of Practice
Taxonomy:
Knowledge/Comprehension

150.

1. **Use of an individually fitted spinal orthosis (a brace) is generally successful in halting or slowing the progression of most curvatures while the child reaches skeletal maturity.**
2. Surgery is required only for severe scoliosis.
3. Exercises have been proven to be of limited use with scoliosis, although they do help to prevent atrophy of spinal and abdominal muscles.
4. This treatment has not proven to be effective.

CLASSIFICATION
Competency:
Foundations of Practice
Taxonomy:
Knowledge/Comprehension

151.

1. **Emergency contraception pills stop or delay the release of an egg from the ovary. They should be taken within 72 hours of unprotected sex in order to be effective.**
2. It does not stimulate menstruation.
3. It will not prevent a fertilized ovum from developing but may stop it implanting in the uterus.
4. It does not terminate a pregnancy and will not work if the woman is already pregnant.

CLASSIFICATION
Competency: **Foundations of Practice**
Taxonomy: **Knowledge/Comprehension**

152.

1. Mild analgesia
2. Muscle relaxant
3. Mild analgesia
4. **Commonly prescribed for treatment of moderate to severe pain**

CLASSIFICATION
Competency: **Foundations of Practice**
Taxonomy: **Knowledge and Comprehension**

153.

1. The practical nurse should not be delegating this task.
2. **This response offers correct information and explains why she cannot delegate the task.**
3. Allowing an unregulated care provider to perform this task is irresponsible and constitutes professional malpractice.
4. Taking this action is unnecessary since Mr. Leslie has been performing suctioning safely for some time.

CLASSIFICATION
Competency: **Collaborative Practice**
Taxonomy: **Critical Thinking**

154.

1. **Research has shown that positioning infants in the supine position for sleep has reduced the mortality from SUIDS by 50%.**
2. This action will help the infant's general health but has not been proven to have a significant effect on SUIDS.
3. It was previously believed that placing children in the prone position would prevent asphyxia. This belief has been discredited.
4. This action may be recommended for high-risk premature infants who have a history of apnea, but it was not part of the public awareness campaign.

CLASSIFICATION
Competency: **Foundations of Practice**
Taxonomy: **Knowledge/Comprehension**

155.

1. This action places the nursing responsibility on the wife and does not solve the problem.
2. Mr. Morgan has refused the medication because of the adverse effects, not the taste.
3. This action could be considered a threat.
4. **The pharmacist may be able to recommend or the physician may be able to prescribe a different medication that will not cause digestive distress.**

CLASSIFICATION
Competency: **Professional Practice**
Taxonomy: **Application**

156.

1. Discomfort is a late sign.
2. Discharge becomes foul smelling only after there is necrosis and infection; it is not an early sign.
3. Pressure is not an early symptom because the cancer must be extensive to cause pressure.
4. **Any abnormal vaginal bleeding may indicate cervical cancer.**

CLASSIFICATION
Competency: **Foundations of Practice**
Taxonomy: **Knowledge/Comprehension**

157.

1. This term does not refer to involvement of lymph nodes.
2. Estrogen contributes to tumour growth; supplements are not indicated.
3. **Estrogen receptor–positive (ER-positive) tumours have a more dramatic response to hormonal therapies that reduce estrogen.**
4. This term is unrelated to metastasis.

CLASSIFICATION
Competency:
Foundations of Practice
Taxonomy:
Knowledge/Comprehension

158.

1. **Cardiac nitrates relax the smooth muscles of the coronary arteries so that they dilate and deliver more blood to relieve ischemic pain.**
2. Although cardiac output may improve because of improved oxygenation of the myocardium, this is not a basis for evaluating the drug's effectiveness.
3. Although the dilation of blood vessels and a subsequent drop in blood pressure may occur, this is not the basis for evaluating the drug's effectiveness.
4. Although superficial vessels dilate, lowering the blood pressure and creating a flushed appearance, this is not a basis for evaluating the drug's effectiveness.

CLASSIFICATION
Competency:
Foundations of Practice
Taxonomy:
Application

159.

1. This action will not necessarily provide reassurance. The parents have a need to actually see for themselves that their child is stable.
2. This action is therapeutic but unlikely to reduce the parents' anxiety; seeing their child would be more therapeutic.
3. **This action provides the best reassurance, as long as the parents know what to expect in the postanaesthetic care unit.**
4. There is an immediate need to reduce the parents' anxiety; time away will not meet this need.

CLASSIFICATION
Competency:
Collaborative Practice
Taxonomy:
Application

160.

1. Never give injections, take blood samples, or start intravenous lines in the access site arm; this could damage the shunt.
2. Same as answer 1.
3. **Do not take the blood pressure or put pressure on the access arm to prevent damage to and preserve the internal arteriovenous shunt.**
4. It is important to palpate the AVF for a thrill (vibration). It may indicate a clotted access if the vibration is not present when the AVF is palpated.

CLASSIFICATION
Competency:
Foundations of Practice
Taxonomy:
Critical Thinking

161.

1. HIV can be transmitted in vaginal fluids during unprotected vaginal intercourse, but this is not the most high-risk behaviour.
2. HIV may be transmitted via oral sex with either gender, but this is not the most high-risk behaviour.
3. HIV transmission depends on sexual behaviour, not sexual orientation.
4. **Anal intercourse is an extremely high-risk behaviour because HIV may enter the bloodstream via small tears in the fragile lining of the anus.**

CLASSIFICATION
Competency:
Foundations of Practice
Taxonomy:
Critical Thinking

162.

1. People respond more positively to policies when they understand them. Just instituting policies without providing education about them is less effective.
2. **Education would increase employees' awareness of environmental issues and help them to understand the importance of the "green" initiatives.**

CLASSIFICATION
Competency:
Professional Practice
Taxonomy:
Critical Thinking

3. This strategy is not practical.
4. This action is valuable, but employees may not use the containers if they are not educated about and do not "buy into" the program.

163.

1. The surgeon's action constitutes abuse and should be reported, but reporting it is not the practical nurse's first action.
2. **The practical nurse's first action when encountering abuse is to intervene and speak up.**
3. This action may be taken but is not the practical nurse's first action.
4. Intervention is best when it is immediate. Due to the abusive behaviour, the practical nurse should not confront the surgeon in private.

CLASSIFICATION
Competency:
Professional Practice
Taxonomy:
Critical Thinking

164.

1. Milk contains fat and protein—both of which require a longer digestion time—and lactose, which is a disaccharide.
2. Bread contains carbohydrates, which require a longer time to digest because they must be converted to simple sugars.
3. Chocolate bars do not contain the high proportion of simple sugars found in orange juice; they also contain fat, which takes longer to digest.
4. **Fruit juice has a higher proportion of simple sugars, which are quickly absorbed and are then readily available for conversion to energy.**

CLASSIFICATION
Competency:
Foundations of Practice
Taxonomy:
Critical Thinking

165.

1. **Sleeping on pillows raises the upper torso and prevents reflux of the gastric contents through the hernia.**
2. This action would have no effect on the mechanical problem of the stomach entering the thoracic cavity.
3. Increasing the contents of the stomach before lying down would aggravate the symptoms associated with a hiatal hernia.
4. The effect of antacids is not long-lasting enough to promote a full night's sleep; also, sodium bicarbonate is not the antacid of choice.

CLASSIFICATION
Competency:
Foundations of Practice
Taxonomy:
Application

166.

1. This action evaluates fluid balance and is best performed over a 24-hour period.
2. **Residual volume indicates whether gastric emptying is delayed. Depending on agency policy and physician or dietitian decision, if residual volume exceeds 500 mL, feedings may be withheld.**
3. No longer considered reliable, this action was a method used for evaluating the placement of the nasogastric tube.
4. Although weighing the client regularly is important in evaluating overall nutritional progress, it cannot provide information about absorption of a particular feeding.

CLASSIFICATION
Competency:
Foundations of Practice
Taxonomy:
Critical Thinking

167.

1. Liver abscesses may occur as a complication of intestinal infections. They are not related to portal hypertension or cirrhosis.
2. An intestinal obstruction is not related to portal hypertension or cirrhosis. It may be caused by manipulation of the bowel during surgery, peritonitis, neurological disorders, or organic obstruction.
3. Perforation of the duodenum is usually caused by peptic ulcers. It is not a direct result of portal hypertension or cirrhosis.

4. **The elevated pressure within the portal circulatory system causes elevated pressure in areas of portal systemic collateral circulation (most important, in the distal esophagus and proximal stomach). Hemorrhage is a possible life-threatening complication.**

CLASSIFICATION
Competency:
Foundations of Practice
Taxonomy:
Knowledge/Comprehension

168.
1. This factor is a "red flag" but is not the most indicative finding.
2. This factor is a possible sign of neglect but is not a confirmation of abuse.
3. This factor is a definite risk factor for this infant for neglect, but it is not the most indicative finding.
4. **Previous fractures without adequate explanation in a child under 1 year of age is highly suggestive of abuse.**

CLASSIFICATION
Competency:
Ethical Practice
Taxonomy:
Critical Thinking

169.
1. This manifestation describes psoriasis.
2. This manifestation is alopecia areata. It is a benign condition with an unknown cause, but the client usually has a complete regrowth of the hair.
3. These manifestations are normal in an aging person and are commonly known as liver spots.
4. **This manifestation describes malignant melanoma.**

CLASSIFICATION
Competency:
Foundations of Practice
Taxonomy:
Critical Thinking

170.
1. Sterile water is a hypotonic solution, which may be absorbed by body tissues.
2. Isotonic, not hypertonic, solutions are used because they are similar to body fluids.
3. **Although other solutions may be ordered, irrigations of the bladder usually employ sterile normal saline (0.9% NaCl), which is a solution of approximately the tonicity of normal body fluids.**
4. Similar to answer 1 and tap water is not sterile solution. You do not want to instill unsterile solutions into the bladder cavity.

CLASSIFICATION
Competency:
Foundations of Practice
Taxonomy:
Application

171.
1. **An honest nurse–client relationship should be maintained so that trust can develop.**
2. This action is punitive and will not assist the practical nurse in working with Mr. Beauclerc to stop smoking.
3. Through this action, the practical nurse is deferring professional responsibility to another health care provider.
4. This action does nothing to establish communication about feelings or motivation behind the client's behaviour.

CLASSIFICATION
Competency:
Professional Practice
Taxonomy:
Critical Thinking

172.
1. Each province and territory is responsible for registering its nurses.
2. **This description accurately describes the role of the Canadian Nurses Association.**
3. This description describes a nursing union.
4. Each provincial, not federal, government delegates regulation to a provincial college of nurses.

CLASSIFICATION
Competency:
Professional Practice
Taxonomy:
Knowledge/Comprehension

173.
1. It is obvious that things are not right, and Ms. Serena would be tired.
2. This comment does not deal with the mother's concerns.
3. This question may be interpreted as criticism and could make Ms. Serena feel defensive.
4. **This comment acknowledges Ms. Serena's feelings. An open-ended, unbiased question provides an opportunity for the practical nurse to collect as much data as possible.**

CLASSIFICATION
Competency:
Collaborative Practice
Taxonomy:
Critical Thinking

174.
1. This is not a sign of physical abuse.
2. This is not a sign of neglect.
3. This is not a sign of financial abuse.
4. **Isolation from family and friends is a sign of emotional abuse.**

CLASSIFICATION
Competency:
Professional Practice
Taxonomy:
Knowledge and Comprehension

175.
1. Frequent breastfeeding is recommended.
2. This action may be recommended for mild hyperbilirubinemia since the sun will help to decrease the bilirubin in the blood. However, because the extent of the hyperbilirubinemia is not known, this treatment may be inadequate.
3. A glucose and water mixture is to be avoided in jaundiced breastfed infants because it will decrease the amount of breast milk they drink.
4. **The degree of jaundice is determined by serum bilirubin measurements. Although most newborn jaundice is benign, this cannot be determined without an actual level.**

CLASSIFICATION
Competency:
Foundations of Practice
Taxonomy:
Critical Thinking

176.
1. This emotion cannot be assumed from the situation described.
2. **Changes in self-image and family role can initiate a grieving process with a variety of emotional responses.**
3. Same as answer 1.
4. This emotion may be present, but it is only part of his general loss of independence.

CLASSIFICATION
Competency:
Foundations of Practice
Taxonomy:
Critical Thinking

177.
1. Herpes zoster is potentially contagious to anyone who has not had chickenpox.
2. **Herpes zoster is caused by activation of the varicella-zoster virus, the virus that causes chickenpox. Mrs. Hoagy is potentially contagious to anyone who has not had chickenpox.**
3. Same as answer 1.
4. Same as answer 1.

CLASSIFICATION
Competency:
Foundations of Practice
Taxonomy:
Knowledge and Comprehension

178.
1. This is less than the normal adult urine output expected per day.
2. **This is the normal urine output expected per day.**
3. This is more than the normal adult urine output expected per day.
4. Same as answer 3.

CLASSIFICATION
Competency:
Foundations of Practice
Taxonomy:
Application

179.
1. Immobilization of the wrist would achieve this outcome. In addition to the wrist bones being aligned, the hand must not move at the wrist. Only an elbow cast can accomplish this.

2. The elbow is immobilized to prevent pronation and supination of the wrist.

3. A longer cast is not easier to manage.
4. This response does not answer the question, and "provide support" is vague.

CLASSIFICATION
Competency:
Foundations of Practice
Taxonomy:
Application

180.

1. This is not effective for relieving acute episodes; it takes hours for the desired effect to occur.

2. This is a treatment for life-threatening allergic (anaphylaxis) reactions.

3. This is not effective for an anaphylactic emergency treatment.
4. Same as answer 3.

CLASSIFICATION
Competency:
Foundations of Practice
Taxonomy:
Critical Thinking

181.

1. Justice involves treating others equitably and with fairness.
2. Nonmaleficence involves doing no harm whether intentionally or unintentionally.
3. Autonomy involves the recognition that people have a right to make their own choices and take action based on their own personal beliefs.

4. The practical nurse is demonstrating beneficence for what is best for the client balancing against risk and harm. She is working to understand the client's needs and then working actively to meet those needs.

CLASSIFICATION
Competency:
Ethical Practice
Taxonomy:
Application

182.

1. This information is correct. Sexual intercourse is not more taxing than climbing two flights of stairs.

2. This response avoids answering the client's partner's question.
3. A wait of 4 to 6 months is unnecessary.
4. Jogging may not be possible for the client and is not an accurate reflection of when relations may be resumed.

CLASSIFICATION
Competency:
Foundations of Practice
Taxonomy:
Application

183.

1. The showers will help thin the secretions. A fever would indicate infection, which would require antibiotic therapy.

2. It is unrealistic to ask Mr. Phillion not to swim if he is part of a competitive team. Taking over-the-counter medications may disqualify him from the competition.
3. Frequent nose blowing may irritate the lining of the nasal passage and will not help the sinusitis.
4. It is unlikely that Mr. Phillion would be able to keep his head out of the water during competitive swimming.

CLASSIFICATION
Competency:
Foundations of Practice
Taxonomy:
Application

184.

1. Presence of other diseases such as diabetes and depressions increase the risk of poor nutrition.

2. Age-related gastrointestinal changes such as reduced saliva production and decreased esophageal and colonic peristalsis affect maintenance of nutrition.

3. Although Canada offers Old Age Security to older persons, this payment is sometimes not sufficient to cover food expenses.
4. Metabolic demands are decreased, but this does not equate to older persons getting adequate nutrition.

CLASSIFICATION
Competency:
Foundations of Practice
Taxonomy:
Application

185.
1. Turning onto the unaffected side will not splint the chest wall.
2. The hands may be used, but the semi-Fowler position provides no support to the chest wall.
3. **This method is best. Turning onto the affected side splints the chest wall and reduces the stretching of the pleura.**
4. Deep breathing needs to be encouraged; fluid intake will help, but secretions are not indicated in the question.

CLASSIFICATION
Competency:
Foundations of Practice
Taxonomy:
Application

186.
1. A newborn will likely not regain his or her birth weight by this age.
2. Same as answer 1.
3. **A newborn is most likely to regain birth weight by 10 to 12 days. This guideline is important for parents who are anxious concerning infant feeding and growth.**
4. A newborn should have regained his or her birth weight before the age of 14 to 21 days.

CLASSIFICATION
Competency:
Foundations of Practice
Taxonomy:
Knowledge/Comprehension

187.
1. This response would make the client wonder if the nurse had any knowledge or understanding of his diagnosis.
2. This response cuts off any further communication of feelings; it ignores what the client has expressed to the nurse.
3. **Sitting down with the client indicates a willingness to talk and to give attention in a relaxed manner.**
4. This response does not provide the client an opportunity to discuss his suicidal feelings.

CLASSIFICATION
Competency:
Collaborative Practice
Taxonomy:
Application

188.
1. This health care provider will not have the necessary triage skills.
2. Same as answer 1.
3. The respiratory therapist is trained in airway management and general first aid measures but does not have the necessary advanced triage skills.
4. **The paramedic is trained in triage and emergency first aid. It is within the scope of practice for the paramedic to provide appropriate care to casualty victims.**

CLASSIFICATION
Competency:
Professional Practice
Taxonomy:
Critical Thinking

189.
1. **Having the client dress appropriately helps keep her more in touch with reality.**
2. This approach may cause the client to be a target of ridicule by the other clients.
3. This approach could be perceived as punitive.
4. This approach may not be acceptable to the client and does not help her to make appropriate clothing decisions.

CLASSIFICATION
Competency:
Foundations of Practice
Taxonomy:
Application

190.
1. This action is an option, but it is unlikely to have any effect.
2. This action is an option, but it is not the most professional one.
3. **Advocating healthy public policy is the foundation of health promotion. Nurses should persuade decision makers to adopt options that preserve the *Canada Health Act*.**

CLASSIFICATION
Competency:
Professional Practice
Taxonomy:
Critical Thinking

4. This action is an option and may assist to develop a network of like-minded individuals. However, they still need to bring their concerns to the local government.

191.

1. This approach is an option, but research has shown abstinence education does not reduce the number of unwanted pregnancies.
2. This approach is an option; however, in most societies, it is women who take the responsibility for effective birth control.
3. This approach serves to reduce unwanted pregnancies after the fact and may not be an ethical option for some clients.
4. **Research has shown there are fewer unplanned pregnancies when contraceptives are readily and easily available.**

CLASSIFICATION
Competency:
Foundations of Practice
Taxonomy:
Critical Thinking

192.

1. **The first step in the nursing process is to validate data. Asking this question will provide the practical nurse with specific information on the severity of the vomiting.**
2. This question will be asked but is not the first question.
3. Same as answer 2.
4. Same as answer 2.

CLASSIFICATION
Competency:
Foundations of Practice
Taxonomy:
Critical Thinking

193.

1. Gonorrhea is common. The increasing rate and number of gonorrhea cases are a serious public health concern for Canada and around the world.
2. **Gonorrhea is a reportable sexually transmitted infection.**
3. Usually, a single dose of medication is sufficient to cure the client.
4. Gonorrhea does not cause permanent damage to the testes.

CLASSIFICATION
Competency:
Foundations of Practice
Taxonomy:
Application

194.

1. This complication may occur as a consequence of severe respiratory distress syndrome.
2. This complication is not a primary concern unless severe hypoxia occurred during labour; it would be difficult to diagnose at this time.
3. This complication may be a problem, but generally the air passageway is well suctioned at birth.
4. **Immaturity of the respiratory tract in preterm infants can be evidenced by a lack of functional alveoli; smaller lumens, increasing the possibility of the collapse of the respiratory passages; weakness of respiratory musculature; and insufficient calcification of the bony thorax, leading to respiratory distress.**

CLASSIFICATION
Competency:
Foundations of Practice
Taxonomy:
Critical Thinking

195.

1. High blood pressure during pregnancy is one of the symptoms of preeclampsia, not hypotension.
2. **Proteins are seen in the urine due to temporary damage of the kidneys' filtering process.**
3. Sudden weight gain of 7.5 to 12.5 kilograms (3 to 5 pounds) may be an indicator of preeclampsia.
4. This is not a sign of preeclampsia.

CLASSIFICATION
Competency:
Foundations of Practice
Taxonomy:
Knowledge and Comprehension

196.

1. This therapy does not remove the virus.
2. **Raising the CD4 count and reducing the viral load are the purposes of the therapy. This answer is in language easily understood by Mr. Brankston.**
3. Antiretrovirals do not kill the virus.
4. This statement is not accurate and is too complex an answer for Mr. Brankston.

CLASSIFICATION
Competency:
Foundations of Practice
Taxonomy:
Knowledge/Comprehension

197.

1. The practical nurse does not have competence to manage the heparin infusion and cannot safely care for Mr. Levy.
2. **Consultation with the RN to discuss care transition is required since the practical nurse is not competent in managing the heparin infusion.**
3. The practical nurse can provide aspects of Mr. Levy's care.
4. Same as answer 1.

CLASSIFICATION
Competency:
Professional Practice
Taxonomy:
Critical Thinking

198.

1. **This strategy would provide the staff with the opportunity to be involved in coming to a democratic solution, which may be perceived as a fair approach.**
2. This action may not be perceived by staff as a fair solution.
3. This strategy is often implemented by managers but may not be viewed as a fair approach by less senior members of the nursing staff.
4. A lottery may be an effective solution but only if agreed upon by the entire nursing staff.

CLASSIFICATION
Competency:
Professional Practice
Taxonomy:
Critical Thinking

199.

1. It is important for clients with hypertension to exercise.
2. **This regimen starts with mild exercise and increases as Ms. Pratha increases her fitness level.**
3. This recommendation is unnecessary and may be harmful.
4. Blood pressure is not lower in the evening.

CLASSIFICATION
Competency:
Foundations of Practice
Taxonomy:
Application

200.

1. Assessing the client prior to discharge is important but not as important as assessing the client with breathing difficulties.
2. Assessing the client who prefers personal care before 0800 is important but not as important as assessing the client with breathing difficulties.
3. Assessing the client with cloudy urine is important but not as important as assessing the client with breathing difficulties.
4. **Breathing difficulties are a priority of care and this client should be assessed first.**

CLASSIFICATION
Competency:
Professional Practice
Taxonomy:
Critical Thinking

END OF ANSWERS AND RATIONALES TO PRACTICE EXAM 3

Bibliography

American Psychiatric Association. (2013). *Diagnostic and statistical manual of mental disorders* (5th ed.). Washington, DC: Author.

Arnold, E., & Boggs, K. (2020). *Interpersonal relationships: Professional communication skills for nurses* (8th ed). Saunders/Elsevier.

Assessment Strategies Inc. (2016). *The Canadian Practical Nurse Registration Examination (CPNRE) prep guide* (5th ed.). Ottawa: Author.

Assessment Strategies Inc. (2017). *Canadian practical nurse registration examination blueprint.* Ottawa: Author.

Callahan. B. (2019). *Clinical nursing skills: A concept-based approach to learning* (3rd ed.). Pearson.

Canadian Cancer Society. (2020). *Treatments for testicular cancer.* https://www.cancer.ca/en/cancer-information/cancer-type/testicular/treatment/?region=on

Canadian Mental Health Association. (2020). *Understanding mental illness: Resource manual.* https://cmha.ca/mental-health/understanding-mental-illness

Canadian Nurses Association. (2017). *Code of ethics for registered nurses.* https://www.cna-aiic.ca/~/media/cna/page-content/pdf-en/code-of-ethics-2017-edition-secure-interactive

Canadian Nurses Protective Society. (2018). *Access to cannabis for medical purposes: What every nurse should know.* https://www.cnps.ca/index.php?page=502#nurses

College of Nurses. (Revised 2019). *The standard of care. Entry-to-practice competencies for registered practical nurses* (Publication No. 41042). https://www.cno.org/globalassets/docs/reg/41042_entrypracrpn-2020.pdf#:~:text=In%202019%2C%20CNO%20worked%20as%20part%20of%20the,%28with%20Quebec%20as%20an%20observer%29%2C%20led%20the%20project .

College of Nurses of Ontario. (2012). *Requisite skills and abilities for nursing practice in Ontario* (Publication No. 41078). http://www.cno.org/globalassets/docs/reg/41078-skillabilities-4pager-final.pdf

College of Nurses of Ontario. (2013). *Practice guideline: Working with unregulated care providers* (Publication No. 41014). https://www.cno.org/globalassets/docs/prac/41014_workingucp.pdf

College of Nurses of Ontario. (2017). *Practice guideline: Refusing assignments and discontinuing nursing services* (Publication No. 41070). http://www.cno.org/globalassets/docs/prac/41070_refusing.pdf

College of Nurses of Ontario. (2018a). *Practice standard: Professional standards*, revised 2002 (Publication No. 41006). http://www.cno.org/globalassets/docs/prac/41006_profstds.pdf

College of Nurses of Ontario. (2018b). *Practice guideline: RN and RPN practice: The client, the nurse, and the environment* (Publication No. 41062). https://www.cno.org/globalassets/docs/prac/41062.pdf

College of Nurses of Ontario. (2018c). *The standard of care: Guidance on nurses' roles in medical assistance in dying* (Publication No. 41056). http://www.cno.org/globalassets/docs/prac/41056-guidance-on-nurses-roles-in-maid.pdf

College of Nurses of Ontario. (2019a). *Practice standard: Confidentiality & privacy-personal health information* (Publication No. 41069). http://www.cno.org/globalassets/docs/prac/41069_privacy.pdf

College of Nurses of Ontario. (2019b). *Practice standard: Documentation*, revised 2008 (Publication No. 41001). http://www.cno.org/globalassets/docs/prac/41001_documentation.pdf

College of Nurses of Ontario. (2019c). *Practice standard: Ethics* (Publication No. 41034). http://www.cno.org/globalassets/docs/prac/41034_ethics.pdf

College of Nurses of Ontario. (2019d). *Practice standard: Medication* (Publication No. 41007). http://www.cno.org/globalassets/docs/prac/41007_medication.pdf

College of Nurses of Ontario. (2019e). *Reference document: Profession conduct, professional misconduct* (Publication No. 42007). https://www.cno.org/globalassets/docs/ih/42007_misconduct.pdf

College of Nurses of Ontario. (2019f). *Practice standard: Therapeutic nurse–client relationship*, revised 2006 (Publication No. 41033). https://www.cno.org/globalassets/docs/prac/41033_therapeutic.pdf

College of Nurses of Ontario. (2020a). *Legislation and regulation. An introduction to the Nursing Act, 1991* (Publication No. 41064). http://www.cno.org/globalassets/docs/prac/41064_fsnursingact.pdf

College of Nurses of Ontario. (2020b). *Practice standard: Decisions about procedures and authority* (Publication No. 41071). http://cno.org/globalassets/docs/prac/41071_decisions.pdf

College of Nurses of Ontario. (2020c). *Reference document: Legislation and regulation. RHPA: Scope of practice, controlled acts model* (Publication No. 41052). http://www.cno.org/globalassets/docs/policy/41052_rhpascope.pdf

College of Nurses of Ontario. (2020d). *The standard of care: Nursing during a pandemic.* http://www.cno.org/en/learn-about-standards-guidelines/educational-tools/pandemic-planning/nursing-during-a-pandemic/

Dipchand, A., Friedman, J., Bismilla, Z., Gupta, S., & Lam, C. (2010). *The Hospital for Sick Children handbook of pediatrics* (11th ed.). Saunders.

Dudek. S. G. (2010). *Nutrition essentials for nursing practice* (6th ed.). Wolters Kluwer Health/Lippincott Williams & Wilkins.

Durbin, T., Martin, T., Merritt, K., & Poppel, T. (2018). *Culturally competent preceptorship. International journal of nursing and health care research.* https://gavinpublishers.com/articles/Mini-Review/International-Journal-of-Nursing-and-Health-Care-Research/culturally-competent-preceptorship

Government of Canada. (2018). *Information for health care rofessionals: Cannabis (marihuana, marijuana) and the cannabinoids.* https://www.canada.ca/en/health-canada/services/drugs-medication/cannabis/information-medical-practitioners/information-health-care-professionals-cannabis-cannabinoids.html#a4.1

Government of Canada. (2019a). *Canadian pandemic influenza preparedness: Planning guidance for the health sector.* https://www.canada.ca/en/public-health/services/flu-influenza/canadian-pandemic-influenza-preparedness-planning-guidance-health-sector.html

Government of Canada. (2019b). *Preventing the spread of extensively drug resistant gonorrhea* (Vol. 45 2/3). https://www.canada.ca/en/public-health/services/reports-publications/canada-communicable-disease-report-ccdr/monthly-issue/2019-45/issue-2-february-7-2019/article-2-preventing-spread-drug-resistant-gonorrhea.html

Government of Canada. (2020a). *Canada food guide.* https://food-guide.canada.ca/en/

Government of Canada. (2020b). *Medical assistance in dying.* https://www.canada.ca/en/health-canada/services/medical-assistance-dying.html#grievous

Hales, D., & Lauzon, L. (2018). *An invitation to health* (5th ed.). Thomson Nelson.

Halter. M. J. (2018). *Varcarolis' foundations of psychiatric mental health nursing: A clinical approach* (8th ed.). Elsevier/Saunders.

Halter, M. J., Pollard, C. L., & Jakubec, S. L. (2019). *Varcarolis' foundations of psychiatric mental health nursing: A clinical approach* (2nd ed.). Elsevier.

Health Nexus. (2020). *Breast feeding matters. An important guide to breastfeeding families.* Breast Start Resource Centre. https://resources.beststart.org/wp-content/uploads/2017/01/B04-E_BF_matters_EN_2020.pdf .

Hockenberry, M., Rodgers, C., & Wilson, D. (2021). *Wong's essentials of pediatric nursing* (11th ed.). Elsevier.

Hockenberry, M. J., Wilson, D., & Rodgers, C. (2019). *Wong's nursing care of infants and children* (11th ed.). Mosby/Elsevier.

Huson, H. B., Granados, T. M., & Rasko, Y. (2018). Surgical considerations of marijuana in elective procedures. *Heliyon*, *4*(9), e00779.

Hypertension Canada. (2015). *Accurate measurement of blood pressure: Guidelines.* https://guidelines.hypertension.ca/diagnosis-assessment/measuring-blood-pressure/

Jarvis, C., Browne, A. J., MacDonald-Jenkins, J., & Luctkar-Flude, M. (2018). *Physical examination & health assessment* (3rd ed.). Saunders.

Katsademas, K., & Langille, M. (2020). *Mosby's comprehensive review for the Canadian PN exam.* Mosby/Elsevier.

Keatings, M., & Adams, P. (2020). *Ethical and legal issues in Canadian nursing* (4th ed.). Elsevier.

Leifer, G., & Keenan-Lindsay, L. (2020). *Leifer's introduction to maternity and pediatric nursing in Canada.* Elsevier.

Lewis, S., Bucher, L., Heitkemper, M. M., Harding, M., Barry, M., Lok, J., … Goldsworthy, S. (2019). *Medical-surgical nursing in Canada* (4th ed.). Elsevier.

Lowdermilk, E., Perry, S., Cashion, M. C., & Alden, K. R. (2019). *Maternity and women's health care* (10th ed.). Mosby/Elsevier.

Marshall-Henty, J., & Bradshaw, J. (2011). *Mosby's prep guide for the Canadian RN exam. Practice questions for exam success* (2nd ed.). Mosby/Elsevier.

National Council of State Boards of Nursing (NCSBN). (2020). *2022 Regulatory Exam-Practical Nurse (Rex-PN). Test Plan.* Chicago: Author.

O'Toole, M. (Ed.), *Mosby's dictionary of medicine, nursing, and health professions* (10th ed). Elsevier/Mosby.

Pagana, K. D., Pagana, T. J., & Pike-MacDonald, S. A. (2019). *Mosby's Canadian manual of diagnostic and laboratory tests* (2nd ed.). Elsevier.

Perry, A. G., Potter, P. A., Ostendorf, W., & Cobbett, S. (2019). *Canadian clinical nursing skills and techniques.* Mosby/Elsevier.

Perry, S., Hockenberry, M. J., Lowdermilk, D. L., Wilson, D., Rhodes Alden, K., & Cashion, M. C. (2018). *Maternal child nursing care* (6th ed.). Mosby.

Potter, P. A., Perry, A. G., Stockert, P., & Hall, A. (2019). *Canadian fundamentals of nursing* (6th ed.). Elsevier.

Public Health Agency of Canada. (2018). *Joint statement on safe sleep. Preventing sudden infant deaths in Canada.* https://www.canada.ca/en/public-health/services/health-promotion/childhood-adolescence/stages-childhood/infancy-birth-two-years/safe-sleep/joint-statement-on-safe-sleep.html

Registered Nurses Association. (2007). *Nursing best practice guidelines: Embracing cultural diversity in health care: Developing cultural competence.* https://rnao.ca/bpg/guidelines/embracing-cultural-diversity-health-care-developing-cultural-competence

Registered Nurses Association of Ontario. (Revised 2008). *Nursing best practice guidelines: promoting asthma control in children.* https://rnao.ca/sites/rnao-ca/files/Promoting_Asthma_Control_in_Children.pdf

Registered Nurses Association of Ontario. (2011). *Nursing best practice guidelines: Preventing and mitigating nurse fatigue in health care healthy work environments best practice guideline.* https://rnao.ca/bpg/guidelines/preventing-and-mitigating-nurse-fatigue-health-care

Registered Nurses Association of Ontario. (2012). *Nursing best practice guidelines: Promoting safety: Alternative approaches to the use of restraints.* https://rnao.ca/sites/rnao-ca/files/Promoting_Safety_-_Alternative_Approaches_to_the_Use_of_Restraints_0.pdf

Registered Nurses Association of Ontario. (2013). *Clinical best practice guidelines: Assessment and management of pain (2013)* (3rd ed.). https://rnao.ca/sites/rnao-ca/files/AssessAndManagementOfPain_15_WEB-_FINAL_DEC_2.pdf

Registered Nurses Association of Ontario. (2016). *Clinical best practice guidelines: Delirium, dementia and depression in older adults: Assessment and care* (2nd ed.). https://rnao.ca/sites/rnao-ca/files/bpg/RNAO_Delirium_Dementia_Depression_Older_Adults_Assessment_and_Care.pdf

Registered Nurses Association of Ontario. (2017). *Clinical best practice guidelines: Adult asthma: Promoting control of asthma* (2nd ed.). https://rnao.ca/bpg/guidelines/adult-asthma-care

Sealock, K., Seneviratne, C., Lilley, L., & Snyder, J. (2021). *Lilley's Pharmacology for Canadian Health Care Practice* (4th ed.). Mosby.

Skidmore-Roth. L. (2019). *Mosby's drug guide for nursing students with 2020 update* (13th ed.). Mosby/Elsevier.

Skidmore-Roth. L. (2021). *Mosby's nursing drug reference* (34th ed.). Mosby/Elsevier.

Sorrentino, A., Remmert, L., & Wilk, M. (2018). *Mosby's Canadian textbook for the support worker* (4th ed.). Elsevier.

Stuart. G. W. (2013). *Principles and practice of psychiatric nursing* (10th ed.). Mosby.

Turner. S. (2019). *Mulholland's the nurse, the math, the meds: Drug calculations using dimensional analysis* (4th ed.). Elsevier.

University Health Network. (2017, Updated 2018). *Vancomycin resistant Enterococcus (VRE). Information for patients, families and visitors at UHN.* https://www.uhn.ca/PatientsFamilies/Health_Information/Health_Topics/Documents/Patient%20VRE%20Q+A.pdf

Waddell, J. I., & Walton, N. A. (2020). *Yoder-Wise's leading and managing in Canadian nursing* (2nd ed.). Elsevier.

Appendix

Entry-Level/Entry-to-Practice Competencies for Licensed/Registered Practical Nurses in Canada

Adapted from College of Nurses of Ontario Entry-to-Practice Competencies for Registered Practical Nurses (2019), Canadian Council of Practical Nurse Regulators Entry-Level Competencies for Licensed Practical Nurses (2019), and British Columbia College of Nursing Professionals Entry-Level Competencies for Licensed Practical Nurses (2019).

ASSUMPTIONS

The following are a set of assumptions that are understood to apply to the practice of practical nursing in Canada and to the Entry-Level/Entry-to-Practice competencies listed.

- The foundation of practical nursing is defined by:
  - entry-level/entry-to-practice competencies
  - professional nursing standards of practice of the regulatory authority
  - nursing code(s) of ethics and ethical standards
  - scope of nursing practice applicable in the jurisdiction
  - provincial, territorial and federal legislation and regulations that direct practice
- Licensed Practical Nurse (LPN)/Registered Practical Nurse (RPN) practice is built upon the four concepts of person, environment, health and nursing, and is grounded within the context of the current Canadian health care system, primary health care and emerging health trends.
- LPNs/RPNs possess competencies that are transferable across all areas of responsibility (e.g., direct care, administration, education and research).
- LPNs/RPNs are active participants in health promotion, illness prevention and harm reduction activities.
- LPNs/RPNs practice in any setting or circumstance where health care is delivered.
- Requisite skills and abilities are required to attain the LPN/RPN entry-to-practice competencies.
- LPNs/RPNs practice autonomously, safely, competently and ethically along the continuum of care in situations of health and illness across a client's lifespan.
- LPNs/RPNs practice in situations of varying complexity and work collaboratively with the health care team to maximize client outcomes.
- LPNs/RPNs demonstrate leadership by fostering continued self-growth to meet the challenges of an evolving health care system.
- LPNs/RPNs follow a systematic approach to deliver safe, competent and ethical care by using the nursing process.
- LPNs/RPNs advocate for the implementation and use of evidence-informed practice.

1. PROFESSIONAL PRACTICE

LPNs/RPNs adhere to practice standards and an ethical framework. They are responsible and accountable for safe, competent and ethical nursing practice. They are expected to demonstrate professional conduct as reflected through personal attitudes, beliefs, opinions and actions. LPNs/RPNs focus on personal and professional growth. LPNs/RPNs are expected to use knowledge, critical thinking, critical inquiry and research to build an evidence-informed practice.

1. Demonstrates accountability and accepts responsibility for own decisions and actions.
2. Practices autonomously within legislated scope of practice.
3. Displays self-awareness and recognizes when to seek assistance and guidance.
4. Adheres to regulatory requirements of jurisdictional legislation.
5. Practices within own level of competence.
6. Initiates, maintains and terminates the therapeutic nurse–client relationship.
7. Provides client care in a non-judgemental manner.
8. Adapts practice in response to the spiritual beliefs and cultural practices of clients.
9. Supports clients in making informed decisions about their health care, and respects their decisions.
10. Engages in self-reflection and continuous learning to maintain and enhance competence.
11. Integrates relevant evidence into practice.
12. Collaborates in the analysis, development, implementation and evaluation of practice and policy.
13. Integrates continuous quality improvement principles and activities into nursing practice.
14. Demonstrates a professional presence, honesty, integrity and respect in all interactions.
15. Demonstrates fitness to practice.

16. Maintains current knowledge about trends and issues that impact the client, the RPN, the health care team and the delivery of health services.

17. Identifies and responds to inappropriate behaviour and incidents of professional misconduct.

18. Recognizes, responds and reports own and others' near misses, errors and adverse events.

19. Distinguishes between the mandates of regulatory bodies, professional associations and unions.

2. ETHICAL PRACTICE

LPNs/RPNs use ethical frameworks (e.g., Code of Ethics, ethical standards) when making professional judgements and practice decisions. They engage in critical thinking and critical inquiry to inform decision-making and use self-reflection to understand the impact of personal values, beliefs and assumptions in the provision of care.

20. Establishes and maintains professional boundaries.

21. Takes action to minimize the impact of personal values and assumptions on interactions and decisions.

22. Demonstrates respect for the values, opinions, needs and beliefs of others.

23. Applies ethical frameworks and reasoning to identify and respond to situations involving moral and ethical conflict, dilemma or distress.

24. Obtains knowledge of and responds to the *Calls to Action of the Truth and Reconciliation Commission of Canada.*

25. Preserves the dignity of clients in all personal and professional contexts.

26. Advocates for equitable access, treatment and allocation of resources, particularly for vulnerable and/or diverse clients and populations.

27. Advocates for clients, especially when they are unable to advocate for themselves.

28. Adheres to the duty to provide care.* (ON/BC only)

3. LEGAL PRACTICE

LPNs/RPNs adhere to applicable provincial/territorial and federal legislation and regulations, professional standards and employer policies that direct practice. They engage in professional regulation by enhancing their competence, promoting safe practice and maintaining their fitness to practice. LPNs/RPNs recognize that safe nursing practice includes knowledge of relevant laws and legal boundaries within which LPNs/RPNs must practice.

29. Practices according to legislation, practice standards, ethics and organizational policies.

30. Practices according to relevant mandatory reporting legislation.

31. Recognizes, responds and reports questionable orders, actions or decisions made by others.

32. Adheres to the duty to report.

33. Protects clients' rights by maintaining confidentiality and privacy in all personal and professional contexts.

34. Respond to the clients' right to health care information in adherence within relevant privacy legislation.

35. Documents according to established legislation, practice standards, ethics and organizational policies.

36. Obtains informed consent to support the client's informed decision-making.

4. FOUNDATIONS OF PRACTICE

LPNs/RPNs use critical thinking, reflection and evidence integration to assess clients, plan care, implement interventions, and evaluate outcomes and processes. Foundational knowledge includes: nursing theory, health sciences, humanities, pharmacology and ethics.

37. Completes comprehensive health assessments of clients across the lifespan.

38. Selects and uses information and communication technologies (ICTs) in the delivery of client care.

39. Researches and responds to relevant clinical data.

40. Engages in evidence-informed practice by considering a variety of relevant sources of information.

41. Comprehends, responds to and reports assessment findings.

42. Formulates clinical decisions consistent with client needs and priorities.

43. Identifies nursing diagnoses.

44. Develops the care plan with the client, health care team and others.

45. Implements nursing interventions based on assessment findings, client preferences and desired outcomes.

46. Responds to clients' conditions by organizing competing priorities into actions.

47. Assesses clients' health literacy, knowledge and readiness to learn.

48. Assesses, plans, implements and evaluates the teaching and learning process.

49. Provides information and access to resources to facilitate health education.

50. Evaluates the effectiveness of health education.

51. Applies principles of client safety.

52. Engages in quality improvement and risk management to promote a quality practice environment.

53. Evaluates the effectiveness of nursing interventions by comparing actual outcomes to expected outcomes.

54. Reviews and revises the plan of care and communicates accordingly.

55. Assesses implications of own decisions.

56. Uses critical thinking, critical inquiry and clinical judgement for decision-making.

57. Demonstrates professional judgement in using ICTs and social media.

58. Recognizes high-risk practices and integrates mitigation strategies that promote safe care.

59. Applies strategies to prevent, de-escalate and manage disruptive, aggressive or violent behaviour.

60. Recognizes and responds immediately when a client's condition is deteriorating.

61. Demonstrates knowledge of nursing theory, pharmacology, health sciences, humanities and ethics.

62. Applies knowledge of pharmacology and principles of safe medication practice.* (ON/BC only)

5. COLLABORATIVE PRACTICE

LPNs/RPNs work collaboratively with clients and other members of the health care team. They recognize that collaborative practice is guided by shared values and accountability, a common purpose or care outcome, mutual respect, and effective communication.

63. Engages clients in identifying their health needs, strengths, capacities and goals.

64. Communicates collaboratively with the client and the health care team.

65. Provides essential client information to the client and the health care team.

66. Promotes effective interpersonal interaction.

67. Uses conflict resolution strategies to promote healthy relationships and optimal client outcomes.

68. Articulates own role based on legislated scope of practice, individual competence and care context, including employer policies.

69. Determines their own professional and interprofessional role within the team by considering the roles, responsibilities and the scope of practice of others.

70. Advocates for the use of Indigenous health knowledge and healing practices in collaboration with the client.

71. Demonstrates leadership, direction and supervision to unregulated health workers and others.

72. Participates in emergency preparedness and disaster management.

73. Participates in creating and maintaining a quality practice environment that is healthy, respectful and psychologically safe.

74. Fosters an environment that encourages questioning and exchange of information.

75. Initiates and fosters mentoring relationships.

76. Applies the principles of team dynamics and group processes in interprofessional team collaboration.

77. Demonstrates formal and informal leadership in practice.

78. Organizes workload, assigns/coordinates nursing care, sets priorities and demonstrates effective time-management skills.

79. Prepares client and collaborates with health care team in transition and transfer of responsibility of care.* (ON/BC only)

Scoring Sheets

COMMON ERRORS WHEN FILLING IN SCORING SHEETS

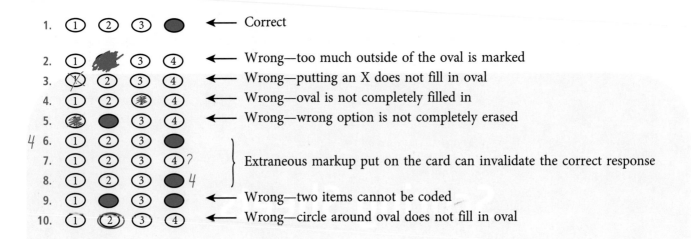

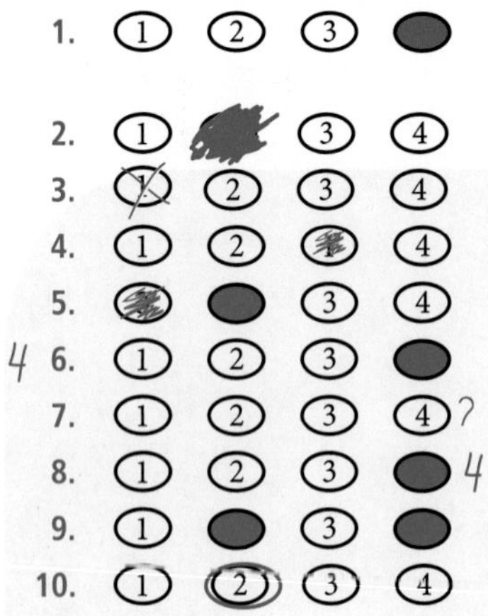

1. ← Correct
2. ← Wrong—too much outside of the oval is marked
3. ← Wrong—putting an X does not fill in oval
4. ← Wrong—oval is not completely filled in
5. ← Wrong—wrong option is not completely erased
6.–8. } Extraneous markup put on the card can invalidate the correct response
9. ← Wrong—two items cannot be coded
10. ← Wrong—circle around oval does not fill in oval

EXAM 1 SCORING SHEETS

CASE-BASED QUESTIONS

1.	1	2	3	4
2.	1	2	3	4
3.	1	2	3	4
4.	1	2	3	4
5.	1	2	3	4
6.	1	2	3	4
7.	1	2	3	4
8.	1	2	3	4
9.	1	2	3	4
10.	1	2	3	4
11.	1	2	3	4
12.	1	2	3	4
13.	1	2	3	4
14.	1	2	3	4
15.	1	2	3	4
16.	1	2	3	4
17.	1	2	3	4
18.	1	2	3	4
19.	1	2	3	4
20.	1	2	3	4
21.	1	2	3	4
22.	1	2	3	4
23.	1	2	3	4
24.	1	2	3	4
25.	1	2	3	4
26.	1	2	3	4
27.	1	2	3	4
28.	1	2	3	4
29.	1	2	3	4
30.	1	2	3	4
31.	1	2	3	4
32.	1	2	3	4
33.	1	2	3	4
34.	1	2	3	4
35.	1	2	3	4
36.	1	2	3	4
37.	1	2	3	4
38.	1	2	3	4
39.	1	2	3	4
40.	1	2	3	4
41.	1	2	3	4
42.	1	2	3	4
43.	1	2	3	4
44.	1	2	3	4
45.	1	2	3	4
46.	1	2	3	4
47.	1	2	3	4
48.	1	2	3	4
49.	1	2	3	4
50.	1	2	3	4
51.	1	2	3	4
52.	1	2	3	4
53.	1	2	3	4
54.	1	2	3	4
55.	1	2	3	4
56.	1	2	3	4
57.	1	2	3	4
58.	1	2	3	4
59.	1	2	3	4
60.	1	2	3	4
61.	1	2	3	4
62.	1	2	3	4
63.	1	2	3	4
64.	1	2	3	4
65.	1	2	3	4
66.	1	2	3	4
67.	1	2	3	4
68.	1	2	3	4
69.	1	2	3	4
70.	1	2	3	4
71.	1	2	3	4
72.	1	2	3	4
73.	1	2	3	4
74.	1	2	3	4
75.	1	2	3	4
76.	1	2	3	4
77.	1	2	3	4
78.	1	2	3	4
79.	1	2	3	4
80.	1	2	3	4
81.	1	2	3	4
82.	1	2	3	4
83.	1	2	3	4
84.	1	2	3	4
85.	1	2	3	4
86.	1	2	3	4
87.	1	2	3	4
88.	1	2	3	4
89.	1	2	3	4
90.	1	2	3	4
91.	1	2	3	4
92.	1	2	3	4
93.	1	2	3	4
94.	1	2	3	4
95.	1	2	3	4
96.	1	2	3	4
97.	1	2	3	4
98.	1	2	3	4
99.	1	2	3	4
100.	1	2	3	4

EXAM 1 SCORING SHEETS

INDEPENDENT QUESTIONS

101. ① ② ③ ④	126. ① ② ③ ④	151. ① ② ③ ④	176. ① ② ③ ④
102. ① ② ③ ④	127. ① ② ③ ④	152. ① ② ③ ④	177. ① ② ③ ④
103. ① ② ③ ④	128. ① ② ③ ④	153. ① ② ③ ④	178. ① ② ③ ④
104. ① ② ③ ④	129. ① ② ③ ④	154. ① ② ③ ④	179. ① ② ③ ④
105. ① ② ③ ④	130. ① ② ③ ④	155. ① ② ③ ④	180. ① ② ③ ④
106. ① ② ③ ④	131. ① ② ③ ④	156. ① ② ③ ④	181. ① ② ③ ④
107. ① ② ③ ④	132. ① ② ③ ④	157. ① ② ③ ④	182. ① ② ③ ④
108. ① ② ③ ④	133. ① ② ③ ④	158. ① ② ③ ④	183. ① ② ③ ④
109. ① ② ③ ④	134. ① ② ③ ④	159. ① ② ③ ④	184. ① ② ③ ④
110. ① ② ③ ④	135. ① ② ③ ④	160. ① ② ③ ④	185. ① ② ③ ④
111. ① ② ③ ④	136. ① ② ③ ④	161. ① ② ③ ④	186. ① ② ③ ④
112. ① ② ③ ④	137. ① ② ③ ④	162. ① ② ③ ④	187. ① ② ③ ④
113. ① ② ③ ④	138. ① ② ③ ④	163. ① ② ③ ④	188. ① ② ③ ④
114. ① ② ③ ④	139. ① ② ③ ④	164. ① ② ③ ④	189. ① ② ③ ④
115. ① ② ③ ④	140. ① ② ③ ④	165. ① ② ③ ④	190. ① ② ③ ④
116. ① ② ③ ④	141. ① ② ③ ④	166. ① ② ③ ④	191. ① ② ③ ④
117. ① ② ③ ④	142. ① ② ③ ④	167. ① ② ③ ④	192. ① ② ③ ④
118. ① ② ③ ④	143. ① ② ③ ④	168. ① ② ③ ④	193. ① ② ③ ④
119. ① ② ③ ④	144. ① ② ③ ④	169. ① ② ③ ④	194. ① ② ③ ④
120. ① ② ③ ④	145. ① ② ③ ④	170. ① ② ③ ④	195. ① ② ③ ④
121. ① ② ③ ④	146. ① ② ③ ④	171. ① ② ③ ④	196. ① ② ③ ④
122. ① ② ③ ④	147. ① ② ③ ④	172. ① ② ③ ④	197. ① ② ③ ④
123. ① ② ③ ④	148. ① ② ③ ④	173. ① ② ③ ④	198. ① ② ③ ④
124. ① ② ③ ④	149. ① ② ③ ④	174. ① ② ③ ④	199. ① ② ③ ④
125. ① ② ③ ④	150. ① ② ③ ④	175. ① ② ③ ④	200. ① ② ③ ④

EXAM 2 SCORING SHEETS

CASE-BASED QUESTIONS

1.	1	2	3	4
2.	1	2	3	4
3.	1	2	3	4
4.	1	2	3	4
5.	1	2	3	4
6.	1	2	3	4
7.	1	2	3	4
8.	1	2	3	4
9.	1	2	3	4
10.	1	2	3	4
11.	1	2	3	4
12.	1	2	3	4
13.	1	2	3	4
14.	1	2	3	4
15.	1	2	3	4
16.	1	2	3	4
17.	1	2	3	4
18.	1	2	3	4
19.	1	2	3	4
20.	1	2	3	4
21.	1	2	3	4
22.	1	2	3	4
23.	1	2	3	4
24.	1	2	3	4
25.	1	2	3	4
26.	1	2	3	4
27.	1	2	3	4
28.	1	2	3	4
29.	1	2	3	4
30.	1	2	3	4
31.	1	2	3	4
32.	1	2	3	4
33.	1	2	3	4
34.	1	2	3	4
35.	1	2	3	4
36.	1	2	3	4
37.	1	2	3	4
38.	1	2	3	4
39.	1	2	3	4
40.	1	2	3	4
41.	1	2	3	4
42.	1	2	3	4
43.	1	2	3	4
44.	1	2	3	4
45.	1	2	3	4
46.	1	2	3	4
47.	1	2	3	4
48.	1	2	3	4
49.	1	2	3	4
50.	1	2	3	4
51.	1	2	3	4
52.	1	2	3	4
53.	1	2	3	4
54.	1	2	3	4
55.	1	2	3	4
56.	1	2	3	4
57.	1	2	3	4
58.	1	2	3	4
59.	1	2	3	4
60.	1	2	3	4
61.	1	2	3	4
62.	1	2	3	4
63.	1	2	3	4
64.	1	2	3	4
65.	1	2	3	4
66.	1	2	3	4
67.	1	2	3	4
68.	1	2	3	4
69.	1	2	3	4
70.	1	2	3	4
71.	1	2	3	4
72.	1	2	3	4
73.	1	2	3	4
74.	1	2	3	4
75.	1	2	3	4
76.	1	2	3	4
77.	1	2	3	4
78.	1	2	3	4
79.	1	2	3	4
80.	1	2	3	4
81.	1	2	3	4
82.	1	2	3	4
83.	1	2	3	4
84.	1	2	3	4
85.	1	2	3	4
86.	1	2	3	4
87.	1	2	3	4
88.	1	2	3	4
89.	1	2	3	4
90.	1	2	3	4
91.	1	2	3	4
92.	1	2	3	4
93.	1	2	3	4
94.	1	2	3	4
95.	1	2	3	4
96.	1	2	3	4
97.	1	2	3	4
98.	1	2	3	4
99.	1	2	3	4
100.	1	2	3	4

EXAM 2 SCORING SHEETS

INDEPENDENT QUESTIONS

101.	1	2	3	4	126.	1	2	3	4	151.	1	2	3	4	176.	1	2	3	4
102.	1	2	3	4	127.	1	2	3	4	152.	1	2	3	4	177.	1	2	3	4
103.	1	2	3	4	128.	1	2	3	4	153.	1	2	3	4	178.	1	2	3	4
104.	1	2	3	4	129.	1	2	3	4	154.	1	2	3	4	179.	1	2	3	4
105.	1	2	3	4	130.	1	2	3	4	155.	1	2	3	4	180.	1	2	3	4
106.	1	2	3	4	131.	1	2	3	4	156.	1	2	3	4	181.	1	2	3	4
107.	1	2	3	4	132.	1	2	3	4	157.	1	2	3	4	182.	1	2	3	4
108.	1	2	3	4	133.	1	2	3	4	158.	1	2	3	4	183.	1	2	3	4
109.	1	2	3	4	134.	1	2	3	4	159.	1	2	3	4	184.	1	2	3	4
110.	1	2	3	4	135.	1	2	3	4	160.	1	2	3	4	185.	1	2	3	4
111.	1	2	3	4	136.	1	2	3	4	161.	1	2	3	4	186.	1	2	3	4
112.	1	2	3	4	137.	1	2	3	4	162.	1	2	3	4	187.	1	2	3	4
113.	1	2	3	4	138.	1	2	3	4	163.	1	2	3	4	188.	1	2	3	4
114.	1	2	3	4	139.	1	2	3	4	164.	1	2	3	4	189.	1	2	3	4
115.	1	2	3	4	140.	1	2	3	4	165.	1	2	3	4	190.	1	2	3	4
116.	1	2	3	4	141.	1	2	3	4	166.	1	2	3	4	191.	1	2	3	4
117.	1	2	3	4	142.	1	2	3	4	167.	1	2	3	4	192.	1	2	3	4
118.	1	2	3	4	143.	1	2	3	4	168.	1	2	3	4	193.	1	2	3	4
119.	1	2	3	4	144.	1	2	3	4	169.	1	2	3	4	194.	1	2	3	4
120.	1	2	3	4	145.	1	2	3	4	170.	1	2	3	4	195.	1	2	3	4
121.	1	2	3	4	146.	1	2	3	4	171.	1	2	3	4	196.	1	2	3	4
122.	1	2	3	4	147.	1	2	3	4	172.	1	2	3	4	197.	1	2	3	4
123.	1	2	3	4	148.	1	2	3	4	173.	1	2	3	4	198.	1	2	3	4
124.	1	2	3	4	149.	1	2	3	4	174.	1	2	3	4	199.	1	2	3	4
125.	1	2	3	4	150.	1	2	3	4	175.	1	2	3	4	200.	1	2	3	4

EXAM 3 SCORING SHEETS

CASE-BASED QUESTIONS

1. (1) (2) (3) (4)	26. (1) (2) (3) (4)	51. (1) (2) (3) (4)	76. (1) (2) (3) (4)
2. (1) (2) (3) (4)	27. (1) (2) (3) (4)	52. (1) (2) (3) (4)	77. (1) (2) (3) (4)
3. (1) (2) (3) (4)	28. (1) (2) (3) (4)	53. (1) (2) (3) (4)	78. (1) (2) (3) (4)
4. (1) (2) (3) (4)	29. (1) (2) (3) (4)	54. (1) (2) (3) (4)	79. (1) (2) (3) (4)
5. (1) (2) (3) (4)	30. (1) (2) (3) (4)	55. (1) (2) (3) (4)	80. (1) (2) (3) (4)
6. (1) (2) (3) (4)	31. (1) (2) (3) (4)	56. (1) (2) (3) (4)	81. (1) (2) (3) (4)
7. (1) (2) (3) (4)	32. (1) (2) (3) (4)	57. (1) (2) (3) (4)	82. (1) (2) (3) (4)
8. (1) (2) (3) (4)	33. (1) (2) (3) (4)	58. (1) (2) (3) (4)	83. (1) (2) (3) (4)
9. (1) (2) (3) (4)	34. (1) (2) (3) (4)	59. (1) (2) (3) (4)	84. (1) (2) (3) (4)
10. (1) (2) (3) (4)	35. (1) (2) (3) (4)	60. (1) (2) (3) (4)	85. (1) (2) (3) (4)
11. (1) (2) (3) (4)	36. (1) (2) (3) (4)	61. (1) (2) (3) (4)	86. (1) (2) (3) (4)
12. (1) (2) (3) (4)	37. (1) (2) (3) (4)	62. (1) (2) (3) (4)	87. (1) (2) (3) (4)
13. (1) (2) (3) (4)	38. (1) (2) (3) (4)	63. (1) (2) (3) (4)	88. (1) (2) (3) (4)
14. (1) (2) (3) (4)	39. (1) (2) (3) (4)	64. (1) (2) (3) (4)	89. (1) (2) (3) (4)
15. (1) (2) (3) (4)	40. (1) (2) (3) (4)	65. (1) (2) (3) (4)	90. (1) (2) (3) (4)
16. (1) (2) (3) (4)	41. (1) (2) (3) (4)	66. (1) (2) (3) (4)	91. (1) (2) (3) (4)
17. (1) (2) (3) (4)	42. (1) (2) (3) (4)	67. (1) (2) (3) (4)	92. (1) (2) (3) (4)
18. (1) (2) (3) (4)	43. (1) (2) (3) (4)	68. (1) (2) (3) (4)	93. (1) (2) (3) (4)
19. (1) (2) (3) (4)	44. (1) (2) (3) (4)	69. (1) (2) (3) (4)	94. (1) (2) (3) (4)
20. (1) (2) (3) (4)	45. (1) (2) (3) (4)	70. (1) (2) (3) (4)	95. (1) (2) (3) (4)
21. (1) (2) (3) (4)	46. (1) (2) (3) (4)	71. (1) (2) (3) (4)	96. (1) (2) (3) (4)
22. (1) (2) (3) (4)	47. (1) (2) (3) (4)	72. (1) (2) (3) (4)	97. (1) (2) (3) (4)
23. (1) (2) (3) (4)	48. (1) (2) (3) (4)	73. (1) (2) (3) (4)	98. (1) (2) (3) (4)
24. (1) (2) (3) (4)	49. (1) (2) (3) (4)	74. (1) (2) (3) (4)	99. (1) (2) (3) (4)
25. (1) (2) (3) (4)	50. (1) (2) (3) (4)	75. (1) (2) (3) (4)	100. (1) (2) (3) (4)

EXAM 3 SCORING SHEETS

INDEPENDENT QUESTIONS

101.	1	2	3	4	126.	1	2	3	4	151.	1	2	3	4	176.	1	2	3	4
102.	1	2	3	4	127.	1	2	3	4	152.	1	2	3	4	177.	1	2	3	4
103.	1	2	3	4	128.	1	2	3	4	153.	1	2	3	4	178.	1	2	3	4
104.	1	2	3	4	129.	1	2	3	4	154.	1	2	3	4	179.	1	2	3	4
105.	1	2	3	4	130.	1	2	3	4	155.	1	2	3	4	180.	1	2	3	4
106.	1	2	3	4	131.	1	2	3	4	156.	1	2	3	4	181.	1	2	3	4
107.	1	2	3	4	132.	1	2	3	4	157.	1	2	3	4	182.	1	2	3	4
108.	1	2	3	4	133.	1	2	3	4	158.	1	2	3	4	183.	1	2	3	4
109.	1	2	3	4	134.	1	2	3	4	159.	1	2	3	4	184.	1	2	3	4
110.	1	2	3	4	135.	1	2	3	4	160.	1	2	3	4	185.	1	2	3	4
111.	1	2	3	4	136.	1	2	3	4	161.	1	2	3	4	186.	1	2	3	4
112.	1	2	3	4	137.	1	2	3	4	162.	1	2	3	4	187.	1	2	3	4
113.	1	2	3	4	138.	1	2	3	4	163.	1	2	3	4	188.	1	2	3	4
114.	1	2	3	4	139.	1	2	3	4	164.	1	2	3	4	189.	1	2	3	4
115.	1	2	3	4	140.	1	2	3	4	165.	1	2	3	4	190.	1	2	3	4
116.	1	2	3	4	141.	1	2	3	4	166.	1	2	3	4	191.	1	2	3	4
117.	1	2	3	4	142.	1	2	3	4	167.	1	2	3	4	192.	1	2	3	4
118.	1	2	3	4	143.	1	2	3	4	168.	1	2	3	4	193.	1	2	3	4
119.	1	2	3	4	144.	1	2	3	4	169.	1	2	3	4	194.	1	2	3	4
120.	1	2	3	4	145.	1	2	3	4	170.	1	2	3	4	195.	1	2	3	4
121.	1	2	3	4	146.	1	2	3	4	171.	1	2	3	4	196.	1	2	3	4
122.	1	2	3	4	147.	1	2	3	4	172.	1	2	3	4	197.	1	2	3	4
123.	1	2	3	4	148.	1	2	3	4	173.	1	2	3	4	198.	1	2	3	4
124.	1	2	3	4	149.	1	2	3	4	174.	1	2	3	4	199.	1	2	3	4
125.	1	2	3	4	150.	1	2	3	4	175.	1	2	3	4	200.	1	2	3	4